CMT and Me

An intimate 75-year journey of love, loss and refusal to surrender to a disabling disease

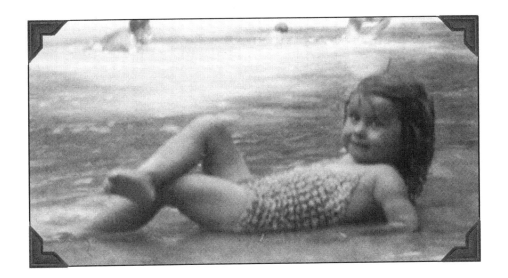

LINDA D. CRABTREE

CMT and Me: An intimate 75-year journey of love, loss and refusal to surrender to a disabling disease

by Linda D. Crabtree C.M., O.Ont., O.M.C., LL.D.

ISBN: 978-1-7750582-0-5.

Cover design and back cover photo: Natalie Stickles – fivebyfivedesignstudio.com
Front cover photo: Linda at Queenston Heights wading pool (circa 1944)
Cover watercolour leaves – Linda Crabtree
©Linda Crabtree.

All photographs copyright Linda Crabtree with exceptions listed at end of text in Photo and Art Credits.

linda@lindacrabtree.com

Introduction to CMT and why this book

As a child I wrote short stories. As an adolescent, as so many young girls do, I kept a diary. In 1963 when I ventured forth on crutches to begin studying art in a strange city, every new experience was recorded. I have been keeping track of my life with words now for 55 years and the sagging shelves in my office chock full of journals and binders of photos attest to a full and varied life albeit lived with a neuromuscular disease that is slowly taking away my independence. The creative force in me is very strong. I am constantly looking for ways to express myself and writing has proven to help me understand the world around me and my place within it. Give me a blank piece of paper and you'll either get back a drawing or 500 words. Here, I write about my family, those I have loved and love, and my journey with this crazy disease that affects so many people but still remains misunderstood and often undiagnosed.

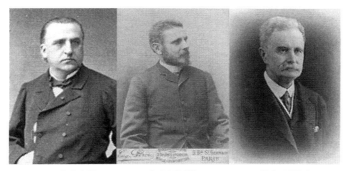

CHARCOT   MARIE   TOOTH

What is CMT? Charcot (pronounced *shahr-KOH*)-Marie-Tooth disease is named after three physicians: Dr. Jean-Martin Charcot and his student, Dr. Pierre Marie of France, and Dr. Howard Henry Tooth of the United Kingdom who discovered it in 1886.

CMT is a genetic, progressively debilitating neuromuscular disease that usually begins by affecting a person's ability to walk. It can then go on to affect any part of the body served by the peripheral nervous system, including hands, voice, breathing and a myriad of other bodily functions. It is estimated that CMT affects one in every 2,500 people.

When the local university agreed to take my journals and personal papers for their archives, I wondered how anyone would ever make sense of them and began writing this book to bring some order to the chaos that has been 75 years in the making. I do not write simply about CMT, but first about my life as a woman and then what it means to be a woman with a disability.

Table of contents

Dedication

To my husband Ron who keeps me going, to my family whom I miss more than words can say and to everyone world-wide who lives with CMT.

1

A hard start

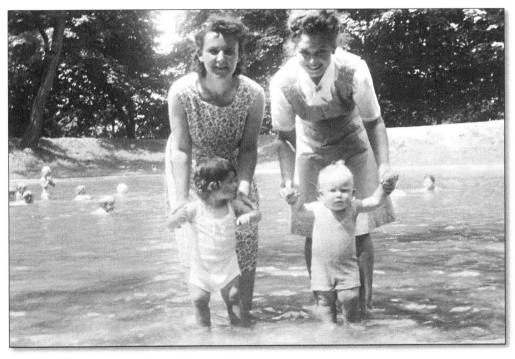

Dorothy and Linda (left) with Myrtle and Ann in the wading pool at Queenston

Imagine two young mothers sitting on the lawn beside a large circular cement wading pool, their 16-month-old daughters happily splashing about in the warm water.

The place is Queenston Heights, Ontario, very near Niagara Falls. The year: 1943.

One of the mothers gets up and walks into the dry part of the pool where her daughter, Linda, has just stepped. The little wet footprints are flat. Her daughter was born with high arches just like her own. Why are they now flat?

From that day on there was something wrong with Linda.

I am Linda and my journey begins when I was born to a couple, Dorothy and Floyd Crabtree, who met while they were in high school and only 15 years old.

Floyd was a stocky young man with a kind, round face and a shock of dark hair that sometimes fell over his forehead. He wore glasses, was almost blind without them.

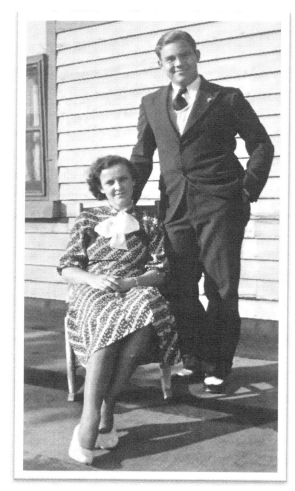

Dorothy and Floyd – courting days

And he would walk Dorothy home every school day before he did his paper route on his bike, whistling as he went.

Dorothy was slight and pretty but shy. She lived with her mother, Clara, and older sister, Madeline, in a big double house that

had been in the family for years and had seen many relatives pass in the big front upstairs bedroom. That room was reserved for guests, births and deaths. She was born up there.

The couple courted for eight years and married in 1939 when they were 23 and 24. Mom was eight months older than Dad and from the photos I have, they were a dapper looking twosome.

Mom learned how to sew from my grandmother and there were plenty of hand-me-downs from Madeline. Mom could sew anything from simple pillowcases to evening gowns and slipcovers, and she did it beautifully.

Her older brother, Bruce, had died of appendicitis at age 15. Her father, Harry, a piano tuner, had died young at 55, also of appendicitis. Clara didn't like to be alone and when Harry was off in the country, tuning pianos, Mom was the one person she could count on being there. They were very close.

Mom and Dad's first home was an apartment in a home that my grandfather Art Crabtree, a builder, had owned, and then they moved to an apartment building he had just finished. I spent my first three years in that second-floor apartment.

A happy young man, Dad had musical

talent. His mother, Stella, saved enough out of the grocery money to buy him saxophone lessons and he soon learned how to read music and play the clarinet as well. He also had a lovely falsetto voice and enjoyed being on stage. These talents, a head for

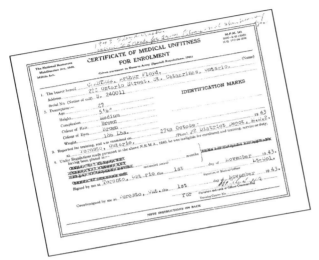

Dad's WW II unfitness certificate

figures, and a strong work ethic would serve him well all his life.

I was born to the happy couple in April 1942. Dad was working in the office of a car dealership and Mom was at home.

Men were being called up to serve in the Second World War and, in October 1943, Dad was summoned to Toronto for an Army fitness examination to see if he was eligible. I have his Certificate of Medical Unfitness for enrolment. My mother wrote this on the back of it, "Floyd Crabtree found ineligible for enrolment and training service or duty as his eyes were not strong enough -

Toronto Nov. 1, 1943. When the war went on he was reclassified and while we were waiting for a telegram telling him to report to Toronto for active duty, Japan surrendered and the war was over. Thank God."

When my brother, Ronald, was born in late April 1945, I had just turned three. I was walking and wore little white boots. But carrying baby Ronald up and down stairs and helping a three-year-old navigate the steps as well saw my parents move down to a first-floor apartment. I often asked to be carried and "Pick me up! Pick me up!" was a constant

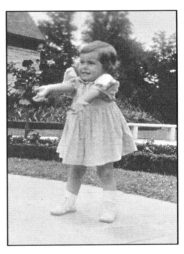

Pick me up! Pick me up!

plea. No one knew why. And when Mom had Ronald in the carriage, I'd want to ride along with him, especially if we were walking the six blocks to her mother's place. Six blocks there and six back were like a marathon for me. With a new baby and a three-year-old having trouble walking, Mom was exhausted most of the time and the photos I have of her show it.

The Second World War was over and so was

the rationing of sugar, tea, coffee, butter and meat. Before we moved downstairs, Mom gave me her ration books to play with. I tore all the little coloured coupons apart and I still remember letting them flutter like pastel rain from the top floor down the stairwell to the back door.

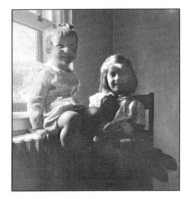

Waiting on the rad for Dad

Now, Dad worked just two blocks down the street at McKinnon Industries, which became General Motors some years later. He could walk home in ten minutes. And on winter afternoons when it was dark by 4:30, Ronald and I would climb up on the radiator under the front window, press our faces to the cold glass and wait. The streetcar would glide by on its tracks, clickity-clack, clickity-clack, heading downtown, its connection to the overhead wire flashing sparks into the dark. And always, just after 5, he'd come home, his brown great coat buttoned up with a white silk scarf tucked in at the neck and his fedora at a jaunty angle, wearing leather gloves that were a Christmas present, and trousers tucked into galoshes. The excitement never waned. He always came and we always waited, watched, and then announced with great gusto to Mom, who would be fixing supper in the little kitchen just behind us with its steamed-up window, "Here comes Dad!"

The doorframe of that kitchen was also what I hung onto for dear life as Dr. Vogel, our pediatrician, tried to give me my vaccinations. All children at that time were immunized against whooping cough, small pox, tetanus and diphtheria. I disliked needles and I really didn't like Dr. Vogel. He had a great bushy mustache and I didn't like it when he put his ear to my chest to hear my heart. He was stiff, old and, to me, frightening. I'd hang on to that doorframe and scream blue murder.

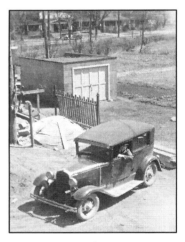

Dad's first car

But what about those flat feet?

I know Mom and Dad were concerned, but what to do about it? I was regularly trucked off to doctors in Hamilton and Toronto. The back seat of Dad's Ford Model A was my favourite place to lie down and look out the window. The seats were brown plush and as I looked up I knew where we were by the tops of buildings, as we'd pass them so regularly on our way to yet another doctor. The rhythmic jiggling

10

and putt-putt of the car never failed to put me to sleep. That car was Dad's first and I can still recall him putting a new tar paper roof on it when he sold it years later. Dad saved his money for what he thought were the truly important things in life, like a home and family, and having a fancy car wasn't one of them.

Each new doctor would have me parade up and down the cold hardwood floor of his examining room, dressed only in my little white underpants. Then I'd be lifted onto the examining table and he'd run a sharp tool up the bottoms of my feet. I found out later, that was to elicit the Babinski sign. If, when the tool was run from my heel up my foot, my big toe went up, it could mean I had a central nervous system problem. All I knew was it hurt and my toes didn't budge. Then he'd prick my feet and legs with a pin to see if I felt it, or he'd strike a tuning fork on something and put it to my legs and feet to see if I could feel the vibrations. Yes, I felt everything. I always wondered why one doctor didn't tell the other that I felt everything. Why did they have to keep on poking and pricking me?

Finally, a diagnosis was given. I'd had polio. But, my mother argued, I had never been

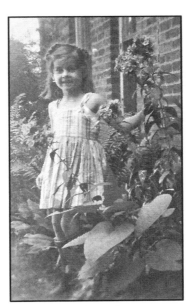

Braces on, hanging onto a phlox stem and knees bent for balance but still smiling

sick. No more answers came. That wouldn't be the only misdiagnosis we'd be given in those frustrating early years.

Dr. Vogel thought perhaps exercises would help strengthen my feet and ankles. Every night Mom would lift me onto the bathroom counter and we'd work my ankles left and right, left and right. Then I was to touch her finger with my foot on the left, on the right. Curl my toes down, then up, down, up. I could do the exercises for a while, however in time I could no longer make my ankles, feet and toes move voluntarily. Even with regular exercise I wasn't getting stronger. I was getting weaker.

Why? No one knew.

My walk became what the doctors called an equinus gait: I walked with a high step like a horse. I had developed complete foot drop. My ankles couldn't lift my feet up to clear my toes off the floor. I had to lift my dangling foot from the thigh and then slap it down hoping the heel would hit first. It was an awkward way to have to walk and I often fell because I tripped over my own feet or nothing at all.

A local orthopedic specialist, Dr. Robinson, watched me walk. He prescribed ankle-high, lace-up leather boots with metal braces that fastened below my knees and ran down the side of my leg to a lock protruding from the sole of my shoe to hold my foot up as I took a step. They were hot and heavy but I could walk better in them. I didn't complain. I could feel my mother and father's anguish seeing their firstborn in braces. I remained stoic, said nothing and just took whatever came.

Getting my feet into those boots became a regular morning struggle. They laced down the front and my foot would drop into the open boot, but I still had to push it down into the toe. As I did, my paralyzed toes would curl under. The end result was that walking was very painful. Off would come the boots and we'd begin all over again. Mom tried using a shoe horn and putting powder and slippery tissue paper in my boots, anything to help my foot slide in without my toes curling under. Some mornings my feet slid in like they were buttered. On others, my toes curled again and again. By the time we got them on, it would be too late for school and we'd both be in tears; mom out of sheer frustration and me because she was crying.

While we lived in the apartment I was able to get to Memorial Public School by cutting through our neighbour's rear garden into a small field, then under a wire fence strung over a deep ditch. Once that was accomplished, there were several sets of railroad tracks to navigate before I'd reach the sidewalk, only a block from the back entrance to the schoolyard. It sounds dangerous but really it was close enough to my grandmother's porch that I could see her hanging laundry on the line.

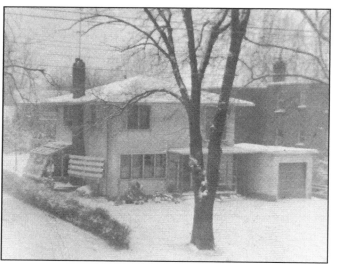
Our new home at 221 Ontario Street

Then, in 1949, my parents built a house at #221 Ontario Street, almost across the road from the apartment at #222. Ontario Street in St. Catharines was, and still is, a main artery to the Queen Elizabeth highway that leads to Hamilton, Toronto and Niagara Falls. It was, and still is, very busy.

Now, my school was two long blocks away and I had to cross a busy road. For a skinny little kid of seven in grade two, or even twelve in my final grade there, it was a long way to go in leg braces. I dreaded crossing the road but I had to do it. The traffic was fast and it was hard for me to climb curbs onto the grass boulevard. If I miscalculated I'd fall backwards so I had to cross at

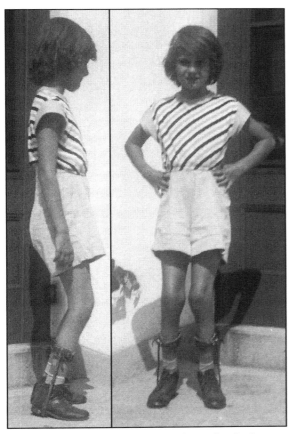

In my braces with my knees bent for balance

driveway curb cuts, but they also posed a problem. If they slanted too much my knees would give out and I'd fall. And once across the road I couldn't keep my momentum going enough to push myself up a sharply slanted curb cut. I never did find two driveways on corresponding sides of the street where I could get down easily and still have enough momentum left after crossing the road to mount the curb on the far side. When I look back, these were

pretty strange tasks for a youngster to be worrying about but they were with me every day of my life, four times a day, for five years until I completed grade six.

Speaking of grade six: our teacher, Mr. Orr, also the principal, would begin most mornings by drawing a circle of numbers on the blackboard and in the middle of the circle he'd put a number from 4 to 12. When he called your name, you'd stand beside your desk and multiply the number he pointed to in the circle by whatever number was in the centre. I was always petrified that I'd be called on, because I not only had to call out the answers at his speed (which wasn't mine) but I had to hang onto my desk so I wouldn't fall over or stand there with my knees bent to keep my balance. I'm still anxious when faced with mathematics, although I really do quite well.

Several times while on my way home for lunch, one of my metal braces broke and I couldn't walk. I had to stand where I was until I was missed or ask someone on their way past our house to knock on the front door and ask my father to come and get me. He walked home each day for lunch from the office and I came home for lunch from school in the opposite direction. Standing in someone's driveway, trying to balance in the gravel on a broken brace, praying that my father was on his way, was something I'll never forget. Because my balance standing still was so poor, I had to either bend my knees or keep moving and in the middle of the driveway there was nothing to touch to help me keep my equilibrium. To keep my knees bent for 15 minutes while standing still was excruciatingly difficult. I'd start to sweat and swallow hard. I couldn't move because if I did, my knees would buckle or I'd lose my balance and have to take a few steps and then settle into my bent knee stance again. Once exhausted, the result was that I'd be down on the gravel. I had to keep those knees bent. I'd look at the gravel wondering if it would be better to fall knees first or hands first; which part of my anatomy did I want bits of gravel embedded in?

After what seemed like forever I would see my father coming to my rescue. He'd lift me up in his arms, squeeze me and carry me the remaining long block home on his arm like Bob Cratchit carrying Tiny Tim in *A Christmas Carol*. I felt safe and loved. I also knew that I wouldn't be able to go back to school until my brace was welded together again.

I usually walked to school alone as I always left home almost too late to get to school on time. I liked school but because I was often sick, or more likely just exhausted, I was never able to keep my attendance up enough to do really well. When I was there for any length of time, say three weeks, I excelled and began to love it, only to get sick again or have a brace break, take time off and fall behind once more.

I think you can tell by now that public school isn't a fond memory. I remember walking up the dirt path to the playing field that I crossed to get to the back entrance, having to take a run at a small hill and then line up to go into school every morning. Each year a different line, each line a challenge for me in my braces with huge divots of grass usually attached to them that they'd pulled out as I crossed the field.

As I stood in line, I'd either have to keep moving to keep from falling over or touch the kid in front of me to keep my balance. But what if the kid in front of me didn't want to be touched or didn't understand? That was always a problem unless someone I knew was in my class. If there was no one to touch and I stood too long with my knees bent, I'd be almost too exhausted to walk into the school. What a dilemma for a little kid!

Mom would pay for my friend, Joyce, to go to the Saturday movies with me so I would have someone to touch for balance while we waited in line to get in. For once, my disability proved an asset; we loved going to the movies together. Joyce wouldn't likely have been able to come up with the price of a ticket if Mom hadn't pitched in to supply me with a "stabilizer."

At school, weather permitting, one afternoon a week the entire class would go out back to play baseball. I always went with them but had to sit alone on the sidelines, so I began bringing a garter snake or two in my pocket with me to keep me company. I thought it was a terrific idea. Most of the girls in the class and the teacher didn't agree.

My pal Joyce excelled at sports and I was her coach, so to speak. I encouraged her, cheered her on until my throat was raw and was truly delighted when she won ribbon after ribbon at the school's annual field day event.

Each day when school was out I'd have to jump down out of the side door of the classroom, a drop of what was likely 18 inches (there's a step there now) but seemed like a mile to me, then go down that bit of a hill into the huge playground that I cut through each way to school. The dirt path through the playground was dug deep from boys on bicycles getting up momentum on the top of the hill then roaring down as fast as they could, pedaling like crazy, and then coasting all the way to the end. The only way I could quickly get through the playground in my braces without risking a fall was to take that path. That meant dodging the bicycles.

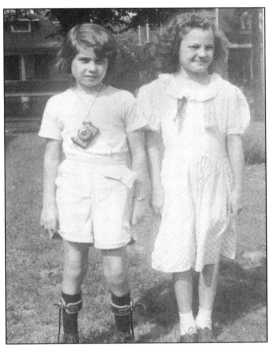

Me with my camera and Joyce wearing her field day ribbons

There was one boy, Brian, who refused to let me walk the path. He constantly teased me and threatened to run me over with his bicycle. I was very afraid of him. You'd call it bullying today.

Just before I was to move on to junior high school I had a confrontation with Brian when he wasn't on his bike. I remember kicking him hard with my brace. I can still see the tears in his eyes. I felt sad that I'd hurt him and was sure the police would be at our door to arrest me for hurting someone so badly.

About 30 years later we met in my orthopedic surgeon's office. He recognized me and told me he had a bone infection in his leg. I wondered if my kick had done it and came to the conclusion that he was no longer my worry.

Was it any wonder that every time I finally reached the corner of the lawn of our big house I breathed a deep sigh of relief? I was safe! I had calculated driveway slopes and

15

curb cut heights, braved traffic, dodged bicycles, pushed myself uphill, balanced in line for what seemed like forever and then had to do it all over again to go home for lunch and then yet again in the afternoon. And always, in the back of my mind, I knew from experience that I could fall for absolutely no reason at any given time and take the skin off my hands and knees. Once on our soft green lawn, I could crawl or even roll to the house if I fell. I say "roll" because my knees were so badly bruised from falling that crawling was sheer torture.

You might wonder why my mother didn't walk or even drive me to school. I don't think it ever occurred to her; parents didn't walk their kids to school back then much less drive them. We were taught not to talk to strangers and to come straight home. She had my brother, who was three years younger, to look after, a meal to put in the oven and, as far as everyone was concerned, I could look after myself. No one asked me how I felt about it all and I think if they had, I wouldn't have known what to say; that was just the way it was. That's what I had to do every day and I did it.

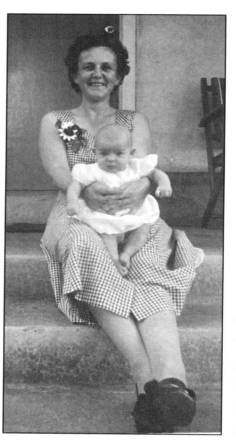

Mom and baby Kathie

One day in May 1954, the 28th to be exact, I was almost home from school for lunch when my Aunt Audrey pulled up beside me in her car. She was headed the opposite way. After rolling down the window she said, "Your mother is in the hospital. You have a baby sister. Your father will get you lunch." And with that she was off to the hospital to see Mom.

Wow, I thought, a baby sister. I was 12. A diagnosis of Duchenne muscular dystrophy had been given for me at one time, as well as polio. Duchenne usually affects boys but every now and then a girl would show up with it too. Most didn't survive much past age 12. Somewhere along the line my mother told me that she and Dad decided to have another child because they were pretty sure they'd lose me. She later denied that and said we were all planned for from the beginning but, whatever the reason for the pregnancy, the result was Kathie and she was one of the best things that ever happened to us.

16

2

Fun and friends

Although it may sound like it, my childhood wasn't all angst and drama. I had a good deal of fun as well.

When we lived in the apartment, Mom had gone down the street to visit a woman who had what seemed like quite a few children at home. She had asked if their daughter, Joyce, who was

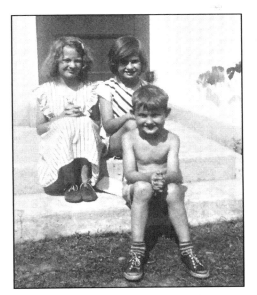

Joyce, Linda and Ronald in front

about my age, and one of the boys, Bruce, could come up and play with me from time to time. They did and we got to know each other. Joyce was my first friend.

I think I was about five when I told Joyce and Bruce that it was my birthday and there was going to be a party. It wasn't my birthday and there was no party. They went home and came back that afternoon dressed in their Sunday best carrying little gifts. I was caught in a lie. My mother sent them home with her apologies and I got a stern talking to.

When it really was my birthday in April, Mom went next door to the neighbours' place and cut some branches off a spirea bush that hadn't leafed out yet. She stuck brightly coloured sugared gumdrops on the ends so it looked like a candy tree. I thought it was beautiful and that she was the most creative, greatest mother on earth.

The people next door were an older couple, Mr. and Mrs. Burrell. Their daughter, Olive Whitfield, with her two sons, Grant and Rodney, lived with them. The house was a tiny, slightly off kilter, one-storey brick cottage. Their back door led out to a huge, typically English, perennial garden at least four times as long as the house and behind that they grew vegetables next to the railroad tracks that I crossed every day on the way to school. The Burrells guarded their garden. No children were allowed, except for the two boys who lived there and, for some reason, we rarely saw them.

Joyce, Bruce and I had to cross their garden to get to the homes of our playmates, Billy Rutherford and Mary Embleu. We had a backyard layout in our minds that let us play hide and seek and travel way down the block without ever going on the street. It was exciting; we'd play out there until it got too dark to see and our mothers were calling us home for bed. Old Mr. Burrell would rush out the backdoor of their cottage, swinging a broom as we darted through his bearded iris, but he was never fast enough to catch us, not even me in my braces.

I remember being given my mother's beautiful porcelain-headed baby doll and trying to walk carefully with it along the side of the apartment building. Naturally, I fell, and the head shattered into pieces. Mom took it in stride. She had likely figured that would happen but gave it to me anyway. I was absolutely devastated.

Most of all I remember the fun. The running and, yes, the falling. But the games and hideouts under lacey white spirea and quince bushes with their lovely rosy flowers and beneath back porches, peering through diamond-shaped lattices at dusk, were magical. I hid in a garbage can once and the

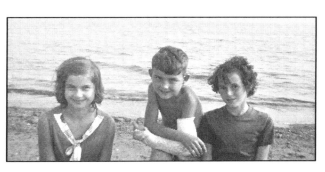

Me, Ronald in cast for a broken arm after a fall from a tree and JoAnne Urlocker at the beach

stink just about did me in. They finally found me after what seemed like ages.

Four girls lived across the road from us but Mom didn't want me crossing at such a tender age. It wasn't until we built the new house at #221 and moved across the road that I got to venture down the street to play with Margot and Martha Neilson and JoAnne Urlocker and her younger sister, Mary. Martha and Margot lived in a house my grandfather had built and my grandparents and Dad and aunts and uncles had lived in for several years. My grandfather, would build a house, the family would live in it while he was building another, then he'd sell the one they were living in and everyone would move into the new place; sort of like present-day house flipping. JoAnne and Mary lived in a grand house beside the one that Granddad built, in a location that had once been the original farmhouse on the land that now held likely 40 or more homes. It was imposing; the lot rose from the sidewalk some six feet and the house had bay windows, a large screened-in porch on the south side and vast lawns around it.

It was while playing at JoAnne's that I

became fascinated with a toy copier called a hectograph. It was nothing more than a gel pad you wrote on with a fluid pen. When you pressed paper onto the reversed pad, whatever was written came off on the paper and you could make a few copies. My budding entrepreneurial spirit kicked in. I talked JoAnne into working up a neighbourhood newspaper with me and we began selling subscriptions. Naturally, nothing came of it but it was a shade of things to come.

One summer day, after we'd moved across the road to the new house, JoAnne's mother called Mom to ask her if it was safe for her daughters to play with me. Could she catch whatever I had? I guess it was understandable during that time of polio but it dampened my enthusiasm for the girls on the west side of the street. I also had a feeling that their mothers didn't want Joyce in their homes. So it was either the four down the street or Joyce and Bruce across the road who lived upstairs over a convenience store with numerous siblings and their parents in a two-bedroom apartment backing on the railroad tracks. I chose Joyce and we spent most of our time together.

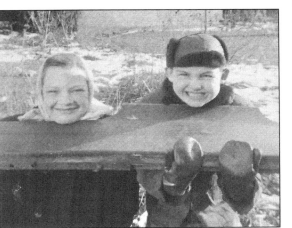

Joyce and Ronald hamming it up

On hot summer days Joyce and I would play Monopoly on the front lawn, with the seeds from the huge elm tree overhead fluttering down on us. We'd bounce balls up against the chimney at the side of the house and I got pretty good at keeping three and even four balls going like a juggler. The bonking sound drove my father nuts.

Joyce, Bruce, my brother Ronald and I built a fort beside the house from packing crates we'd lugged home from Pilkington Glass just across the tracks. It was a real structure with walls, a roof and a cardboard floor but not tall enough to stand up in. Lying on our backs looking up at the sun filtering through the cracks in the walls, we'd smoke (we didn't inhale) milkweed silk. My father knew what we were doing in there and told us that we'd set the fort on fire as well as the house if we didn't stop. We stopped.

In the winter, we built snow forts and had a marvelous time pelting each other with snowballs.

I kept snakes in the basement window wells that I'd catch down the old Welland Canal embankment just two blocks from our house. Those were the snakes I'd take to school in my pockets. It was down that canal bank that I learned about trees and vines, small animals, reptiles, insects and just about anything not human, although I did see a naked man sunbathing down there once when I was picking wild raspberries for Dad's lunch.

I couldn't stand up very well to go down the steep, narrow path that led to the canal and was warned by my mother not to go near the water. Even though there was a high chain link fence at the bottom that no one was supposed to climb, a body was usually found every year in Port Dalhousie where the canal ended at Lake Ontario.

A model church complete with four and Kensington Place, receives a little crosses was made of snow by Edward help from Linda Crabtree, 221 Ont. Duguay, 19, of 230 Ontario Street, and his and Joyce Hallett, 228 Ontario St. He brothers, Albert, 16, and Wilfred, 15. Ed- he modelled it on the lines of a chu ward, shown here putting finishing touches used to attend at Island River, N.B to the church at the corner of Ontario St. Photo, Standard Engraving.

A newspaper clipping shows a snow church the French-Canadian boys who lived across the road below the Hallett's built in the field next to our house. Joyce and I were just props for this photo but we often built snow forts.
pc2.1

When there was no garden in that patch, the weeds were shoulder high and we played hide and seek in them. When it was mowed in mid-summer, we gathered up the dried weeds and made a fort, or played baseball on the mowed field. I learned the hard way that the remaining weed stubble could pierce skin if you fell on it, so I refused to run bases but I could pitch. Once I threw a decent ball and it was hit back, square between my eyes. I had two shiners from that one but wore them as badges of honour. I could play baseball!

When it came time to ride a two-wheeled bicycle, Mom took me up to the schoolyard so I could learn to balance. The grass was soft and if I fell I couldn't hurt myself. But it was also so thick I didn't have the strength to pedal through it so we soon gave up on that idea. The street just beyond Mr. Maroney's garden was very quiet and had grassy treed islands down the middle. Starting there, Joyce and Bruce would take turns riding my bike all over the neighbourhood while I waited on one of the islands. It wasn't as hard-hearted as it sounds. Between each one of their trips

When my parents built the house across the road from the apartment, they bought two lots: one on the corner and the one beside it. They didn't build on the corner lot but rented it out to Mr. Maroney, who planted it as a large vegetable garden. We were supposed to stay out of it but it became a prime place for catching butterflies, running between the rows and just plain having fun.

they'd get me on my bike and push me; I'd lose my balance, begin to fall off, and they'd catch me and help me off. Then they'd go again. But one day they got me on it, gave me a push and, I took off. I had it! I was balancing and I didn't come back. The only trouble was that I knew how to steer, pedal and now balance, but I didn't know how to stop or get off. I couldn't point my toe down to the road. Out of desperation, I quickly figured out that I had to ride up beside a curb where I could put my foot out on the raised concrete. It was either that or ride forever through the streets of Thairs, Kensington, Woodruff and Queen Mary Drive.

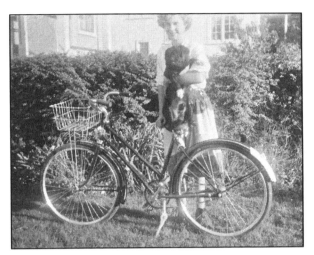

Me holding Gus behind my beloved CCM Cadet bicycle

After that my CCM Cadet three-quarter-sized two-wheeler became my wings and the two big blocks behind our house became the neighbourhood I rode through almost every day. I remember riding past a long row of poplar trees that had just leafed out and thinking what a terrific birthday present Mother Nature had given me. I didn't care about the weather as long as there were leaves on the trees. I was probably 12 years old. I still feel that way.

***

A huge happening in our young lives was when Mom got us a dog. One late Saturday morning when Dad was golfing, she packed us all in the car and off we went to the Lincoln County Humane Society shelter. We looked at all kinds of dogs barking up an almost unbearable racket in a long, cage-filled, cement brick building that echoed every plea from every pooch tenfold.

We didn't have a say, really. She picked the quiet one that wasn't lunging at the wire or barking. In fact, he was cowering in a back corner. We could hardly see him. The Humane Society fellow reckoned he'd been beaten. He was a black lab/terrier mix with short legs ending in small white and black spotted feet that pointed outward like that of a ballet dancer in repose. He had a long body, a white flash on his chest, a lovely head with big soft brown eyes and floppy silky ears. His most distinguishing feature was a jutting lower jaw with four small crooked teeth poking out, and no other teeth to speak of. No one knew how old he was. We didn't care. He was a dog. Our dog. We loved him from the minute we brought him home and slowly, with much patience, we began to gain his trust. We named him Gus.

When Dad got home he saw us all on the front lawn with Gus. "Whose dog is this?" he asked. "He's ours," we all said with conviction and absolute joy. "We'll see about that," Dad said as he climbed the front porch steps two at a time. Whatever was said between Mom and Dad didn't change a thing. I think Dad would have liked a purebred dog with a little more class but Gus was just the best, classiest dog in the whole world as far as we were concerned. Kissing his feet sent him running in frenzied circles – it was really funny to watch – and then we'd turn him over and kiss his belly. The look on his little black mug was that of a small entity who had died and gone to a blissful doggy heaven. He was often called "Gussersbeshaberandbeshovers." Don't ask me why but Joyce and I had all kinds of crazy names for him.

Gus wandered the neighbourhood and always came home, but many years after he joined our household he became deaf. One wintery day he was let out and didn't come

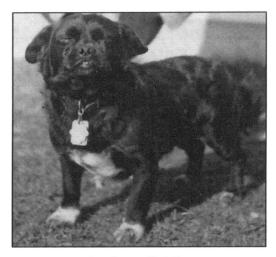

Our beautiful Gus

home. A knock on the front door and a stranger told us that he thought our dog had been hit by a truck. Sure enough, Gus had been crossing Ontario Street after a heavy snowfall that dampened the sound of oncoming traffic and he most likely didn't hear the transport truck gaining on him. I hope he died instantly.

Mom wrapped his little body in a blanket and brought him home where he stayed in the freezer in the garage until we could give him a decent burial in the backyard when the ground thawed out. For years after his demise, we saw little Guses all over the neighbourhood and as far away as the Armenian section of town, way past General Motors. That little fellow was a closet Don Juan. Who knew!

***

Our parents weren't the kind who played with their children. Sure, they likely played patty-cake with us when we were tiny but we didn't remember that. Did their parents play with them when they were kids? Likely not. Dad's father was a hard-working and, most likely, hard-drinking, asthmatic Englishman who built houses by day. When he died, the mayor wrote to my grandmother saying how much he would miss his good friend, but play with his kids?

I doubt it. Dad's mom was a hard-working housewife with four children to look after. Mom's dad, the piano tuner, was away a great deal and her mother was heavily involved with the church. I don't think anybody had the time or inclination to throw a ball around with the boys or dance a jig with the girls. Kids made their own fun and played with their siblings and neighbouring children back then and it was the same for us.

When our dad wasn't working at the office, he was playing saxophone and clarinet two or three nights a week at the bandstand in Port Dalhousie with Bruce Anthony's dance band. Mom was interested in art and antiques.

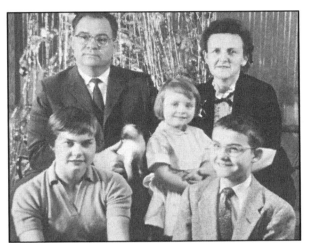
The Crabtree family at Christmas 1955

I don't remember playing with either of my parents, ever. As long as we were happily at play with our friends, they were happy.

All five of us did go on a short summer vacation once to Turkey Point on the north shore of Lake Erie when Kathie was still in diapers. I remember it as a week of fly and mosquito bites, sunburn, and Ronald being afraid to get into a canoe. We never went on vacation together as a family again. That was enough for Dad; he preferred to spend any spare time he had on the golf course and who could blame him.

***

I am forever grateful to my mother for not protecting me as a child with a disability. Left to my own devices, I made friends, lost friends, even fought with friends; played with dolls and broke dolls; pushed a doll carriage, played with a dollhouse, rode a tricycle, tried unsuccessfully to skate with ice skates and roller skates, learned to ride a bicycle, played baseball, played house, hide and seek, blind man's bluff; built straw, snow and wooden forts (depending on the season); explored nature, played board games, and learned to play hop-scotch and marbles (Dad brought home some ball bearings from GM and everyone wanted to win them from me).

I got dirty, wet and occasionally hurt but it was all part of growing up and no one should have to miss out on all of that if they can help it.

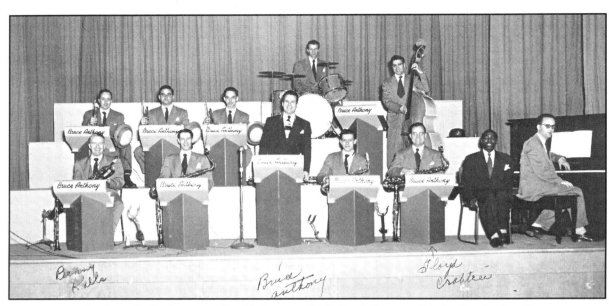

Bruce Anthony's Orchestra – Dad is just to the left of the vocalist in the dark suit - pc2.2

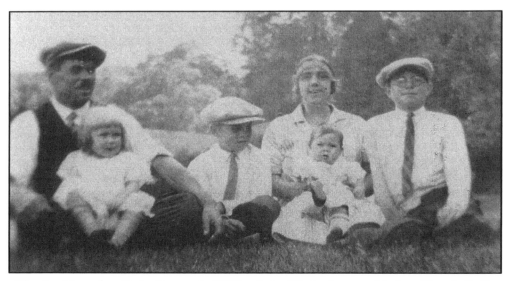

The Crabtree family in the early 1920s: Art with Audrey on his lap, Floyd, Stella with baby Irma, and Omer

3

Those early teens

Eager to find out what was wrong with me, at age 12, my parents took me to Dr. Omar Younghusband, my father's doctor and a friend of the family. He had heard my father talking about me while on the golf course and was pretty sure that I had Charcot-Marie-Tooth (CMT) disease. From what I understood then, some of the members of his family had it and because of that he recognized my high-stepping walk, my inability to move my ankles, feet and toes, and my lack of balance. But he wasn't sure as it was usually inherited from a parent and my parents seemed just fine.

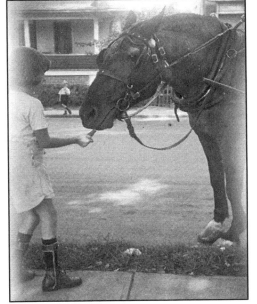

Feeding the breadman's horse

There was almost no information available on CMT at the time and I think Mom and Dad decided to just carry on. What else could they do? There was no treatment or cure that they knew of. The physiotherapy prescribed when I was younger had only resulted in my becoming weaker, despite my mother's determination to keep at it. I can't imagine the disappointment she must've felt as I grew weaker and weaker, nor can I imagine the frustration both Mom and Dad must've experienced not knowing what was taking away their daughter's ability to walk.

Nothing was easy about being a young teenager in leg braces. All the kids who passed grade six from Memorial Public School had to go many miles to Queen Mary Senior Public School for grades seven and eight. The school was almost brand new, very modern and had no steps, except for one room that had a little stage built into it so we could each give a speech to our classmates several times a year.

In speech class, the last name "Crabtree" came up in the alphabetical list fairly fast. I'd research my topic thoroughly, prepare my talk for several weeks and shake like a trembling aspen when I had to finally ask for help to climb the three steps to the stage and stand there, knees bent, to give my talk. I still know more about pearls than the average Joe.

I've always intensely disliked trying to memorize anything. Einstein once said something like, "Never memorize anything that you can look up." I agree. I know where to find most things I need. And committing things to memory doesn't always work well with me, especially when

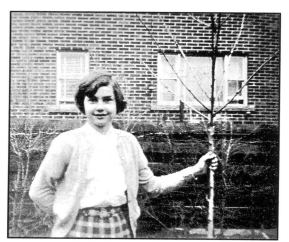

Early teens – me and tree

trying to recollect it. The terrible surges of anxiety I feel, in the days and weeks before I'm on stage, stress me out so badly it simply isn't worth the effort. Even if I have a written script in front of me, my atrophied fingers won't let me turn the pages. I visibly shook during my little speeches back then and still avoid public speaking although I have done a fair bit of it in my time.

Aside from public speaking, getting to my new school became the most difficult part of those two years at Queen Mary. It was too far to walk so Mom drove me many times. There was a school bus but waiting across the road from the house for it in freezing rain, snow and slush proved to be a

new kind of torture. My knees, bent to keep my balance, and lower legs would turn blue, and I couldn't feel my thighs.

When the bus finally did come, I had to almost throw myself at the bottom step, fling my books and purse up onto the floor of the bus, grab at the handrail and pull myself up one step at a time. Often I'd have to lean on the top step with my hands. I simply didn't have the strength to make it up those three steps in one go.

If the bus driver stopped the bus too far away from the curb for me to make my move onto the bottom step, the hike up was impossible to manage. The driver had to jockey back and forth to get closer to me, or go further down the street and pull alongside the curb, or leave me where I stood. I never knew from one morning to the next if the driver would be new and wouldn't know my limitations. If I couldn't get to school, all of my homework would have been for nothing and once again I'd lose out on learning.

I absolutely loved science class and, through Mr. Scott, developed a love for tropical fish and all things aquatic, insects (that attachment has waned over the years), plants and mammals. Art classes also suited me to a T and I was very much at home in the school library, taking home books and writing copious book reviews.

Mr. Scott came into class once with his fly undone. Georgina Koski and I were both in the front row and, looking back and forth, tried to figure out how to tell him. I'm not sure how we did it but we succeeded. We didn't laugh at him but tried to clue him in and that felt very grownup.

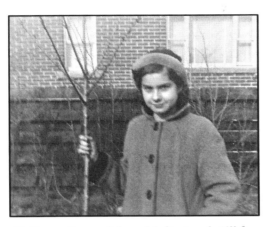

Notice a theme? I couldn't stand still for a photo without touching something for balance. Many years later Mom wrote on the back of this photo, "Tree must need to be held up." She'd forgotten I couldn't balance.

Music class was something I dreaded. Ms. Parks tried to teach us to read music. I was away from school so much I missed most of it. When I was there, I became part of her routine that involved each student standing and reading the musical notes on the black (green) board by singing it out loud. I'd simply freeze. I had no idea what those notes sounded like. None. I still can't read music. Later in life I had an opportunity to talk to Ms. Parks, as she was a dear friend of a neighbour. I told her how much anxiety her class had caused me and she was surprised that I hadn't enjoyed it. She and Mr. Orr, who loved math quizzes, should have gotten together.

It was also while at Queen Mary that I threw my leg braces in the closet. I was a teenager now and hated being different. The metal braces and leather boots were heavy. I could walk better without them, albeit with complete foot drop. Soft lightweight moccasins became my everyday footwear, with clear plastic rain boots over them in winter. It wasn't a good solution but Mom had given up trying to persuade me to wear the boots and braces. I was developing attitude and had a mouth on me.

When I needed eye glasses to see distances, my aunt took one look at me and said they didn't look so bad. As far as I was concerned, glasses were just one more thing on top of all the other things that made me different and ugly. I pulled myself upstairs by the railing, stumbled to my bedroom and flopped on my bed sobbing. I think it was then and there that I decided the boots and braces definitely had to go. I was certain that I was going to fail at everything, no one would ever like much less love me and life was the pits.

Growing up is hard to do, especially when you are different.

4

The '49 Meteor

My teen years were ones of growth and enlightenment, earned the hard way. I think many can relate to that, especially if a disability is factored into a pattern of mixed emotions and moods, which included angst, curiosity, fear and self-loathing.

I was new to life and didn't really know how to cope with my disability or my changing body. Neither did my parents.

The high school most of the kids in our neighbourhood attended was old. It had steps up to the front and long flights of stairs everywhere. I was still wearing light moccasins most of the time and the braces remained in the closet. In order to alleviate the stress and difficulty of climbing stairs, I was sent to Grantham Secondary School, a modern high school further away that had only two floors. My classes would be kept to the ground floor. It was ideal but too far to walk and public transportation to it didn't exist. My mother drove me every day. We had a beautiful new yellow Pontiac convertible so I arrived in style, but what a chore that drive must have been for her. Mind you, I don't remember ever hearing her complain but she did have three-year-

old Kathie to take along with us and Ronald to get off to school as well.

My brother and his friends used to change in the garage to go swimming in our pool. One day when Mom was driving me to school she noticed that there was a police car behind us. He eventually burped his siren and Mom pulled over, certain that she hadn't broken the speed limit or done anything wrong. Maybe a taillight was out? After inspection, it turned out there was an entire set of clothes on the roof of the car. One of my brother's friends had likely gone home in his bathing suit and just left everything on the top. Later we told Dad what had happened and everyone had a good laugh at our brush with the law. We never did find out who left their clothes behind.

***

Mom and Dad would occasionally go out for the evening when they felt I was old enough to stay at home with Ronald without a babysitter. They'd give us 50 cents and after they left Ronald would go across the road, over the tracks and behind the gas station to Louie's Variety store. I loved to stuff half a bag of Lever's potato chips in my mouth, add a couple of long draws of Orange Crush, give it all a few chews and produce what I considered junk food heaven.

One night I asked Ronald to bring me home a cola and then decided that I was going to mix myself a drink. We all knew where Dad kept the hard liquor and it wasn't long before I had one drink and then another. We laid down under the cranked up hi-fi listening to Dad's LPs and I bedazzled Ronald with my rendition of Julie London's *Cry Me a River.* We both did calisthenics on the living room rug, with me asking Ronald to stand on my rock-hard stomach. The boy was enamored with his older sister and we had some good times together, but that night when the bell to the locked side door rang and I had to go down two steps to open it for my parents, I was obviously having trouble. When I finally unlocked the door, my mother took one look at me and turning to my father said, "My God, Floyd, I think our daughter is drunk."

I was having such difficulty walking that nothing much else was said and I think it was then that it dawned on Mom and Dad that their daughter wasn't such an angel after all. Under their scowls, I could detect a slight hint of amusement. I went straight to bed and the next morning found out for the first time in my life what a hangover felt like. That was punishment enough.

***

Grade 9 was fine. I was taking Latin and

French and enjoyed it all. I was still in serious work mode and thought of school as something I could do well. I was 14 for most of that year and pretty naïve.

Grade 10 was another thing. I was taking the same electives and assigned the same classes but nothing seemed to click. I failed my year. I was so ashamed of myself that I could have crawled into a hole and died. The worst part was that my mother would have to drive me all the way to that school for an extra year.

Eventually we found several older male students who lived only a couple miles from us who had cars and, for a fee, would drive me to and from school. The pressure was off Mom.

Just to lighten the load, for my second try at grade 10, I switched to the Commercial program. Even though it was up a half flight of stairs, I was able to make it and excelled. Rapid calculation, bookkeeping, letter writing, shorthand and business machines all made my head spin, but I was good at writing and could do math in my head.

I soon found out that Maureen and Jan and the rest of the girls in Commercial were considerably more worldly than those studying Latin and French. I'd never even heard of blue ointment for crabs but I learned all about it in Commercial class. And that wasn't all: makeup, dating and sex were the standard topics before and after lessons.

And it wasn't long before I discovered boys. I had a crush on Bobby, who had one time lived in our neighbourhood and was now on the basketball team. I'd wait by the hallway to the gymnasium locker room hoping that he would say a few words to me after practice but he usually pushed past me.

I also joined the school yearbook team and with my little Brownie camera went to some of the dances, always sticking to the sidelines while snapping pictures of my classmates living it up on the dance floor. No one ever asked me to dance even though I knew I could because I danced all the time in my room at home. The fact that it was a flat-footed dance and that my chances of falling were pretty good, staying off the dance floor was likely a smart move. At times I probably felt sorry for myself but I think I always made the best of whatever situation presented itself and, because I was curious about almost everything, I never got bored.

***

I'm not sure how we met, but Lee, a lovely petite blonde, asked me if I'd like to meet her boyfriend and his friend during lunch at school. They had a car!

The car was a '49 dark blue Meteor and it belonged to, well, I'll call him Blaine.

I can't recall how long it was before we were going out on double dates. At long last, I had a boyfriend.

We'd go swimming in the big pool at a local resort. I still remember the snow blowing in the broken window of the women's change room. But once we hit that lovely warm water it was heaven. The fact that I had complete foot drop and very thin legs from the knees down didn't seem to bother anyone and I was in my element. You can't hurt yourself if you fall in the water.

My body was developing. I had perky breasts, shapely hips and weighed 118 pounds. I was also becoming smart-assed and belligerent. Hey, I was 15.

I took my first drag of a cigarette in the back of that '49 Meteor when Blaine was filling it up at a gas station. I thought I'd choke to death. I bought mascara at the five and dime, outlining my eyes and coating my eyelashes like a badge of honour. I was rebelling. When my mother took it away from me, I learned to burn a match on a mirror and used the soot for the same look. I loved it. She said my eyes looked like two piss holes in the snow.

I smoked Matinee cigarettes in my bedroom and blew the smoke out the holes in the bottom of the storm window until one day when my father was walking home from work for lunch and happened to look up to see smoke curling up the side of the house. I think he took the stairs to the second floor two at a time and I was told in no uncertain terms to never smoke in the house again.

I was mouthy. My father actually slapped me across the face one morning when we got into an argument and I told him to f*** off while he was shaving. I needed that. He was a gentle, loving man and I know it upset him terribly to hit me, but it was a knee-jerk impulse on his part and I deserved it. I felt ashamed of myself for having caused him grief. I knew he loved me although he never said it. Every one of us revered Dad and knew how hard he worked to give us everything we needed or pretty well wanted.

No one ever spoke about love in our family, but I believe all of us felt very loved. Having said that, I've often wondered if my brother should've been given more attention as he was growing up. Yes, he had his friends but he didn't have his father's counsel or arm around him. He started to bounce at a very early age, sitting on the couch and rocking back and forth against the back of the couch for what seemed like hours. I think it was a way for him to comfort himself. As I grew older I realized that a great deal of the attention in that family was focused on me, my needs and my disability. My brother needed my father and my father was busy making a living.

Boyfriend Blaine reminded me a bit of Marlon Brando and he had the chutzpah of a Brando character, too. Once when we were in our family living room watching TV with my father, Blaine walked up the TV and switched channels from the golf Dad was into to something else. I watched my father almost explode and rightly so.

By the time I was 15, Blaine and I were having regular sex. I lost my virginity one summer night, lying in the bull rushes where the water meets the beach. After that, we never looked back. We had hot and heavy sex in the Meteor, sex on the beach after everyone had gone home and sex in the woods. One day a hiker happened upon us and I can still see his startled look as he made a swift about face. In retrospect, it was the best sex I've ever had, bar one. I'll tell you about him later.

Blaine also had a motorcycle and a racing green, late 40s model MGB as well as the '49 Meteor. He was handy with cars and kept at least one of them running all the time. We always had wheels and, if we didn't, his mother, who was a widow, had a little Vauxhall we could borrow to run back and forth between his home in rural Niagara farm country and mine in St. Catharines.

I remember the police trying to chase us through an orchard. We were on the motorcycle and they were in a cruiser. They didn't get very far.

That little green sports car had exterior windshield wipers that were linked together; when one moved, the other would follow. They would often fail. I would sit on Blaine's best friend's lap (it was a two-seater) and work the windshield wipers with my right hand stuck between the convertible top and the windshield. When my hand was almost frozen I'd pull it in, massage it, and out it would go again.

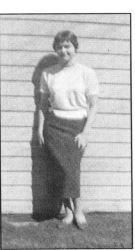

Growing up

Watching Blaine work on his cars in the old garage behind the farmhouse also taught me to change a tire and use a ridge reamer when changing pistons in an engine. I learned all about broken fan belts, exhaust systems and ignitions. If it could go wrong or break, it did. Blaine was a "body man" at an auto repair service centre. Cars were his thing. Thank heaven.

Many a time we'd go "over the river," rain or shine, to Lewiston or Niagara Falls, New York, for beer by the jug in the MGB or the Meteor, when it was running. The US border was maybe 20 minutes away. Customs officials rarely asked us anything except whether we had anything to declare besides "goods consumed." We didn't but we all had to find a toilet fast – beer goes through you quickly after the first jug. We didn't do drugs. There weren't any to do. We didn't smoke pot. There was none of that either. It was a different time then with different ideas about behaviour and definitely looser checks at the border.

I remember making love on a huge bearskin rug in front of a roaring fire while Blaine's best friend looked on. Making out in the MGB was a feat of calisthenics but we made do. Life was fun and sex was an entirely new dimension I hadn't realized even existed.

I also remember the many times I wrote "IWB" (intercourse with Blaine) on my calendar so I could track the dates we had sex. I wasn't on the pill. I wasn't supposed to be having sex. I was far too young according to convention but no one asked me if we were sexually active. We were doing what many red-blooded teenagers would do.

Often we didn't have money for condoms or it was either $5 worth of gas or a trip to the drug store. Without gas you didn't go anywhere, so we used condoms when we could.

***

Sweet 16 slipped by.

My parents, especially my father, really disliked Blaine and the fact that he had wheels. He was three years older than me and cocky as hell. We could be anywhere doing anything and they'd never know.

Often forbidden to see Blaine, I'd sneak around the corner and meet him with his car or motorcycle there. One time I hopped on the motorcycle and off we went. Very few wore helmets in those days. About a half mile from home he took a cutoff near General Motors and the front wheel went into a huge hole. I flew off the back and ended up in a deep puddle. I was wet and stunned but not hurt. After changing, I was back in the saddle again and off we went. Nothing kept us apart. He was working and had money. And he had me.

5

Up to other things

After easily passing grade ten Commercial, it was decided that I would try to go to the local high school about 12 blocks away, the one with the steps everywhere.

Mom drove me mornings and a mental map (of low curbs and driveway cuts that I could manage) saw me get home in one piece most days. I

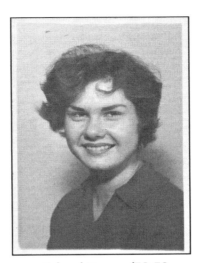

School Days – '58-59

sometimes had help up the school's front steps and sometimes made it up them myself but dreaded every try. The courage it took to throw myself up even a small flight of steps knowing that at any second I could end up lying on the cement was gut-wrenching. And even if I did get myself up the three steps of the front of the school, there was still the step at the door and then the flights of stairs inside. It. Just. Never. Ended.

This was the era of huge zippered binders that held everything from subject notebooks to pencil cases and cosmetic bags. We'd pile our textbooks on top of the binder and carry it on our hip or hug it in front of us, our arms wrapped around it.

The principal had one very short leg and wore a boot with a high lift to even him out. "Could I please have a locker on the first floor?" I asked. I couldn't carry my binder and books up the stairs, as I needed both hands on the railing to pull myself up. I thought that if anyone could understand my request the principal could, but the answer was no. He did finally assign one of the fellows on the football team to meet me right after class and he'd run my binder and books up or down to the classroom where I was supposed to be next. Later I wondered what that football player had done to merit such humbling punishment.

I can't tell you how many times I fell down those stairs. In their haste, other students would just brush by me on their way down and I'd lose my balance and be hanging onto the railing for dear life. And it didn't help that the railings started two steps up and ended at the step before the landing.

What was I supposed to do when the railing ran out? If I let go I went down a flight of hard terrazzo steps to land in a bruised, bleeding crumpled mess at the bottom. Sometimes I was rescued, sometimes I was given a hand up to a landing … and sometimes I wasn't.

I liked that school and made some friends but the stress of trying to get around the building was making me wonder if I could continue. I was still going steady with Blaine and still had an active sex life.

English literature was my love. I didn't, however, do too well in the Commercial classes. I was terrible at typing because I couldn't make my fingers hit the keys independently. Shorthand was a bust. I wasn't fast enough, although I still remember some of it. The keys on the business machines were too hard for me to push and I had to look to see where my fingers were. The other kids could just put their hands on the keys and they'd hit what they expected to. I'd hit anything but.

Mr. Groh, my business machines teacher, lived just three blocks from us and said he'd pick me up in the mornings. That took the pressure off Mom.

My defensive attitude carried over to my typing class and one day I actually threw an assignment on Mrs. Clifford's desk. She told me that if I didn't smarten up I was going to have a very tough future. No teacher had ever spoken to me like that. I took what she said to heart and stopped taking out my hate for the world on unsuspecting others. It wasn't their fault I had a disability. It wasn't mine, either. It just was.

Rapid calculation, spelling and filing were easy. The Dewey Decimal System was a breeze. My English was good. I could write and I was well-spoken but I wasn't enjoying life at school. There was nothing there for me. Everything I really liked, except English class where we studied Shakespeare, was outside of school.

I began to think that I was going to fail Grade 11 just as I'd failed 10. The weather was getting meaner, the trees dropping their leaves. Every day was a real struggle just to get into the school and then praying I'd get to my classroom through the press of kids without falling or being flattened up against a wall. But trying to navigate those stairs, and often failing, was the final straw. Slowly, I mentally descended into "quit school mode" and, once there, there was no turning back.

I'd had several sessions with Mrs. Forsey, the guidance counsellor, and liked her. I wanted to do something in the natural sciences, but since I was in the Commercial stream she suggested that I should become a librarian. That was about all she could see ahead for me.

My body image was shaped like a bowling pin: no arms, no legs. If anyone had asked me to draw myself that's what they'd have gotten.

Finally, just before Christmas exams, and having given my situation a lot of thought, I sat on the top step of the stairs leading down to the basement office in our home, where my father did his secretary/treasurer work for the Musician's Union (AF&M) Local 299 (his third job after General Motors and his big band gigs), and asked him if I could quit school, telling him why. He said that if I could find a job I could quit school, likely never thinking that I'd ever find one.

***

Dad's third job taught me a lot, as I watched him collect dues from musicians, make out receipts and spend hours at night on the books. Every two years he would put out an update for the little loose-leaf booklet that members carried to find a sideman or pull together a trio, quartet, or dance band from among fellow musicians. Punched printed pages would sit on a long narrow table that Dad had Uncle Omer make. Dad, along with Ronald, me, and even Mom at times, would start at one end and go around the table collecting and collating pages as we went. Then we'd stack each group of pages in a little crisscrossed pile. We must've stacked thousands of those little piles and eventually each little bundle of pages was wrapped in a small strip of paper explaining what it was, tucked in an envelope and sent

out to every one of the musicians in the local. Dad had a machine called an Addressograph that took piles of small address forms. When he put an envelope in the machine and pulled the handle down, ink was forced through gauze on the little form, onto the envelope. That's how he addressed the hundreds of envelopes that were sent out regularly.

There was a Musicians' Union convention every two years and as Ronald and I grew older, Mom and Dad would go with Joe Phelan, the local's President, his wife Alma and sometimes other members of the executive. They'd fly down to San Francisco, Chicago, Detroit or some other large city in the United States for 10 days, leaving us with a kindly older woman who was more like a grandmother than anything else.

Mom always brought me back something to wear that you couldn't find in Canada. I remember a turquoise V-neck sleeveless cotton top with ties at the shoulders that looked fabulous with my summer tan.

Ronald and I would cross the day off on the calendar each night when they were away. And we'd wait by the window or on the front porch the day they were expected back, imagining the airplane landing and their drive home from Toronto. Finally, when the car pulled into the driveway, we ran to greet them. Yes, we were excited and couldn't wait to see what they'd brought us

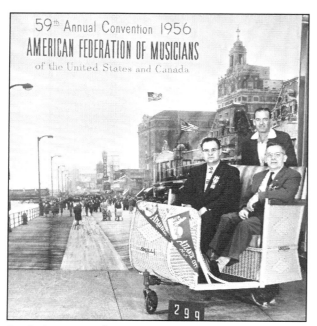

Dad, Secretary/Treasurer; Joe Phelan, President and Jack Stunt, Vice President (behind) of AF of M, Local 299, in an official convention photo taken at Atlantic City in 1956.

but mostly we were just happy to have everyone back home the way it should be.

Dad usually worked down in the basement office two or three nights a week after supper. It was a job he had taken on and he did it to the best of his ability, just like everything else he did. He had a mortgage to pay off and a family to support. His superior work ethic really impressed me and emulating Dad has seen me accomplish much throughout my life.

Another example of something Dad taught me was in a blue exercise book, found 40 years after he died. From September 15, 1938 to the end of April 1945, Dad recorded every engagement he played, and often where, and with remarks. Samples following, as he wrote them:

September 23/39 - Friday night 9 pm - 2 am 9 piece orchestra at the Welland House for St. Catharines District Tennis Clubs. Played a good job

amount made $4.50

The next night he recorded the same hours and the same pay, only this time in Niagara Falls. On it went, almost every Friday night and many Saturday nights and sometimes both. He mainly played with local dance bands led by Bruce Anthony, Clarence Colton, Murray Morton or Wilf Wheeler, but once in a while he had a chance to play with an out-of-town band if they came to the area for a special engagement and needed sidemen.

Nov. 25/38 - Friday night 9 PM - 1 AM - 8 pieces at Oddfellow's Hall on James Street for Lightning Fastener dance. Played fair job for a very rowdy crowd. Girls had very little on.

amount made $4.00

Sometimes each member of the orchestra received so little you'd hardly think it worthwhile.

At Foxhead Niagara Falls 9 - 12:30 Oct. 14/39 *$1.00*

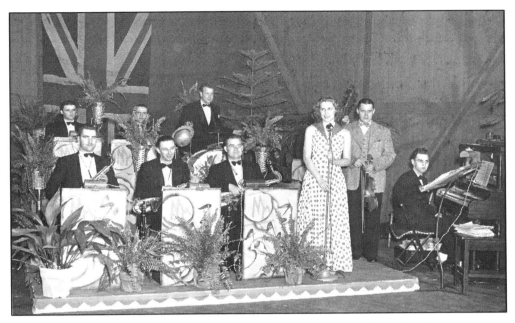

Murray Morton's Orchestra – Dad is just to the left of the singer

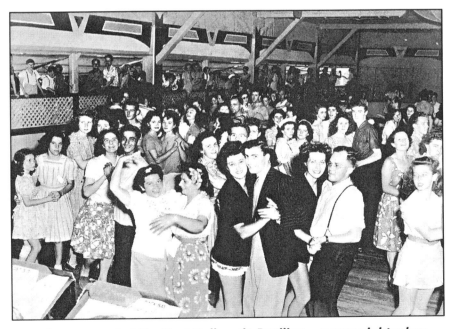

A dance crowd at the Port Dalhousie Pavilion – a rare night when Dad wasn't playing as Mom and Dad are just behind the couple in the dark jackets in front – pc5.1

But as little or as much as it was, Dad kept playing and adding up the gigs on each page of his little blue book, carrying the totals forward. As the years went by, musicians were paid more, likely due to the influence of the union, and by 1944 he had made $2,765 playing sax and clarinet and sometimes filling in for a missing vocalist, for crowds all over Niagara and as far away as Crystal Beach on Lake Erie. He was bound and determined to give us our own home and he'd saved enough to buy a building lot and apply for a mortgage to build the home we now lived in. The mortgage was $6,000 at 4.5% payable over 20 years.

By example, I learned from Dad that if you wanted something badly enough, the way to get it was to work hard and save. In time, that lesson would serve me well.

Dad wasn't perfect by any means but I like to think he at least came close. He had a healthy set of lungs and a naturally loud laugh that would make people turn around and look at him when he let loose. I recall one afternoon when the whole family took my grandmother Crabtree to see *Golden Girl* starring Mitzi Gaynor, a movie about the life of Lotta Crabtree, darling of the American stage during the California Gold Rush. Grandma was ever so proud when the lady in the box office let her in free of charge after we all told her that Grandma was a Crabtree. Something in the movie hit Dad as hilarious and his booming laugh

rattled the rafters. When I was very young I used to duck because everybody would look at us, but as I got to know him I was proud of him and loved that laugh. When he was laughing, we were happy.

At night when we were all in bed he'd sometimes fart so loud we'd all hear it, and each in our respective bedrooms with a full wall of closets between each room, would begin to snicker and snort. A good laugh with Dad was always a great way to close our eyes on the day.

If anything, Dad's one fault was not being around enough. And, when he *was* around he was usually busy looking after something in the house or working downstairs in his office. There wasn't much time for play but I still remember him doing his clog dance in the kitchen, the change in his trouser pockets chinking time and then his arms going around Mom's waist as she stood over the sink washing dishes. He'd nuzzled her neck and she'd feign embarrassment but we all knew they were in love and it was wonderful to see.

Dad was definitely the head of the house, there was no question about it. He was the breadwinner and he made it possible for us to live the privileged lives we grew up to know but I often wonder what price providing us with that lifestyle cost him.

***

If Dad was the head of the household, Mom

was the heart. She was the one who doled out dishes of strawberry covered vanilla ice cream on hot summer days to all the kids in the backyard and bandaged skinned knees while hugging sobbing shoulders and drying tears. She made the house a safe haven for us and we knew as long as we didn't get too rowdy or break anything, everything would be fine. When things did get a little out of hand, Mom, and sometimes Dad, would speak to us but I don't ever remember being spanked or sent to my room. A word was enough.

Mom had many interests and I think keeping house was the least of them. She often let dishes pile up and everything wasn't dusted regularly, but far more importantly we were surrounded and influenced by the beautiful paintings she produced, the antiques she collected and sold, the colourful perennial garden she cultivated in the backyard, and the flowers whose scent wafted into our living room during the winter from the greenhouse on the south side of house. On Sunday mornings when

Dad was off golfing, she'd often take us out to the woods to explore. In the woods, I learned more about nature and wondered more about God out there than I ever did at Sunday school. I think Mom had her priorities straight.

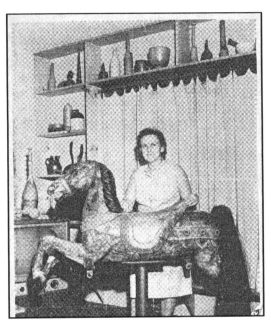

A photo from an article in The Standard dated August 16, 1962 with the heading, "Mrs. Crabtree – Antique Collector, Artist, Gardener." That's the carousel horse she worked on in the kitchen for a couple of years. Our living room had shelves full of antique jugs, mashers, irons and other vintage utensils. – pc5.2

And I've never forgotten her last words as we'd leave the house on a cold winter's day. With a smile in her voice, she'd shout "Got-lotz-on-ya?" from wherever she was in the house. With that we knew she knew we were going out and that she cared how we fared.

***

Back at school, about a week after Dad had given me the okay to leave, I spotted a message on the bulletin board next to the guidance counsellor's office. The Standard, our local newspaper, was looking for someone to work in the morgue (library), where they kept back issues of the paper, clippings filed in categories so the reporters would know what had been written about local issues, photographs and lead engravings, and cardboard cuts that were used to put an ad or photo in the paper. All the newspapers

41

since 1891 were on microfilm. They needed someone who could spell, file, type (I could – sort of) and make some kind of order out of the local news in each of two daily editions. I could do all of that.

A phone call got me a Saturday appointment for an interview with Larry Smith, the editor-in-chief. Dressed in an avocado green shirtwaist dress with two crinolines under the skirt, my tiny waist and ample bosom filling out the top, I wore my auburn hair long, shiny and curled. I didn't really know it but at 17 I had definitely bloomed. As I high-stepped to clear the floor with my toes, my knees hit the crinoline and it popped the skirt up but I just kept going. He asked me to sit, and I handed him my filing and spelling certificates and a letter from the guidance teacher. I must have looked and sounded pretty good, or else he was desperate. In any case, I got the job, and my guidance counsellor's suggestion came true. I was going to be working in a library.

When I got home and told my parents, they were flabbergasted. Their little girl had a job. I felt so grownup, I was bursting. The pay was terribly low: something like $34 a week but that didn't matter, I was working.

Quitting school was a quiet sort of sad affair: I just cleaned out my locker, said goodbye to the few friends I could find, and signed out. It was over. Years and years of continually trying to succeed, trying to keep up, trying, trying. Over.

The job was easy for me and I loved it. The morgue was at the back of the building on the second floor. There was an elevator. A long line of dark green filing cabinets held hundreds of file folders and thousands of dated clippings on everything from the War of 1812 to city sewer backups and my favourite: Hobbies and Oddities. Anything strange or obscure that absolutely wouldn't fit in any other category, let's say a carrot that looked like a two-headed dog, was tucked in there. I was also responsible for date stamping, then clipping and filing the work of our reporters as it appeared in the two editions of the paper every day. I also kept huge boards of pristine newspapers by the month; these were sent out to be microfilmed and I looked after the microfilm machine and drawers of film.

The reporters and editors were a diverse lot: Fred Whitelock, the sweet old editorial writer whose office shared the three-quarter wall between us; and Marj McKay, the Women's page editor, who brought her little dog, Missy, to work in a basket; and Larry Perks, the brusque city editor I tried to stay away from as much as possible. The fellows in Sports were Jack Gatecliffe and Gerry Wolfram, who really didn't pay much attention to the new kid in the back room; the photographers were: all-business Don Sinclair and joking, mustachioed John

McTaggart, who told me to make sure I had a cola around just in case his diabetes began to do him in.

My quitting time was 5 p.m. and most of the reporters drifted out by 3 or 3:30; the city desk staff and wire editor, who started early, were gone by 3:00 for sure. As the day wore on, John and I and any of the reporters still working would gather in editorial: a large room full of desks, each topped with a black metal Underwood typewriter.

One particularly fun day, likely on a dare, I ended up on McTaggart's lap, and he quickly squeezed the back clasp on my bra causing the padded cups to climb up over my breasts. Suddenly, under a bright orange sweater, I had four boobs. There was no way I could get myself back in so, red-faced, I headed to the ladies' room to take off the bra, turn it around, do it up in front, turn the clasp around to the back and pull up the straps; all the time with my sweater tucked under my chin. My hands were too weak to do it the way other women did or the graceful way they did it in the movies. I returned to the office having learned my lesson: Don't get too familiar with the men because they knew tricks I hadn't even thought of.

That was the late 50s. Today that would be cause for a complaint to human resources or more, but back then it was something to laugh at; I was one of the boys except I wasn't a boy. Yes, it was demeaning and I felt it. I've never forgotten it. But nobody thought much if it and I doubt if anyone would have been told to stop. I'd likely have been told to stay off photographer's laps.

***

Blaine and I spent that New Year's Eve together and I slept over at his mother's farmhouse. I spent most of the morning in his bed when his mother went to church. I swear I saw a little light go ping in my brain when we had sex that morning in his little room tucked under the eaves. That ping, or whatever it was, turned out to be my worst nightmare just when I was moving on with my life.

I think one of the most difficult things I've ever had to do was to tell my mother that I was pregnant.

6

Casting call

I don't mean to take my pregnancy lightly but it wasn't something I had to go through. As soon as my parents knew what had happened they went into action, or rather, my mother did. I have no idea what my father did; he was so disappointed he didn't speak to me for months. Perhaps if he'd been more a part of my life it wouldn't have happened, but I can't fault him for trying to make a living for all of us and being absent from home most of the time.

Dr. Younghusband, the same one who had diagnosed me at 12, sat me down in his office and asked me how I felt about my pregnancy. What could I say? A tiny bit of me wanted to keep the baby but most of me didn't. He began the paperwork to have it aborted. Those were the days when you had to have a written piece of paper from two doctors saying you would be in mortal danger if you went through with the pregnancy. I don't think my health was really at stake but coping with a child at 17 and not being able to walk, balance, or use my hands adequately, pretty well meant it would be my mother's to rear and she already had a five year old at home. And what if the child had CMT? There was

definitely a chance and that posed a whole new list of what-ifs.

I know that millions of CMT children have been born, and have been reared by wonderful women who have CMT, but at that time and place, it wasn't going to be me. Simple as that.

Before I knew it, an appointment was made for me to have a D&C, a legitimate name for a dilation and curettage procedure to remove the lining of the uterus that also succeeded in doing away with the embryo.

I had no one to talk to. My mother was in "go" mode and my father was silent. I got up the courage one day to walk into the editor-in-chief's office and asked him if I should go ahead with the procedure. I didn't tell him why. "How the hell would I know," he said. I dearly needed a best friend.

As it turned out, both of my best friends, Joyce and Lee, were in the same boat. Joyce and I had grown apart but I later learned she also had a child and gave her up for adoption. She then had a son when married to her first husband. And Lee, being Catholic, was married in the basement of her church and had the baby … a girl. She went on to have two more girls and is now the proud grandmother of 10 and great-grandmother of 11.

My relationship with Blaine was winding down with a screech. His mother and my parents had it out on our front lawn and the upshot was that my parents blamed her for not keeping an eye on us. She couldn't have kept an eye on us if she'd tried. We were having sex over a 30-mile radius, ranging from Vineland to the Welland Canal: terrific hot and heavy sex in the woods, the orchards, the backseat of his MGB and his '49 Meteor. I painted the torn ceiling cloth of the Meteor blue so I'd have something nice to look at while on my back. Hi mom was a widow, a teacher, very religious, and, I think, somewhat afraid of her adopted son. We were out of her control, out of anyone's control.

The medical procedure over, I went back to work. Blaine and I saw each other one time after that. He was living in the US, just over the border, and he picked me up and we drove back stateside. Parked on a side street, staring at the tall old houses in front of us, we discussed our future. I had a job. He was going to stay in the US and join the military. There were tears. Would we ever see each other again? We said we would, but the shock of what had happened pulled

our relationship sharply into focus and it was clear we were going our separate ways.

The abortion affected me in many ways: I thought everyone knew. They didn't. I hated myself for disappointing my parents. They forgave. Even my father began talking to me after a couple months. My mother said something like it was her first grandchild. That moved me. I'd never looked at it that way. And I wasn't the same carefree spirit after that – just a disillusioned one.

Now 18, girlfriend, Carol Harris, a lovely blonde with beautiful big, blue eyes (my mother called them Bette Davis eyes) and I, would get our hair done after work together at the Leonard Hotel, go to dances at the UAW (United Auto Workers) Hall and play bingo at the Royal Canadian Legion. All good fun.

And, I was also enjoying the attention of several young men including a recent addition to the photographers' roster at the paper. I'll call him Liam. He'd drive me home after work and maybe take a detour to the A+W for a root beer but I was also seeing a fellow from Niagara Falls, New York, and a local man that I liked very much.

The fellow from the Falls, Bob, was an engineer and in the military reserves. One night when we were on our way back across the border to his part of the world for a whistle dog (a hot dog with melted cheese and crispy bacon on it) at a drive-in, he suggested I take a look in the glove box of the Corvette he drove. I opened it and there was a ring box. I remember a sinking feeling in my stomach. I opened the box and there was an engagement ring with the smallest diamond I had ever seen. If I'd have loved him, it wouldn't have mattered what size the diamond was or if there even was one, but I didn't love him. I couldn't imagine living in a trailer on work sites in God-knows-where with someone I admired but didn't love.

I strung him along and the next time he went away on manoeuvres he arranged for his best buddy, also a "Bob" who drove a Corvette, to take me out. I made out with his best friend, who looked like a movie star. Of course, on his return, his friend told him everything and that was pretty well the end of that with both Bobs. Was his friend really a friend if he made moves on me? Who knows. It may have been some kind of a test but all it proved was that I was out for fun, not marriage. Shallow, yes, but I knew what I didn't want.

Another boyfriend, David, was one of those fellows who was always prepared. I loved that. He didn't smoke, but I did, so he'd always have cigarettes in his jacket pocket. His car always had plenty of gas in it. He had a job. He taught me how to play cribbage. And he'd take me dancing even though he

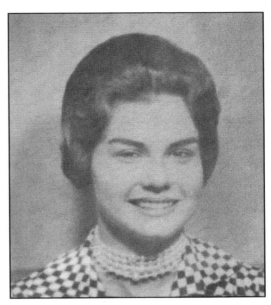

The working girl, age 19, taken in a photo booth after I'd had my hair done

knew I might end up sitting on the dance floor at any given time.

One of my most cherished memories is putting on my white islet dress with the deep neckline, high collar, short sleeves and a skirt full enough to take two crinolines under it. Small one-inch heels and a white clutch bag completed the package. We were going dancing at The Plantation over the river. I think it was a Saturday or Sunday afternoon. The place was empty. He filled the jukebox with quarters and we hit the dance floor. I loved to dance but fell when I tried some of the tricky dance steps I'd seen on American Bandstand. A twirl often saw me off balance enough to end up on my behind or my knees. He'd get behind me, put his arms under my armpits and pick me up almost without missing a beat.

That afternoon, with just the two of us having a ball dancing, laughing and thoroughly enjoying each other, has stayed with me for more than 50 years. I loved him for accepting me as I was. Our relationship began to get serious. I talked to my mother and she suggested I could do better. Again, my feelings weren't strong enough to commit. We were both very young.

Liam and I would sometimes go out on a Friday night but he'd never really take me anywhere but the back roads to have sex in the back seat. I hadn't learned. We didn't go to the movies, to a restaurant, a concert or the theatre. Every so often we'd go out to visit our photographer colleague John, the one with the nimble fingers, and Midge, his exotically beautiful wife. They had a small menagerie of dogs, cats, goats and donkeys that I just loved. Liam talked politics. I wasn't interested in politics. We really had very little in common. I just loved being with him. He had beautiful strong hands, a great head of dark wavy hair and a perpetual tan thanks to his Scottish background.

He'd taken on the additional job of doing all the reprints at the paper: the photos that appeared in the paper that readers could order. During the Henley Regatta, a huge annual rowing event in our city, there were hundreds of 8x10 black and white prints rolling off the dryer into my waiting hands. We worked together in the darkroom, he

exposing and enlarging the images and dodging to bring the best out of each exposure before he slipped it into the developer and me taking it from the developer to the stop, then the wash, and then onto the dryer belt.

We'd have gone through all of the orders beforehand to calculate how many we'd need of each and it didn't take too long before we had everything sorted, stamped on the back with the date and paper's name, and, with its pink order form firmly attached, in a neat manila envelope ready to go.

Those many hours in the darkroom were heaven to me. We were busy doing something we both enjoyed. And I was being useful to him. He didn't so much as kiss me in the darkroom. It was a place for work. Was I a pleaser, or what?

What he did do was take my disability seriously. A good friend of his, Bob Gledhill, was studying medicine at McGill University in Montreal and Liam talked to him about my CMT and my ungainly equinus (drop foot) gait. Bob said he knew a young doctor who was living in California but was moving up to Canada, to St. Catharines, because he was marrying a local girl. That orthopedic surgeon, Dr. Edward Blair, had been trained to do a Lambrinudi triple arthrodesis – an operation that would fuse my foot so it would no longer point downward. I was now pretty well walking on my ankle bones.

After an initial assessment and x-rays, Dr. Blair suggested that, as well as my feet, he'd fuse my ankles to better stabilize my feet in a weight-bearing position. The procedures would take four operations, one on each foot and ankle, and I'd be in a plaster cast for six months at a time for each operation. Yep, that's right, six months times four! If things worked out well, he could do the other side while the bones were still fusing on the other ankle or foot. I could possibly be in two casts, one to the thigh and one to the knee at the same time. The timeframe was two years at the most.

It didn't take a great deal of thought for me to make up my mind. I wanted this. My walk was the same as it had been when I first lost all strength and movement in my ankles, feet and toes at around age four, except now I was bigger and taller. If you've ever seen a stroke victim walk, lifting a floppy foot high off the ground, that was me times two. I had visions of me gliding along like a swan in the water. No more high-stepping. I asked that my heels be fused so I could wear an inch and a half heel. He agreed. But as the operations proceeded, I realized that my feet were pretty flat and, as a result, I could only wear a half-inch heel.

While sitting in bed on the warm summer night before my first operation, I painted a watercolour of my feet. I knew I'd never see them again as they were for the first 19 years of my life.

7

To the bone

The Hotel Dieu Hospital was only two blocks up the street from home. That's where I was to go for my operations. My room was on the fifth floor overlooking Ontario Street. The night before the surgery, my leg was shaved to the groin, scrubbed with an orange antiseptic and wrapped in sterile cloths. I was given a sleeping pill to get me through to the morning.

I was scared. As much as I thought I was prepared for this, and as much as I was looking forward to having a new way of walking, the realization that an operation on the bones of my feet was imminent saw me shaking like a leaf. As I was rolled down the hall into the operating room, my teeth were chattering and I was buzzing with vibration caused by sheer anxiety. Everyone thought I was cold. Uh-uh! I was petrified and my nervous system was on overdrive.

An anesthetic was administered through a needle in my arm and I was out for the count.

When I awoke, maybe five or six hours later, the pain was incredible. No one, not one soul, had warned me that bone surgery was one of the most painful procedures you can undergo. I was given morphine and fell asleep. When I woke up again, the pain was back and I was told I had to wait two more hours before I could have another shot of morphine. I lay there moaning and rocking my head back and forth, back and forth, trying to take my mind off the incredible pain I had at the site of the operation - pain that was so bad I was immobilized, pain that invaded my soul. Two hours is a long time to wait, especially if it's two hours of incredible agony every four hours.

My mother was always there; at least at the beginning, anyway. She would sponge me down to keep me cool, try to get me to drink and talk to me to try to take my mind off the pain. Now when I have pain and measure it against the pain I felt the first two or three days after those operations, there just isn't any comparison. On a scale of 1 to 10, it was a roaring 20.

It took about three days for the site of the operation to settle. After that I was usually sitting up and eating, washing myself, and conversing with the nurses and Dr. Blair. He told me that during those first three days he had given me enough morphine for an adult male and I was still having pain. God help me, I thought, I still have three more operations to go.

I soundly cursed out a buxom physiotherapist who came roaring into my room two days post-op and said, "Let's get you out of bed, young lady," as she proceeded to try to swing my foot, which still felt like jelly held together with staples and screws, out from under the covers. No one was going to touch me when I hurt so bad that I pleaded to be put out of my misery at least four times day and night. No one.

Morphine is a strange drug. It sends you to la-la land and you feel wonderful: floaty and unworldly, until it wears off. After the first three or four days I was allowed morphine as needed. When my morphine wore off, as I was supposed to be weaning myself off it to go home, I was a different person. An entire vase of long-stemmed roses was launched at the tiniest nun I'd ever seen. She'd had the nerve to ask me how I was doing.

My ex-boyfriend Bob sent a dozen red roses, the same ones I threw at the nun, which I thought was pretty nice of him considering, and Liam was there off and on. Having those men in my life made me feel more like an adult or at least less like a kid.

After 10 days I was drug free, peeing on my own, and allowed to go home. We hadn't really worked out how I was going to get around and the hospital sent me home in a wheelchair and also gave me a pair of crutches, but our house had steps up to the main floor and steps to the second floor. I soon learned how to manoeuvre around on crutches and Mom put casters on the legs of two footstools.

I could get into the house on my crutches and then sit on a footstool and propel myself into the kitchen and living room and to the base of the stairs leading up to the second floor and the main bathroom and my bedroom. I soon learned that getting up to the second floor was quite a chore, so I would come down in the morning and my sister Kathie, who was seven by then, would go up and down for me if I needed anything. She was the greatest kid. I used to take out a lot of my anger on her and called her "child of the devil," but, in reality, she was patient and kind to me during the entire time.

Mom and Dad would let me stay up late to watch TV downstairs and I remember trying to bum up the steps backwards and drag my cast quietly so I wouldn't wake up the rest of the house. It wasn't easy and I wasn't always quiet but they put up with me.

Operations two and three went off without a hitch but the cards and flowers stopped as friends lost count of my surgeries. I'd always have a plant in my hospital room so I'd have something green and growing to look at and, in particular, to keep me company. Hospital rooms can be very lonely places. I couldn't very well show up on admission day with my suitcase, a portable radio (to keep up with the Cuban Crisis) and a plant, but I could order one from a florist to be delivered to myself with no questions asked. And by then I could say my morning Hail Marys along with the nun on the intercom speaker on the wall above the foot of my bed just like all good Catholics, even though I wasn't Catholic.

In order to protect myself against over-zealous physiotherapists and cleaning staff who thought nothing of jostling the bed with the handle of their mop or their behinds as they washed the floor, I began looking for a private nurse. As luck would have it, I found Sylvia, a recent nursing school graduate who wasn't much older than me. We got along very well and she understood why and what I needed during those first three or four postoperative days when I was a hurting, vulnerable mess. Having her in my corner greatly lessened the anxiety I experienced before each operation and made my recoveries much easier. We are still friends.

***

I have to tell you how we ended up with the swimming pool I mentioned a while back. In 1957, when I was 15 and Mom was

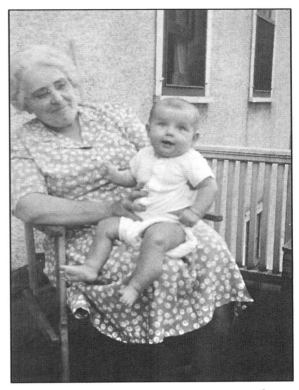

Clara (Nanna) holding me at 4 ½ months

driving me to Grantham, my mother's mother died. Beautiful Clara, the woman who had rocked me in her arms on her front porch and bought me all manner of wonderful doll house furniture along with what must have amounted to pounds of nougat from the downtown Laura Secord candy shop, was gone. I watched my mother standing in front of the living room windows, staring out onto Ontario Street, tears streaming down her face. Some 50 years later I would know how she felt.

Clara had left my mother a small house not more than four or five blocks from ours. Mom and Dad decided to sell the little

53

house and use the money to put a swimming pool in our backyard, thinking that exercising in water might help me. My uncle Omer, who had taken over the family construction firm from my grandfather, had gone from building gas stations to installing swimming pools and he was asked to figure out what would work for us. The result was a beautiful 14' x 28' peanut-shaped, turquoise fiberglass pool situated not more than 20 feet from the house.

After every operation, I had to learn to walk again and the best way to do that was in the pool. Just like my dating days, when I played in the pool at Prudhomme's with Lee and our boyfriends five years before, I knew I couldn't really hurt myself if I fell in water. If the timing was right and it was warm enough to use the pool, Liam would sometimes come over and work with me in the water so that I would eventually become weight bearing on my newly constructed foot or ankle.

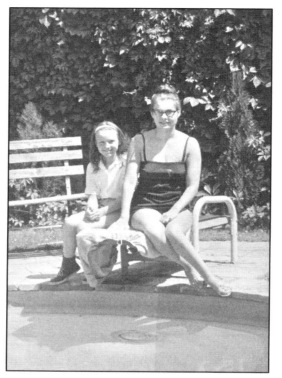

Kathie and me on the diving board

***

Operation four was another thing. Dr. Blair kept taking x-rays; something was wrong.

I'd been in one cast or another for almost two years and I wanted my life back. During that time, I had taken up knitting and made a big black sweater four times, maybe five, each time pulling it out and starting all over again. I think that black sweater and all that black wool represented my mood fairly well. I wasn't really miserable, I think I was more stoic than anything else, just as I'd been as a child. I felt suspended in time but I had signed up for this and there was no going back.

***

One hot Saturday afternoon I sat on the lounge out back and watched my brother, sister and their friends having a ball in the pool. I guess I'd just had enough because I slowly put my knitting needles and the huge ball of black wool down beside the lounge, turned myself sideways, gathered my crutches up under my armpits and headed for the pool. Before anyone could stop me, Kathie was yelling, "Mom, Linda is in the water!" I had crutched to the side of the pool, lifted my arms up from the crutches and let myself free fall into the water. It felt wonderful. I stayed there for a few minutes knowing that the plaster cast would be ruined, but somehow, I felt justified. There's only so much a girl can take. Once I was lifted out and dried off, Mom call Dr. Blair. He would meet us at the hospital. The cast had to be taken off, the incision cleaned and a new cast put on. No one said anything to me, no one gave me hell, and I don't think anyone blamed me. It was my third summer in plaster and I think everyone was simply relieved that they weren't me.

I had counted on four operations and only four. The news that the heel on my right foot had fused too far to the outside meant that I needed a fifth operation. That meant another six months in a cast and a hold on all of my plans. To say I was devastated is an understatement. I'd spent my 19th and 20th year in plaster and was now looking at spending most of my 21st the same way.

The operation took place in the early spring. I remember my mother and father coming down to the living room where I was watching television on the eve of my 21st birthday. They both wished me a happy birthday and Mom gave me a solitaire diamond ring that I didn't know she owned. The diamond had been in my grandfather's 25-year Odd Fellows tie pin and my grandmother Clara had it mounted in a ring setting. I could tell that it had been worn for many years as the shank was so thin it looked like it would come apart at any time, but it was a wonderful present, something my mother cherished and a part of our family's past. Although I've had it reset, I still wear that diamond 54 years later.

***

As the months passed and it looked as if this surgery was going to be a success, I started thinking about what I was going to do with my future. I didn't really want to go back to the newspaper. Liam had moved on to Montreal; in fact, I had gone to see him several times, cast and all. Usually, I took the train both ways and was always helped on and off by my father when the train arrived here at our century-old station in St. Catharines.

The last time I arrived home by train it was dark, cold and snowing. The train was late and everyone was waiting for it outside the station. It came in, clanging and puffing, then screeched to a halt. The few people who were getting off, got off, but being in a plaster cast up to my thigh I had to wait for my father to come and get me. Dad crossed one set of tracks, climbed up the small step and held out his arms. Hanging onto the side of the train, I let myself down and he had me.

Just at that moment we both realized that another train was approaching in the opposite direction, fast, and it wasn't going to stop. A split-second decision on his part saw my father, with me in his arms, run across the tracks to the safety of the station platform. I can still feel the rush of that other train zooming past us, faster than any train should go in a public area. Everyone on the station platform just stood there gobsmacked, not believing what they had just witnessed.

Dad wasn't exactly what you'd call an athletic type of fellow. He was short and stocky and dressed in a fedora, overcoat and toe rubbers. But I think his decision to run had saved our lives. I don't know if there would have been space between the two trains for us and my stiff plaster leg. What if something we had on had been caught on the other train or if he had tripped or somehow lost his footing going over that other set of tracks? What if, indeed!

***

After two and a half years of surgery, healing, patience and hope, I wanted it all to stand for something bigger; I wanted everything I had experienced to launch me into a new era. I was 21, I had a new pair of feet and, no matter what, it was clearly time for me to move on.

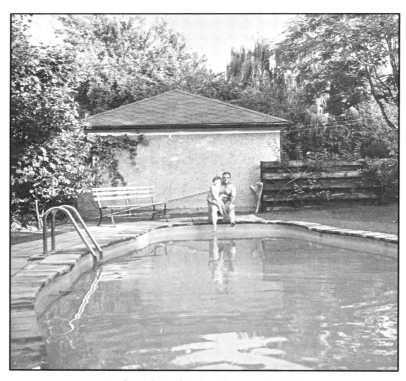

Dad and Kathie by the pool - 1961

8

A new life

I'm not sure how I got to Montreal but ten days after my cast came off I was on my way to a new life. I would be attending Sir George Williams University School of Art and still on crutches because it took a few weeks for the new bone fusions to accept my full body weight.

Before the cast was off, before I knew if I was good to go or not, Mom had dug up trillium and jack-in-the-pulpit from under the huge hemlock trees in the back garden and I'd painted watercolours of them. I'd also drawn sketches of her asleep on the couch in the living room.

As requested, five pieces of artwork were bundled up and sent off to Sir George in Montreal. I also wrote to Parsons School of Design in New York City. I couldn't see myself on crutches alone in New York City but I could see myself in Montreal going to art school with Liam around, if I ran into

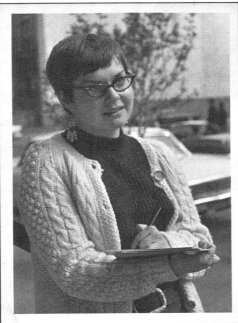

In Montreal

trouble. Fortunately, I was accepted at Sir George.

I had to get away from home. I was ready to leave, more than ready, and I'm sure my parents and Kathie were ready to get their lives back. Two and a half years was a long time to be stuck in the house. When Liam was home he'd take me out to the back forty, but when he wasn't, I was stuck. We were both young and very randy. Making out in the back seat of whatever car he had at the time was a lesson in inventiveness, but we always managed. I was never sure what I meant to him. He never said a word of endearment, never anything for me to hang on to.

***

The YWCA on Montreal's Dorchester (now René Lévesque) Boulevard was to be my home for the school year. When asked by the woman in charge how I liked my room, I replied that it was fine but I'd really like to have the wall colour changed. I'd had enough of institutional green at The Standard to last a lifetime. If I remember right, she snorted. The rooms were painted the same colour every two years whether they needed it or not, she said. I had no say in the colour. Was I naive in thinking my every whim would be met or what?

My room was on the fifth floor overlooking a street and, across the road, a large garage. The room had a single bed, a bedside table, a desk with a chair and lamp, a sink with a mirror over it and a

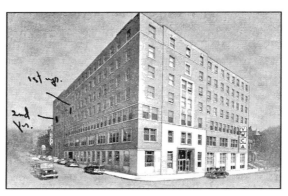

The Montreal YWCA on Dorchester Blvd. My rooms marked on a postcard

clothes closet. The communal toilets, tubs and showers were down the hall. The laundry and TV room were even further down the hall. A luggage room held our suitcases and trunks as very few of us were permanent guests.

The large window in my room had a deep exterior sill that proved to be a great place to keep milk fresh in the winter. You could make tea by boiling water with an immersion heater, dipping the teabag, pour in milk, a few sugar cubes and voila! And Nabisco Shredded Wheat and milk with a little sugar on top for breakfast? What's not to like? In the morning, with only a little ingenuity, you didn't need to go to the cafeteria in the basement and wait in line

for breakfast. Who had time for that? My cafeteria card: blue, the rim surrounded by numbers representing amounts of money that were punched as you purchased, was bought once a month for $20. I ate there so seldom I often sold it.

The only problem I had at the Y was managing the five steps up from the street at either of the two entrances. There was a railing so I managed, but stairs were never easy, particularly when I had my purse and a large artists' portfolio with me. Once inside, there was an elevator and no men were permitted above the second floor. We were secluded and safe from ourselves up there.

***

Soon I was in my element. Because I was on crutches, I was given a key to the elevator at the school. Our classrooms were on Drummond Street in an office building over the Tokay Hungarian Restaurant and a strip bar.

I'm not sure how I made it to school those first few days when I knew no one, but I did. Curb cuts didn't exist back then and I had to manage up the curbs on crutches. Believe it or not, it was easier on crutches than when I could walk on my own, as I may not have had foot drop anymore but I still didn't (and never would) have the muscle strength in my feet, ankles and calves to climb a curb.

Art school cost my mother $215 a year. She paid for everything through her antiques business, or at least I think she did it alone. She was the one who gave me a charge card to the Ogilvy department store and enough money to buy just about anything I needed. I couldn't go nuts but I didn't have to do without either.

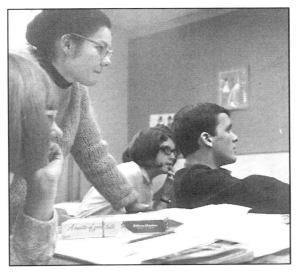

In class- Doreen Benenati, me, Suzanne Binette and Dennis Geden

My classes were in life drawing and art history with Eric Byrd, painting and drawing with Richard Billmeier, advertising design with Alan Harrison, and basic design and graphics with Christopher Lacki. We also took lettering and typography and some took fashion illustration. I didn't.

I remember some of the classes quite well. I wasn't exceptional at anything except perhaps print-making. I could carve a mean linocut. Life drawing classes were interesting: you never knew who or what you'd have standing nude in front of you. I enjoyed painting classes but wish now that I'd listened more and fooled around less. I could use those classes we took on colour and harmony. But it was all good and I was away from home. That was the point, really: to get me back to some semblance of order so I could function without my parents on a new pair of feet.

And I made friends. There were six in our class who soon formed a group and hung around together. Michael Lee from Trinidad was the only one older than me. He was small and gay and just wonderful to hang with. He had the loveliest laugh and his smile lit up the room. I was usually paired with Michael, when he wasn't with his boyfriend. Doreen Benenati was from Verdun, Quebec, and lived at home as did Stewart Marshall and Lynda Moffat. Every school day Lynda would stop by the Y on her way to school and pick me up, giving me an arm like a railing so I could get up the curbs without falling. I still remember her telephone number: OXford 70176, as I called it so many times to tell her not to stop by, I wasn't going to class. I was usually nursing a hangover. Patricia Conley from Grimsby, quite near St. Catharines, and Dennis Geden from North Bay, rounded out our little group.

59

Of the six of us, I know that Stewart and Dennis have made quite a name for themselves in the art world. Stewart lives in British Columbia and has painted gorgeous watercolours while on trips all up and down the North American west coast in his handmade kayak. He is also an avid conservationist. Dennis continues to exhibit his oil paintings in prestigious galleries worldwide and is professor of Fine Art in the Department of Fine and Performing Arts at Nipissing University in North Bay, Ontario. Doreen Benenati was well on her way to becoming well-known for her beautiful posters for the Brome Fair in Quebec and paintings of animals and nature before her untimely death from leukemia in 2000. She left us her son, Stuart.

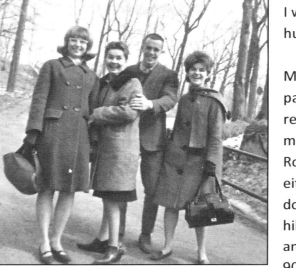

Doreen, me, Stewart Marshall (steadying me) and Pat Conley on Mount Royal

The six of us went on field trips, threw impromptu parties and got very drunk together; we frequented a night club, had a lot of laughs and actually did some art as well. It was the first time in my life that I had been part of a group and it felt wonderful.

There were three years of students and we were, or at least I was, in awe of some of the third-year students. Sid Menkes just floored me. Not only was he wickedly good-looking but he could paint abstract designs that I just loved and he wasn't afraid to tackle huge canvasses. At that time in my life, considering where I was and what I was doing, that was huge.

Montreal is a city built partially on a volcanic-related hill or small mountain (Mount Royal) and the streets either run directly downhill or circle the hill. Remember, my ankles are fused in a 90-degree angle. When I'm horizontal in bed, my toes point to the ceiling. So, when I'm on a hill, my feet don't bend to the slope of the land, the back edge of my heels touch and that's it. If I let my knees go, I crumple on my fusions and, believe it or not, even with all the screws and staples in there, they crack.

Fortunately, art school was horizontal to the Y. I didn't have to go uphill much. Any place else usually wasn't though. Trips "up the mountain" to the park at Mount Royal saw me hanging on to the fellows in our little group and standing sideways. I still had to touch someone for balance or I'd fall. The

60

operations didn't fix that. But bending my knees to stand still was no longer an option because once you bend your knees your ankles flex and mine no longer flexed so I had to keep moving or find something or someone to touch.

I remember falling while crossing multi-laned Dorchester Boulevard. My knees just gave out and I was on my hands and knees on the road. Drivers were revving their engines waiting for the lights to change. I couldn't get up. I looked up and there was a line of cars ready to take off. Did they see me? Was this it? Suddenly, just as the lights changed, an onlooker grabbed me under the arms and carried me to the curb. Close call, yes, but I couldn't let it stop me or I'd never leave my room at the Y.

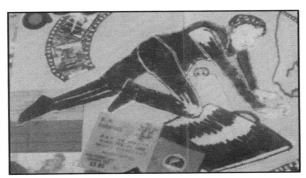

A drawing I did of me down on the road for a collage put together years later – *pc8.1*

With the completion of my first year, I came home for the summer. When I applied at Wallace's, a local dry goods store where my mother had worked before she married, I got a job as the relief switchboard operator. I didn't know how to run a switchboard but figured how hard could it be?

The full-time operator was so relieved to have someone come in to give her

Saturdays and some vacation time off, she taught me the board in an hour. It wasn't what we know now as a switchboard with push buttons that light up to direct your call. This was a vintage beauty, the kind that Lily Tomlin made famous in her "one ringy-dingy, two ringy-dingy" Ernestine sketches. It had cords with metal tips that came out of the base and went into holes in the vertical part of the board at face level. You wore a headset with an ear and mouthpiece. When a call came in you put one cord into the incoming hole and asked what department they'd like. When they told you, you put the cord behind that cord into the department hole, flicked a switch to ring the telephone and your call was connected. When it was finished and they hung up, a buzzer went off and you disconnected both cords. If it was busy, you could have a design of cords all over the board that looked much like a roadmap.

I loved working the switchboard when it was busy. My grip wasn't good, my thumbs barely worked, and extending my fingers to reach down behind to grab a cord was difficult, but I could grip the metal tip between my index and big middle finger,

61

pull it up quickly and, before it slipped back, grab the shaft and plug it in. It may not have been the way I was supposed to be doing it, but it worked.

I still remember the watchword for a shoplifter: Mrs. Grey. Upon being alerted by a salesperson that they'd observed a light-fingered customer, I'd first advise the floor manager and then open the intercom system and say something like, Mrs. Grey in Dept. B., which meant someone was shoplifting in lingerie.

***

During my first and second year, Liam had driven us home several times. It was a long trip, about eight hours straight, and he didn't like stopping. We didn't talk much. He worked at a local advertising firm and was busy with his other interests, which included some of the models he met on the job who had children. Every now and then I'd go to the apartment he shared with Dr. Bob and make stuffed peppers. Sometimes I stayed over, sometimes not. It was a very one-sided romance, mostly my side.

The girls I met at the Y were a good bunch. I particularly remember Bobbi, with whom I shared a double room one weekend just for fun. She was very butch and scared the daylights out of me when she wanted to "play." That wasn't my kind of fun.

Sarah seemed very prissy. We stuffed her keyhole with paper and put plastic wrap on the toilet seats for her. In retrospect, she was likely far more mature than most of us. I recall someone tossing an entire roll of toilet paper over the tub stall wall while I was leisurely soaking. Perhaps it was Sarah wreaking revenge.

And then there was Ilsa. She was a very smart blonde, studying at McGill. How she put up with me and my record player in the next room with only a thin wall between us for an entire school year, I'll never know, but we managed to get along. Also a McGill student, Lynn showed me the ropes: where the laundry room was, how to navigate and find my way in a strange environment. We still correspond.

As often as we could afford it, three or four of us from the Y would make the long trek down to Joe's Steak House for a real feed. I liked my steak blue but warm. I also remember incredibly juicy smoked meat on rye at Ben's Deli. One night, in truth it was early morning, after extricating myself from a bad date and very hungry, I ended up in a cafeteria. My meal on the table in front of me, I looked up and there was Leonard Cohen directly opposite me but two tables away. The rest of the place was empty. We nodded to each other and kept on eating; two people caught up in the slightly sordid ambience of Montreal in the 60s.

***

The second summer, 1965, I stayed in Montreal. My parents had agreed that I could move out of the Y. I knew my way around and wanted to be on my own. But before I moved, my brother Ronald came to visit. He stayed at the small corner hotel across the road and we spent some time together. He had all of Montreal to explore and I left him on his own to do just that. He needed to think. He and his girlfriend were expecting.

Those days were tough. You didn't have the pill and abortion was an impossible ordeal for most. So many married when they were very young and unprepared. He was only 19. He had his whole life in front of him but there was nothing else to be done but to go back and get married. I was a bridesmaid.

***

Rents in downtown Montreal were fairly cheap and I found a one-room furnished bachelor on Mountain Street for something like $85 a month. The only hitch was the eight steps up the front and then another 15 or so inside to my door on the second floor. When I was getting enough sleep, I could do those stairs by pulling myself up by the railing. When I was tired, hungover or worse, they were almost impossible. The apartment was tiny. If you tried to close the bathroom door when sitting on the toilet, you had to put your feet in the shower. There was a tiny half-sized fridge along with a hotplate on the kitchen counter and a chrome dining table that doubled as a desk with two chairs against the inside wall. Two foldout couches took up the rest of the

space. It wasn't much but it was mine and another notch in my freedom belt.

The only window was quite big and overlooked the street. One early morning, around 2 a.m., I watched as a car pulled up to the curb and a man got out, hit a man on the sidewalk on the head, knocking him to the sidewalk, and then proceeded to beat his legs with a baseball bat. It made me sick but served to open my eyes to another side of that cosmopolitan city … a not-so-friendly one. I just lived on the surface.

A fly infestation also hit my little abode. I'd dropped and broken a jar of sweet gherkin pickles on the carpet behind the dining table. I didn't clean up the vinegar well enough and a fly had laid eggs in it that I assume became maggots (I never saw them) that hatched and I ended up with maybe 100 flies on my front window screen all trying to get out. It was pretty disgusting. I told the gang and just about everyone came over to help clean up Crabtree's place.

That big black sweater I'd knit so many times when I was in a cast also came with me and it was pulled out yet again. All of us took turns knitting a long scarf for Geden, who had a suede jacket that didn't really keep him warm enough in winter. He still has the scarf.

My apartment was only two doors from a

French-style downstairs bistro called Chez LouLou – Les Bacchantes. We called it simply, the Bistro. After school, it was a place to go to meet friends and make new ones. Light shone in onto the long bar from the street and there were tables and banquette seats on the mirrored far wall. The washrooms were in the back. Draft beer was served by the tray or, "Une Canadian, s'il vous plait," got you a bottled beer.

Because I lived so close, the Bistro was like going home. I'd pop down after supper on Thursday, Friday and Saturday nights. Doreen who lived at home, and a few others from school who didn't, would sometimes join us. There were also the regulars: Graham, a pianist, who was usually very drunk but fun to listen to; Eddie, billed as a virtuoso of lethargy – who, at 41, had never worked and lived fairly well on $35 a week, provided by his wealthy father in Massachusetts; and David, a lawyer in the financial district, who sold marijuana and buried it in milk bottles in his backyard. David always looked so respectable with his spiffy silk tie, cufflinks and three-piece suit no one would ever suspect he was dealing on the side.

When I "stayed too long at the fair," drinking my beer and smoking my ever-so-sophisticated brown Gitanes cigarettes (I actually liked their taste), I couldn't stand up well enough to walk home. Several early

mornings I pulled myself up the Bistro's steps, turned around, sat down and bummed my way two doors down to my apartment steps, and then slowly hoisted myself backwards up the steps, one by one. I stopped when someone went by, to look as if I was actually meant to be there and perhaps was just sitting on the front steps because I couldn't sleep or it was too hot inside. I don't know if I fooled anyone or not. At the time I didn't really care; my bed was calling and I'd get there any way I could.

And then there was Mickey. Liam knew a lot of people in Montreal and Mickey was one of them. He was working on opening a discothèque and called it the Mousse Spacthèque, which roughly translated to Space Age Froth. I watched as the stainless-steel floor went in and tables with mirrored tops and walls that reflected moving abstract slides, giving the impression that the whole room was moving, were finished. Discothèques were new to Montreal and since this one was just one block over from where I lived and Mickey, who was a tiny fellow with a halo of curly red receding hair above a freckled white constantly worried face, was a friend and didn't mind having me around, I felt welcome. I loved watching the place take shape but once it was open, I never went back. I was more a bistro-type gal than a disco diva.

Pat Conley stayed with me for a while

during my third year, but most of the time I had the tiny place to myself. Mom and Dad had given me a really good portable record player with two detachable speakers. With the speakers in the window, the Mommas and Poppas along with Stan Getz and Dave Brubeck often serenaded my little part of Mountain Street when I was home.

Doreen introduced me to Bell Telephone operator, Shirley, and her friend, Sally, a petite blonde whom you might say was a "working girl." Sally lived in a little, mostly yellow, basement apartment with her daughter, Leah, and a pet rabbit. She smoked marijuana and I remember times in her apartment when everybody was stoned including little Leah, who was just learning to walk. I swear, even the rabbit was hopping strangely.

Doreen and her friends also introduced me

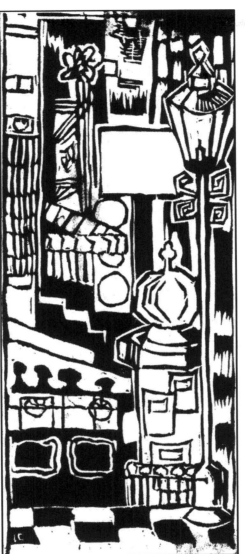

A linocut I did of Mountain Street looking north from my apartment

pc8.2

to the jazz clubs in the Little Burgundy area of the city. Live jazz played by swinging musicians, in an atmosphere so close you could see the rivulets of sweat running down their foreheads, was a life changing experience. I wondered if Dad ever experimented with jazz. I loved it and he likely did as well.

***

During the last few weeks of our third and final year at school, we were required to write a thesis. I left it too late to really do anything meaningful and wound up with a mishmash comparison of the lives of Leonardo Da Vinci and Michelangelo, but I passed my year and was invited to the Art Club on Stanley Street for our graduation ceremony. It was my last year and also the last year for the school. No more Sir George Williams School of Art.

I'm not sure why, but I bought a new dress for graduation. I never wore dresses. Like some of my friends, I was a beatnik, wore black most of the time and my hair straight and long. When I finally got sick of looking after

65

so much hair, I had it cropped short and sassy. My lipstick (when I wore any) was white, eye makeup very dark, and large earrings that looked like miniature beaded trivets hung down to my shoulders.

I think I bought that dress because I absolutely adored the fabric it was made out of. It looked like something from the Arabian Nights to me – orange, purple and red paisley – but it belonged on a wall or a pillow, not on me. I loved to look at it but felt very self-conscious in it. I'd have had a better day and been true to myself in my all

black ensemble.

Graduation day went off without a hitch except for my being so ill-at-ease in my dress. I held onto Geden for balance during the brief ceremony and when I had my certificate in hand, managed to get myself back down the Arts Club stairs and that was the end of art school. Mom and Dad had sent a telegram: WISH WE COULD BE WITH YOU ON YOUR GRADUATION GLAD SOMEONE IN THE FAMILY COULD DO IT LOVE DAD AND MOTHER.

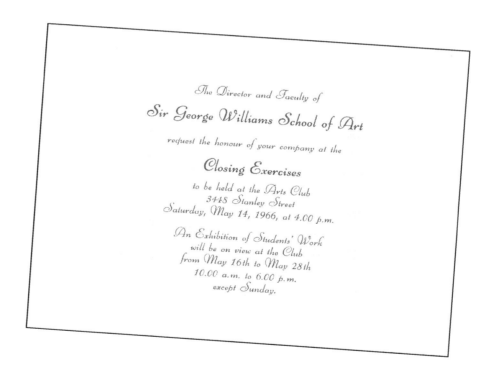

The Director and Faculty of

Sir George Williams School of Art

request the honour of your company at the

Closing Exercises

to be held at the Arts Club
3448 Stanley Street
Saturday, May 14, 1966, at 4.00 p.m.

An Exhibition of Students' Work
will be on view at the Club
from May 16th to May 28th
10.00 a.m. to 6.00 p.m.
except Sunday.

9

Get a job

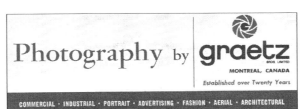

With art school behind me, it was time to find a job. I had a portfolio of artwork but still wasn't sure what would be required of me at a commercial art studio. I applied by letter to several and actually had appointments for interviews, but I always had to call first to see if I could get into the building. Something as simple as a step at the front door would stop me cold and there was no way I could carry a portfolio and climb a step, much less a flight of steps, to a second-floor office.

If it rained I had to take a cab; in fact, I had to take a cab everywhere. It was just that when it rained, everyone took a cab so *my* cab was usually very late or didn't arrive at all.

Finding work, especially in the commercial art field, looked near impossible and it only got worse when I gave up on art studios, tried out for a receptionist's job at a fabric importer and was required to learn a new push-button switchboard. For some reason, it didn't make sense to me and I was told that I needn't come back the next day.

Could I do anything? Was it all just a sick joke ... on me?

Then my luck changed. I landed a job with a company called Graetz Brothers. They were commercial photographers with a studio on Montreal's St. Maurice Street in the older factory district. My job was to work with two whiz Armenian darkroom technicians as they ran off hundreds, sometimes thousands, of prints a day. Remember my darkroom work with Liam at The Standard? Same thing. But these darkrooms were maybe 25 steps up, on the second floor.

Everyday I'd take a cab to work, haul my body up the stairs, and eat lunch up there because there was no way I could do those stairs four times a day. By closing when I was so tired and afraid my knees would give out, I'd sit, bumming it down the steps to go home. On mornings when I felt really rough, I bummed it up the stairs too ... backwards.

It was November by then and I recall running thousands of black and white 8x10 glossy photos off the dryer of a sexy model wearing a white fur bikini, standing beside an elbow-high pyramid of oil cans. The floor got so wet I bought myself a pair of rubber-soled sneakers so I wouldn't slip and fall. It was also my job to stamp the backs of the prints with the Graetz Brothers logo, pop them in large brown 8 x 10 envelopes with a cardboard stiffener and add a mailing label so they were ready for the post. The prints were a Christmas present to gas stations and body shops from the oil distributor.

Finally, the stairs, the water and the monotony got to me and I left.

My next job was at AudioGraphic Presentations, an advertising firm run by a fellow from my hometown of St. Catharines. The business was housed on the second floor of a stately old building and again there were stairs. When they were making commercials, I'd go out and find what was needed for a shoot, use it on the set, and then return it all. They also made continuous filmstrips that could be played on a portable machine to demonstrate a product. You see them at trade shows, but now they are short videos repeated on a computer. These fellows were way ahead of the times and technology wouldn't catch up with their needs for many years. When I wasn't shopping, I was part of the photography, an extra, if you will, in the background, or I was answering the telephone, typing invoices, whatever was needed. It was a full-time job but it didn't

last. One day I arrived at work and the door was locked. A sign said the business was closed; they were filing for bankruptcy.

Liam was working for a large commercial art and photography studio: Arnott, Rogers and Batten, known to most as ARB. He put a word in for me with the audio-visual department and after an interview and a tour of the place, I was hired. My boss was Jim Muir, the production manager, and I was his AV assistant. Expo '67, the World's Fair, would be held in Montreal the next year and there were giant slide shows and rear projection installations to be produced for the Canadian and other pavilions on the new man-made island. The site was becoming more interesting every day with Moshe Safdie's model housing community, Habitat '67, originally built as the Canadian pavilion, growing block atop block; and Buckminster Fuller's geodesic dome taking shape.

I must have mounted thousands of slides during the time I worked there, most of them two pieces of glass sandwiching the film, surrounded with metal. Keeping dust and fingerprints out of the frames was a constantly present challenge and particularly stressful when it was a rush job.

By that time, I'd moved from my one room on Mountain Street to a larger second-floor studio apartment, one block west on Crescent Street. It was brand new, in fact I'd watched it go up, and it still smelled like fresh concrete and paint when I moved in. A huge bonus … there was an elevator.

ARB was downhill, closer to the St. Lawrence River, and I could walk to work if I had the time. But walking downhill was a challenge: if I really got going, I'd pick up speed and couldn't stop. I'd have to hug a utility pole to stop my momentum. Every morning I'd have to wait by the front door of ARB for someone to come along to help me in the door. I couldn't climb the step and grab the door handle at the same time.

One morning on my way to work, downhill, I fell and couldn't get up. Dozens of people walked by me; some even stepped over me. It was humiliating. I was trying my very best but it never seemed good enough. To those people, I was possibly addicted to drugs, alcohol or both. They only saw me down, and down on the street wasn't where most people found themselves at 8:30 in the morning.

I made friends at ARB, especially among the men, and on Fridays we'd go over to the Windsor Hotel after work for a few draft beers, or a gin and tonic if it was payday. They were a talented bunch and I enjoyed their company immensely but I usually went home alone – except for one night, when one of the married men decided he was going to "see me home safely." When I got in the elevator at my apartment building

and he pushed the button, my knees gave out and I crumpled to the floor in a giggling heap. We were too drunk to get me up, so I crawled down the carpeted hall to my apartment. That's something I've never forgotten. Once in, my two budgies, Moose and Alice, were flying from picture frame to picture frame making an awful racket. We left the birds to settle down and attempted to make supper even though it was beyond midnight. After he almost fell into the oven, we decided that neither of us could manage in the kitchen and he soon went home. The next morning, terribly dehydrated and very hung over, I dumped an entire can of frozen orange juice into the blender and just let it go. I chugged the entire thing in five minutes and immediately and violently threw up so forcefully it hit the opposite wall. Serves me right and what a mess it was to clean up.

Hangovers always made me feel so purged. I felt delicate and pure … for about a day.

During my trips to Expo '67, I was invited aboard the HMCS Skeena, which was moored near the Canadian pavilion. It was in the officer's mess that I met Henry, who was stationed in the engine room. He always smelled like oil. But Henry had something else: psoriasis. And it wasn't just in one place; it was everywhere. I was quite sure that spending most of his time down in the bowels of the ship next to a huge bank of engines didn't do him any good, but that was his job. It didn't bother me, after all I wasn't exactly perfect, and I soon learned to apply the tar-based ointment he used to keep the raised plaques on his skin from cracking. That's why he always smelled like oil. He also wasn't to be off the ship all night, so he'd leave my bed by midnight and hail a cab back to the ship. After he left, I'd get the vacuum out and shake the sheets. Hundreds of silver scales would fall like snow to the floor.

I liked Henry. He was kind and he really liked me. After his ship made several trips back to Expo, he began talking marriage, promising me everything he could think of back in his maritime province hometown, including indoor plumbing. Sorry, Henry, but I couldn't see myself living alone, indoor plumbing or not, with my husband gone somewhere on manoeuvres. I'd waited for the ship to come in several times and saw the looks on the faces of the wives. I didn't want to be one of them.

Expo '67 was fabulous. Mom, Dad and Kathie decided to come for a visit. They made the eight-hour drive with a very old, Dutch, pine, flat-to-the-wall cupboard on the roof of their station wagon and the black base of an old cast iron stove in the back. The cupboard has travelled with me ever since and the stove base made an excellent coffee table when it had a slab of white marble, formerly a Victorian washroom stall wall, on it.

Mom knew how to put things together. Her specialty was lamps made from weigh scales, huge old stair balusters, advertising pieces, jugs, oil lamps; you name it, she wired it.

Liam was around, even left his toothbrush, but again we rarely did anything together except have sex … not love … sex. Then he told me he was going back to Ontario. My world dissolved. As much as we both had separate lives, I'd counted on him always being there and I'd somehow hoped we'd end up together.

You know those moments in your life that seem to be engraved in your mind: the ones that never go away? We had one of those in my apartment. I was sitting on my bed by the window and he was across the room, sitting on the edge of the marble coffee table. He was leaving. I was crying. He asked me what I wanted and I said to be married … to him. He said, "Let's give it a try." I was silent. Give it a try. He'd never even said he loved me. The most emotion he'd ever shown me was when I told him I'd been pregnant and for about 20 seconds he thought it was his. When I told him it wasn't, his ardor cooled considerably. He'd been kind and considered me in larger ways: the foot and ankle surgery, the Rolleiflex camera he gave me, the job at ARB; but little things that would have made my heart sing like saying he loved me, touching my face with a gentle look in his eyes, just didn't happen. Kind, yes, but in another way brutal because he'd show up anytime he liked without notice. Because I loved him, I let him into my life and bed far longer than I should have, when deep down I knew there could never be anything more than sex between us.

Give it a try? I looked up at him and said, "You don't really mean that," and it was over. I knew it wasn't going to go any further. I'd met him when I was 17 and eight years later he was still in my life. But not anymore; it was time to let go.

For weeks, I was heartbroken. It was as if someone or something had died. In reality, hope had died and my dreams of a future with Liam were dashed. I should have known it was impossible when, on one of our trips home, he showed me the apartment he had rented in Hamilton. The dining room and kitchen were up a step. A step I simply couldn't manage. He surely wasn't thinking of me ever living there. Why didn't I twig? I did twig; I just tried to ignore it. Was I a project? Someone he took under his wing a long time ago, when we both worked at the newspaper, because I was disabled? Someone he continued to feel

loosely responsible for but not someone to love? I *was* useful, I never said no, but he obviously didn't want to spend the rest of his life with me. He had taught me a great deal and helped me through a very difficult time during my surgery and settling into a strange city. He'd often come up with a solution to a problem I had if I told him about it, but I could never talk to him as an equal. He was five years older than me and those years were too big a gap as far as our education and interests were concerned. I couched everything I said to him and listened to his every word as if it was from God but knew we would never make a go of it. I couldn't be myself around him, couldn't tell him what I really thought, couldn't be silly, couldn't cry … wasn't happy. I had spent far too much time idolizing a man I didn't really know. It happens. Yes, he had given me much but I had given him all I had to give. Me.

Montreal felt empty after Liam left. No matter what I was doing I could no longer imagine him there, working or sleeping or on the job. He was too far away. I had another proposal from a man I'd met at the Bistro and admired but didn't love. I suspect he felt sorry for me and I suspected he was an alcoholic. There seemed to be too many men complicating my life and I'd had enough for the time being. It was time I packed it in and headed for home.

I sublet my Crescent Street apartment to a

large immigrant family, although I was warned not to sublease to people who might build a fire on the balcony to cook their meals. I really didn't care what they did. I just wanted out.

***

Once again, Mom and Dad came with the station wagon and took my furniture to a nice big new one-bedroom apartment on Stephanie Street in Toronto, backing onto the Ontario College of Art and Design (now OCAD University.)

My neighbours were two young boys attending the art school and one taught me the Indonesian art form of wax-resist and dye on cloth, called batik. I loved it. I was still in art mode and made banner installations consisting of hanging yards of nylon and brilliant splashes of printer's ink.

Finally, I found a job at M.S. Art Services/ Film Opticals just three blocks west of my apartment on University Street. I told them I'd been the assistant to a production manager, but thought I knew what he did as he'd introduced me to some of it and felt confident that I could do the job. I didn't really know what I was supposed to be

A brochure from M.S. Art Services Ltd.

doing and I was called in to the boss's office after six months and given the choice of either two weeks' pay or to work out two weeks. I took the pay.

That job had taught me a lot: They did the production work for the studios that made TV commercials and made some themselves. Every product in a commercial was photographed, put back together and air-brushed. None of the instructions, warnings, dietary information you see on a carton or box in a grocery store remained. We did all the cleaning up, all the artwork, the supers (wording that goes over an image) and the titles. My job was to pull all the costs from all the departments together and, in the end, have an invoice ready for the customer.

It wasn't as easy as my boss at ARB had made it look and he actually showed up one day, asking me what I thought it was all about and how could I have misled the people I was working for like that. Stretching the truth to get a job had backfired, big time. This was too close to home.

***

While in Toronto, I met Guy, a friend of an art school buddy. They were both from North Bay. We got along and eventually he moved in. It was partly having him in my life that complicated the job. When there was a rush and everyone wanted everything yesterday, I, along with my crew, was expected to work 12, 15 or even 24 hours straight to get it done. I couldn't and wouldn't do that. And the first thing they had me do there, on my first day on the job, was fire a young girl I didn't even know. What could I do? I needed the job. I'd never fired anyone in my life. Right out of the chute that should have clued me in that this job wasn't going to be my future.

Although I only lived three blocks from work, when it was icy I couldn't leave my apartment and when it was windy my feet would get blown together and I'd trip myself. When I was down, often bloody and bruised, I couldn't get back up. Cab drivers didn't like a three-block fare. Just getting to work and back every day was a struggle.

Guy drank and I drank with him.

When I went to an employment agency looking for another job, Guy went with me. I recall being pulled up a long dark flight of stairs. I was asked to take a typing speed test. Could I file? Yes. Could I spell? Yes. While they graded my typing test, I was asked to watch a film loop on the company and the terrific temporary help they turned out.

Back in the interview room, I was told I was undesirable material. My skills were nil, they couldn't help me and I'd be lucky if I ever found work, anywhere. I asked her to come into the room where the loop was still playing. There I was, in the video right in front of them, at my desk at Audiographic Presentations, obviously able to work. They said nothing. We left.

10

To have and have not

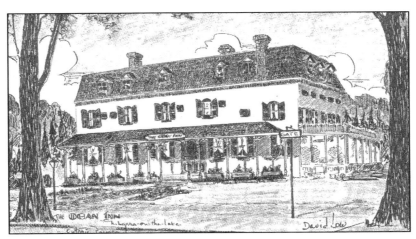

The Oban Inn – Niagara-on-the-Lake, Ontario, in 1968 – pc10.1

Guy and I planned to marry, so I'd sent him home to my parents while I closed up things and sublet the apartment in Toronto. My folks didn't know what to make of this gangly, 6'4" blond. Dad didn't like him right off but Mom was willing to give him the benefit of the doubt. It was fall and the weather was still warm. Mom had bought a collection of African artifacts and a huge olive green tent had been part of the package. They let him stay in the tent in the backyard.

My aunt told me years later that my father had stood at his bedroom window overlooking the backyard and told my mother that if I married that kid with his feet sticking out of the tent door, he'd jump in our swimming pool and drown himself.

We were married on December 15, 1968, in a beautiful old church in Niagara-on-the-Lake, just a few miles from St. Catharines, on a cold, dull Sunday afternoon. I was greatly relieved that my father decided to join us for the nuptials, but still think my mother had a huge hand in that. My sister Kathie and brother Ronald with his wife and their first-born daughter were also there.

No one walked me down the aisle. It wasn't that kind of occasion. We stood together in front of the Anglican minister and the ceremony was over in less than five minutes. After signing the register as a married couple, we were all back out in the cold again. The first thing Guy did was light up a cigarette.

I wore a green turtleneck and the green Joseph Ribkoff suit I'd bought with my earnings from working in the designer's Montreal shipping department on the occasional weekend while at art school. Over the suit was my leather coat with a huge lynx fur collar. Fur was very "in" back then.

After a lovely dinner at the historic Oban Inn, not too far from the church, we all went back to my family home where Guy and I had set up a makeshift living area in the basement.

That night we spent our honeymoon in a bed next to the furnace. Staring at overhead cobweb-draped floor joists, I remember thinking that just two floors up lay my parents. What were they thinking? I couldn't bring myself to go there. They had been as gracious as any parents could be, considering they didn't want me to marry Guy. This wasn't what I'd had in mind for my wedding night, but then I'd never really given it much thought. Wedding gowns, receptions and honeymoons weren't part of my plan for my life, not even with Liam. In my imaginings, I'd always skipped all of that. I just couldn't see myself walking up the aisle in a long white dress, balancing on my father's arm. Perhaps I should have. It might have slowed me down and made me think about what I was really getting myself into. Why was I getting married? Likely because everyone else I knew was married.

I was 27. I didn't want to live with my parents and marriage just seemed like the natural next step.

My father was noticeably quiet during the few weeks after the wedding that we stayed with them. One night during supper I had a long-distance phone call. It was Marc Gallant, an old friend from Montreal. Would Guy and I like to go out to Prince Edward Island (PEI), where I'd work for the new Economic Improvement Corporation? The government had just announced that it was going to set up new departments to build and promote the province. I'd be working in audio-visual wherever needed. I couldn't believe my good fortune. Marc had known me in Montreal through various work associates, had gone back to his hometown in PEI after Montreal, and had sought me out. We'd be out from under my parents' roof. I'd have a job and Guy would likely find one as well. We'd be on our own. The relief around the supper table that night was palpable.

After a train ride to Toronto and an overnight stay at the Royal York Hotel that involved a goodbye party with friends, we boarded an Eastern Provincial Airline 28-seater, twin-engine DC-3, and ended up on PEI in the Gulf of St. Lawrence. We were to stay at The Hotel Charlottetown, an elegant old lady built by the Canadian National Railway in 1931. Our room and expenses were paid for. I was to wait for a phone call to tell me what department I'd be working in and when I'd start.

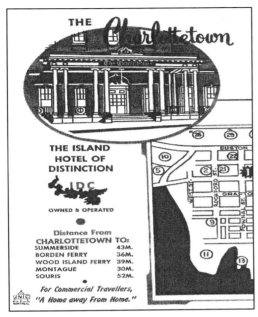

Part of The Charlottetown Hotel restaurant's placemat

We waited and waited. It was winter. I couldn't walk in the snow and ice and my body used every ounce of energy it possessed to fight the cold. I stayed put.

Guy drank downstairs in the bar. We ate all our meals in the dining room or café. I had to let the switchboard operator know everywhere I went and I didn't go far. I remember ordering pizza and, when it arrived, thinking it looked like dog food on a crust … smelled like it too.

Soon the glamour of staying in a hotel wore off. Guy would drink almost every night with some people he'd met in the bar. One

particular friend, Kurt, became a go-between from us to Marc. When Kurt and Guy were drunk enough, they'd go out onto the front circular driveway of the hotel and relieve themselves in the snow. There were huge spotlights pointing up at the building out there. I imagined one exploding in their faces, or worse, from the hot piss hitting the cold bulb.

Something had to give. We'd been in PEI far too long. Something was wrong. I'd never had an official meeting with anyone, had never been told or asked about the job.

Finally, we were notified that the entire program had been cancelled. Our plane fare home would be paid for and we could submit final expenses. That was it. As much as I wanted to work and to begin a new life there, I was relieved. The waiting was over. I could relax.

Before we left, we took a small plane over the island and it was then, for the first time, that I saw pink snow. PEI's soil is dark red. When the dust blows onto fresh snow the snow becomes pink. As I looked down, the snow on each country road was pink on both sides from the red mud being splattered up by tires. The shoreline was fabulous and furious at the same time. Giant dark green waves crashed onto huge black rocks and white seabirds wheeled beneath us. It was a truly beautiful place, but I'd not seen it. I'd spent my days in PEI in a hotel room waiting for a phone call that never came.

Soon we were back where we'd started: in the basement and broke. My mother, bless her, began looking for a place for us to live. I imagine my father had suggested she get us out from underfoot fast. She did. Within days we moved into a first-floor apartment in an old house in the seedier side of town. We were there just long enough for me to find out that the kitchen floor crunched with cockroaches when I walked across it in the dark of night to visit the bathroom and the landlord offered to take the rent out "in trade" if I didn't have the cash. Hours were spent sitting in the front bay window, painting a detailed watercolour of a sweet-smelling cherry blossom branch balanced in a water-filled pop bottle. It was my escape from the reality that was in the rooms behind me.

Guy went out every day to look for some kind of work but usually came home well after any businesses had closed and I knew he'd been drinking. My heart ached for him. I wanted so much for him and us to be happy, but it just didn't happen.

Then Mom found an apartment for us on the lower floor of a Victorian row house in an older but very respectable part of town. I couldn't climb the front steps, there were no railings, but the steps to the side stoop that led to the kitchen had a railing. I could

get in there.

The place was beautiful. The walls were all white and there were high white ceilings, huge sliding pocket doors between the two front rooms that had been the parlour and dining room, hardwood floors, and even a fireplace with a marble surround and mantel. The windows fronting on the street

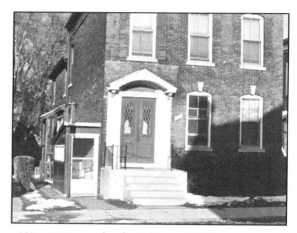

We were on the first floor of this lovely old Victorian townhouse

were almost floor-to-ceiling and there were two huge windows in the second room that looked out to the ivy-covered brick of our neighbour's house. The kitchen was small but adequate and there was another small room beyond that. The bathroom had an old claw-foot tub, a toilet, and pedestal sink. And there wasn't a cockroach in sight.

The front room became my art studio and the room behind it was our living room. Mom contributed her collection of African paddles, spears, mallets and war clubs; they looked fabulous mounted on the white wall

78

over a long grey sectional sofa that came in from the basement at home. The marble-topped coffee table was perfect in that room. Two single beds just fit in the little room in the back that butted up against the apartment behind us. To buffer the sounds of our energetic lovemaking, we glued large grey egg cartons to the wall. When we moved, I'll just bet the landlord loved us for that.

For a while I tried making some money with my art. I made cards, painted canvases, and did large works using found objects like a wall hanging from an old metal hoop, laced with linen string hung with real crystal beads. I batiked silk scarves and cotton by the yard, sewing it into a wall hanging, laced and hung from found wood. Photographs taken of the half-burned-out dance hall at Port Dalhousie, where my father had played in the big bands during the 40s and 50s, were glued to a weather-beaten old grey door. On top of the photos I pasted spike-shaped shards of thick glass that gave the impression that time had broken into the picture.

Being a working exhibiting artist was all well and good, but making money at it didn't happen. We were dependent on my mother. She gave me $20 a week for groceries. Believe it or not, in the early '70s that would actually buy a week's food. She also helped with the rent.

I taught children art at the local YWCA one night a week for $3 a head. It helped. Guy was experimenting with photography and had received a grant to attend school away from home. That time with him away gave me breathing room to explore my own talents, although I was always happy to have him back. But we badly needed a reliable source of income … and soon.

When Alice, my mother's friend who had taken over the newspaper's library when I went for my foot reconstruction surgery, called to say the paper was looking for an editorial assistant and would I be interested, I took a hard swallow, kissed my dreams of being a full-time artist goodbye, and said yes.

***

The Standard was as familiar to me as the back of my hand. I knew there was an elevator to the second-floor editorial department. I didn't have to try to climb stairs. An interview was arranged and they welcomed me back. The pay was $64 a week plus benefits. I was to sit at a reception desk at the entrance of the editorial department, where there was a half ledge separating me from the public.

People would come to that ledge, lean on it or pile their file folders or purse on it, and tell me their concerns or ask for the reporter they wanted to see. I was also to take calls from all of the local undertakers every morning and type out the obituaries on the old see-through, cast-iron Underwood typewriter on my desk. I also typed all the letters-to-the-editor that came in handwritten, and most of them did. I don't think anyone realized that I could only type with two fingers. But two fingers would have to be enough. I needed the job.

There was also a console switchboard on my desk and I was to answer for the editorial department, then switch the calls to the women's or sports department, reporter, city desk or managing editor, or take a message if they weren't in. I'd failed at learning a switchboard in Montreal, but for some reason this one made sense to me and I had it down pat in a day. It was actually fun.

The Standard was a daily newspaper with a circulation of about 45,000. It was the only paper in town, family run, and likely employed about 200 people. The editorial department was a mixture of men and women: the women being in the family department, art and entertainment, and me. The fellows covered the police and fire beats, city council and everything in between. The sports department was a law onto itself. Four fellows worked the hockey, curling, baseball, golf, and rowing in the area. Five or six photographers worked shifts. Everything was bigger and better than when I'd worked there in 1959.

The five-block walk to work was doable in spring, summer and fall, but in the winter I simply couldn't risk it. My balance was terrible and trying to climb a curb impossible unless I was lucky. Not wanting to rely on luck and possibly end up flat on my back in the road, I'd look for driveways and often have to walk down the gutters until I found one I could manage. Eventually I worked out a fairly safe route and, barring any roadwork, usually got to work without falling. In the later years, during the winter months, Betty, the entertainment page editor, picked me up every morning. Alice often drove me home. What a relief that was.

Women didn't wear slacks to work in those days but I finally screwed up enough courage to ask my boss if I could, as I was so cold getting to work and then sitting at my desk that my legs were blue. He reluctantly said yes.

When I did walk to work, my morning journey took me alongside a lovely old home with white wisteria growing up the side of the wall to the roof and by a very old boarded-up convent, then across the road to city hall, through Market Square, then up Queen Street and into the newspaper's front door to the elevator. You'd think I'd feel safe once I got inside but the building was so old the floors had waves in them. If I didn't watch where I was going, I'd stub my foot on the rise of a wave and be down on my knees in a split second.

At one time or another it seemed everyone in town made it down the long dark hall to editorial plus a few who just needed help after too many drinks. I could see those ones leaning on the wall as they made their way toward me. Sometimes I could handle them, other times the nearest reporter took over and it was man-to-man or sometimes woman-to-man.

The people I met as editorial assistant ranged from undertakers and wedding photographers to politicians, cross-country cyclists, actors, natives, artists, local business owners, and regular folks trying to keep something out of the paper or get something in.

***

Guy's back had been bothering him since he'd bent over to pick up a case of beer at the St. Catharines Golf and Country Club, where my father had arranged for him to work before we were married. That ended up with him on Workmen's (now Worker's) Compensation. The back really never got better. He'd try working when he was feeling well, but nothing ever really stuck.

In December 1971, we had gone to Toronto to bring in the new year with our old friends who still lived there. Camped out on the floor in a sleeping bag, I looked at the telephone on the wall and thought about calling my mother and father to say "Happy New Year." This had been a custom of ours since we were old enough to be on our own. Then I thought about how difficult it would be to get up and make my way over all the bodies. I didn't do it.

When we arrived home on New Year's Day around noon, I called my mother and asked her if she had taken the turkey she was going to roast for me out of the freezer.

"Linda, hasn't anyone told you?" she said. "Told me what?" I replied. "Linda, your father died this morning."

He'd had a massive heart attack in bed. My mother had thought he was snoring but when she looked over at him, he was struggling to breathe and turning blue. He was dead by the time the ambulance arrived. He had celebrated his 56th birthday less than three weeks before.

He had told Dr. Younghusband that he was having pain while walking to work and the good doctor said he'd figure out what was causing it even if he had to walk to work with him. He didn't get the chance.

We were all in shock and Mom was devastated. There was no funeral. Brother, Ronald, was asked to witness the burial of Dad's ashes. No one else. The undertaker came to the door looking for payment. Mom broke down in tears. Tributes poured in but there was nothing to hang them on, no service, no anything. We were all simply left in a state of total anguish. Kathie was only 17 but she became Mom's support system for months.

The week between Christmas and New Year's, Dad had arrived at our front door, rang the doorbell, and when no one answered he turned around and went back down the steps to the sidewalk. By the time I got to the door, he was standing there looking up at me, so handsome in his brown ensemble. I was in my housecoat. Guy and I had spent the morning fooling around and I was a mess.

"Do you want to go down to the house in Port Dalhousie with your old father?" he said. I told him I couldn't. I had to take a bath and it would take too long. He walked back to join Mom in the car in our driveway and that was the last time I saw him. Why they hadn't called to tell me they were coming, I'll never know. I've asked "why" about so many things. I guess we all have times in our lives we wish we could do over; loved ones we'd give our eyeteeth to see just once more.

Mom and Dad had arranged to buy me a house in Port Dalhousie. I knew they knew my prospects of having a solid financial future were dim and they wanted me to have some place to live that I could call my own – in my name only. Mom had told me about the house on Canal Street and I was pleased but didn't really think it would happen. When it did, Dad was gone and

because the insurance papers hadn't gone through over the holidays, my mother was in debt $11,500 to pay for it. That doesn't seem like much money now, but in the early '70s it was more than my father made in a year as a Production Manager at General Motors.

The house was old. There was a small boat frozen into the driveway and an ugly grey fire escape from the second floor, zigzagging down the grey sidewall. But it overlooked Martindale Pond and the finish line of the Henley Regatta Rowing course. The location was priceless.

***

Home life was like a rollercoaster. Guy was given and lost jobs so fast our emotions were up one week at the thought of a steady paycheque and way down the next when he was let go. My father, and possibly all of my male relatives plus my mother, had been looking for something he could do well enough to keep at it. Nothing stuck. Finally, he began taking wedding photographs. That's a tricky business. You only have one chance to get it right with no possibility of a do-over.

Every time he went out on a wedding job my heart was in my throat. Would he be drinking on the job? Every time the photos came back from the lab (remember, no digital back then), I'd pray they'd be at least in focus and I could proudly present them to the newlyweds in an album I'd make up of the proofs. They would order blow-ups from those or, for $100, take all of the proofs. Sometimes the photos weren't very good. Once, absolutely nothing turned out. I was devastated. How do you tell a newly married couple they have no wedding photos?

My life wasn't the way I'd hoped it would be. I was raised to work hard and do my very best at absolutely everything, in spite of my inability to get around like other people. I knew Guy was an only child, raised in a good home with smart, loving parents. I also knew that he'd had a brain tumour surgically removed when he was very young. Was his upbringing part of the problem? Perhaps no one ever expected him to succeed on his own. Had everything always been given to him? Was that why he didn't seem to want to grab a job by the tail and do it well and wasn't motivated or showing any enthusiasm? And I could see that he was greatly relieved when each job failed and he could again settle down with his drinking buddies at the pub across the road from the back of the newspaper, where we met Thursday and Friday nights after work. A draft beer was 15 cents. Cigarettes were 35 cents a pack.

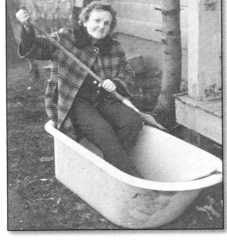

Mom in the tiny tub from the old house

Meanwhile Mom took her grief out on the old house. It needed new wiring, plumbing, heating and insulation. Some walls needed to go and others to be stripped of wallpaper. Battleship linoleum flooring was to be torn up and the old wide pine underneath sanded and several coats of polyurethane applied. The simple wide pine baseboards would get the same treatment.

Mom pulled up flooring, yanked out plumbing, jerried old appliances out the door, stripped everything she could and sanded everything that needed to be readied for painting.

She drove home every night, totally spent and likely in tears. Losing the love of your life in the prime of your life was something she and Dad had probably not given too much thought. He was going to retire in four years, at 60, and together they would head into a life of antiques, golf (more for him than her), and travel. In fact, they had planned a trip to England, had even bought the tickets.

When the gas company cut our home's attic main beam while putting in a new line, she stood firm when they bucked at installing a replacement. It took a few months but we

***

eventually got the main beam replaced with a steel one and Mom had a round table made out of the century-old pine beam. We used that table in the kitchen for years. The wood is at least an inch and a half thick and 18 inches wide. Glue the boards together, scribe out a large circle and cut. Sand the edges, apply layers of protective polyurethane to seal it and sit it atop a simple black wrought iron restaurant table base. No lover of pine could ask for a nicer table. I still have it.

The plan was that we'd have a living room, kitchen, bedroom and bathroom downstairs, and the small apartment upstairs would be rented out to give us money for property taxes and upkeep. I'd had enough of sleeping in the same room where I did everything else. There was a small woodshed on the back of the house with a door into the house. The place had been heated by a woodstove and wood had been piled in there, handy to the kitchen. If we played our cards right, that woodshed could become a tiny bedroom. Two single beds would just fit – if six inches were cut off the foot of mine. After a brief

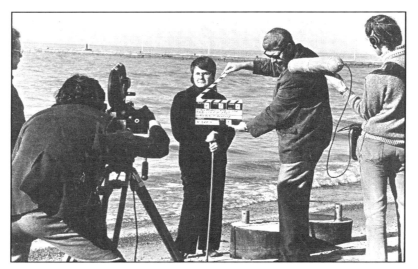

With a CBC film crew on the beach at Port Dalhousie – pc10.2

discussion, it was decided that everything would be done to try to make that little room as comfortable a bedroom as possible.

It took more than a year to get the house in shape. We tried to live in it while it was being worked on, and conditions weren't too bad in the summer when the windows were open, but in the cold weather the odours from paint and varnish and the dust from continual sanding saw me end up with pneumonia – twice.

As if renovating a house wasn't stressful enough, Guy ended up in a full body cast to help relieve the pressure on what had been diagnosed as a "leaking disc." It was a pretty miserable time for all of us.

The producer of a CBC TV show, based in Toronto, called *Of All People* decided that a woman with a disability who wrote obituaries and was renovating an old house would make an interesting subject. A crew filmed us on the beach and in the house. It was a welcomed diversion.

There was an old hotel, The Welland House, just across the road from the back of the newspaper. So that I could work without getting sick, we stayed there for an additional six weeks until the house was finished. The hotel rooms were huge with floor-to-ceiling windows and very high ceilings. Each room had a smaller room behind it for luggage and likely a maid's bed. The bathroom was down the hall. The hotel had been a health spa back during the 1880s and once very grand, but time had definitely worn off the gilt and glamour.

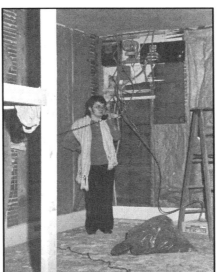

Under renovation

We made our own breakfast in our room every morning to save money. Thursday through Saturday nights, the boom-chugga-boom sound of a local trio could be heard as it wove its way up through the century-old rafters and floorboards from the strip bar downstairs. I always knew where to find Guy.

Alcoholism wasn't in my vocabulary. No one in our immediate family had a drinking problem that I knew of. And, I was

beginning to think that nothing I could do would change things. Guy had a drinking problem and that meant I had a problem.

Because the new house wasn't close to work, a car was needed, but neither of us had a licence to drive. It was thought that Guy would be a shoo-in to get his, but after he failed the driving test twice I decided to go for it and got mine the first time out. My licence was contingent on me always driving with hand-controls, as my ability to lift my foot from gas to brake was nil. I had to slide it over and hope it hit or use my hand to pull my leg and foot over.

My brother found us a little green Mini Minor and, providing Guy could fold his lanky frame into it, we had a car. He could and we did.

The car sat in the driveway until Guy finally passed the driving test on his third try. A friend of mine who used a wheelchair said his father would install hand controls for me and he did. Finally, we had wheels and both could drive. I had no idea at the time how ominous that would be for our future together.

85

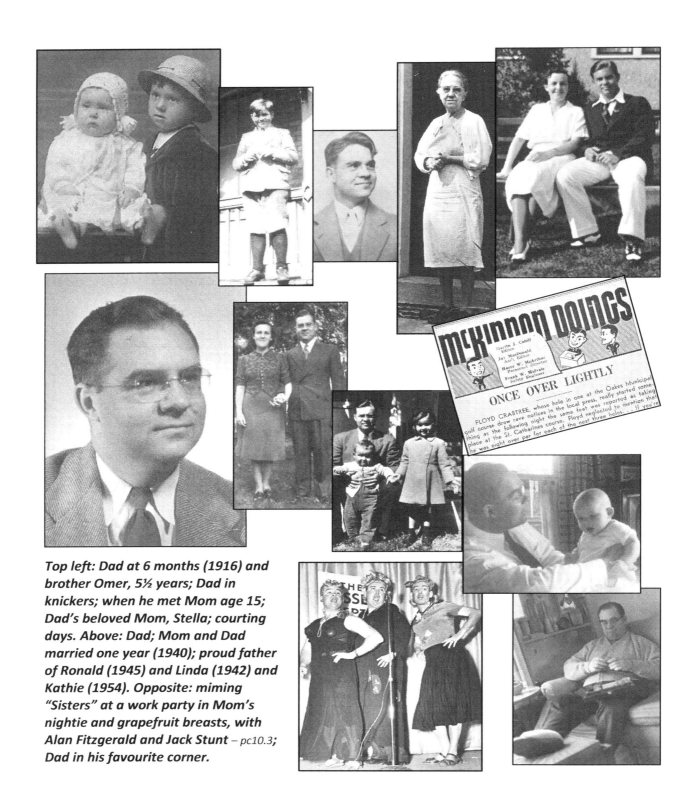

McKINNON DOINGS

ONCE OVER LIGHTLY

FLOYD CRABTREE, whose hole in one at the Oakes Municipal golf course drew rave notices in the local press, really started something as the following night the same feat was reported as taking place at the St. Catharines course. Floyd neglected to mention that he was eight over par for each of the next three holes. . . . If you're

Top left: Dad at 6 months (1916) and brother Omer, 5½ years; Dad in knickers; when he met Mom age 15; Dad's beloved Mom, Stella; courting days. Above: Dad; Mom and Dad married one year (1940); proud father of Ronald (1945) and Linda (1942) and Kathie (1954). Opposite: miming "Sisters" at a work party in Mom's nightie and grapefruit breasts, with Alan Fitzgerald and Jack Stunt – pc10.3; Dad in his favourite corner.

11

A wedding and wondrous ways

To say that life was hectic is an understatement. It seemed not a day went by without some kind of worry, car accident, or incident involving alcohol. Sometimes those happenings were funny and fun – and sometimes not.

***

One Friday night, Ken and Solange (she preferred Sal), Ken's sister and her boyfriend, and the boyfriend's cousin walked into The Mansion House: the bar across the road from the back of the newspaper press building, where Guy and I and some friends had been drinking for the last couple hours. We had spent time with Ken and Sal **before, although** they weren't part of the regular crowd. Ken had taken some kind of drug and by the time we finished bar hopping from The Mansion to Gord's Place to the Austin House, he had had it. One chord of Western music at the Austen and he hit the door and the street like a bomb. He spent the night in jail for breaking a window on the main street. Sal spent the night at our house on my mattress on the kitchen floor. She slept in her clothes and crashed hard, not making a

sound until Saturday morning when we had breakfast together and she left.

A week later Ken and Sal sat down with us at the Mansion and the first thing Guy did was call Ken, "black man." Fortunately, Ken was used to it and they both laughed. He was the handsomest black man I'd ever seen, **with** gorgeous fine features and smooth-as-satin dark chocolate brown skin. Then Sal said they had their marriage license and wanted to get married soon. Their rings **had been** ordered from the jewelers but wouldn't be in until the next day, when they were going to the justice of the peace at city hall. I asked Sal if she wanted to get married in a church and she said yes. They were both Anglican and although he was black and she white, it shouldn't make any difference to anyone and I knew a minister who might be available for an impromptu ceremony: Reverend Maclean at St. Mark's in Niagara-on-the-Lake, the same fellow who had married Guy and me three and a half years before.

"Who's got a dime?" I said, as I stood up to

make my way to the payphone in the pub's lobby to call the rectory. The woman who answered said the Reverend was out but to call back in 15 minutes. It was 9 p.m. by then. At 9:15 I called back and he said that if everything was in order, yes, he didn't know why he couldn't marry them. No, neither of them had been married or divorced. Yes, she was 18 and legal. He was 23. Yes, we could make it in an hour and a half if we moved fast.

So the race, rather wedding, was on. Down to my mother's, who donated a silver band to the cause, and then to sister Kathie's for a zircon ring she didn't wear, and then down to our house in Port Dalhousie to fetch Guy's camera.

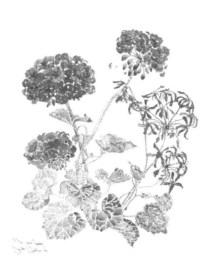

**Plain and Fancy
(geraniums) by Linda**
pc11.1

The bride combed her hair, picked three bright red geraniums from the side porch, we all had a pee and away we went. About a half mile out, Guy suddenly turned the car around. We were running dangerously low on gas and probably wouldn't make it. A full tank saw us on the road again but we were stopped yet again: the bridge was up at the Welland Ship Canal. We waited for a huge ocean-going cargo ship to go through and were off again. We arrived late, yes, but it was still only 10:35. The groom's sister was to meet us with the marriage license under the clock tower on the main street in Niagara-on-the-Lake.

They were waiting **when we arrived** and followed us to the church manse. The men went to the door and shook hands with Reverend Maclean and headed for the church. Both cars were driven through the arched gates and into the gravel parking area of the **nearly** 200-year-old church. The Reverend excused his informal footwear (Hush Puppies) and asked us all to sit down. Ken and Sal went into the back room and 10 minutes later they were back out and we were all given prayer books. We turned to the marriage ceremony and all went through it together. The responses were discussed and within minutes Ken and Sal stood before Reverend Maclean and became man and wife.

The bride wore a blue and black stripped sweater, blue jeans, sneakers and wire-framed glasses. And we can't forget her bouquet of three red geraniums from the pot on my side porch steps. The groom wore a star covered mauve T-shirt, blue jeans and **sneakers, and** sported an elegant Afro haircut. The best man wore a T-shirt, white button fly chino pants and leather open-toed sandals. The maid of honour was radiant in a white T-shirt, jeans and sneakers; her beautiful South African face framed with long black hair.

After the ceremony, Guy went into the small rectory and took a couple of pictures of the newlyweds signing the register. Reverend Maclean showed us where Guy and I were registered and where General Sir Isaac Brock was registered as buried. He died during the War of 1812 at the Battle of Queenston Heights just a couple of miles down the road, where my mother first twigged that there might be something wrong with me.

We all talked for a while and then left to go for a drink to toast the bride and groom at The Prince of Wales Hotel. With all seated at the bar, the best man standing on the bar rail made a toast to the bride. A toast to everyone else and two drinks later it was closing time and we were in the parking lot, everyone thanking everyone else and wishing each other well. The bridal party drove out of the parking lot yelling and happy, waving to Guy who was pissing in the hedge.

I don't know if the marriage lasted. We only saw the couple once again when Guy gave them the pictures he'd taken. I heard the groom's mother was gunning for me.

***

Life wasn't always that crazy but at that

time in my life nothing would surprise me, or so I thought.

Five years into my job at The Standard, and having pretty well mastered the art of obituary writing and deciphering handwritten letters to the editor, I found myself with little to do except a weekly Adopt-a-Pet column, a What's Happening in Niagara column, and a monthly full page of regional resources like helping agencies, blood banks and service club meetings. After spending about an hour reading the hot-off-the-press paper, I was looking for something to do most afternoons.

Janet, a freckled redheaded reporter in her early 40s, whose desk was opposite mine, was beginning to act a little odd. I knew she was a devout Catholic but when she began to wear nothing but black and white, would genuflect beside her desk before she started work and told me that one morning when she cracked an egg into the frying pan a chick plopped out into the sizzling butter, I began to worry about her mental health. On top of that she was beginning to take two or three days off at a time and eventually went on extended medical leave. She had been writing a column on fine art for several years, and we would sometimes talk about what she had written but I knew she really didn't have her finger on the pulse of what was going on in the local art scene.

When her extended leave extended way

past the date she was supposed to return, I asked Larry Smith, the editor-in-chief, if I could fill in for her until she got back. He said I could but it was only on a temporary basis. I was thrilled. At long last I had something I could really get my teeth into, something I loved and could cover with some expertise. I began writing a simple weekly column and as my luck would have it, Janet remained on medical leave long enough for me to beg permission to enlarge the column into an entire weekly art page. I was in my element.

In the early '70s Niagara was just starting to recognize its own artists, thanks to Peter Harris, curator at Rodman Hall, which was our only public art gallery, and several talented artists including Alice Crawley, Janny Fraser, John Boyle, Sandy Fairbairn and artist/poet Dennis Tourbin, who were just beginning to pull together a local artists' cooperative. I like to think that my writing on the local art scene helped to make people aware of the fact that we had some high calibre art being produced in Niagara. People didn't have to go to Toronto or further afield to view or purchase noteworthy pieces. I covered every show and every exhibition at Rodman Hall, interviewed hundreds of artists, was

john b. boyle, canadian artist

pc11.2

asked to judge shows, and wrote about every move we as artists made in the formative years of the Niagara Artists' Center (NAC), of which I was a part. NAC is still active today and a vibrant part of the Niagara art scene.

Several months into my art page, I devised a brazen scheme that would not only get me out of the office but give me a reason to take a vacation: Would the paper send me and Guy (I needed someone with me in case I ran into trouble walking, climbing curbs or taking cabs) to New York City, where I would collect information for a series of articles on art in The Big Apple?

One quiet summer afternoon when there was no one left in the office but me and the editor-in chief, I prepared my notes and asked him what he thought of my idea. To my surprise, he didn't turn me down flat but said he'd take my request to the publisher; he asked how much money I would need for a week in New York City. I had the plane fare figured out and the cost of a hotel and meals, as well as the admission costs to the various galleries, all typed up for him. He promised to get back to me in a couple of days.

I have no idea what was said but, as

promised, two days later he called me into his office to tell me the paper would cover everything except alcohol. I was free to go during a week of my holidays in August. Was I over the moon or what!

Guy and I flew down to New York City, stayed at a pretty horrible hotel and walked from one end of the city to the other. The Guggenheim was made for me; the whole thing is just one huge swirling ramp. At the Metropolitan Museum of Modern Art I was fascinated by a huge water lily painting, one in the series by Monet, and I spent at least an hour in front of Picasso's Guernica, absolutely enthralled. The Frick Museum gave me an overview of the arts such as I'd only seen in art school books. I was particularly taken with the works of James McNeill Whistler on exhibition there, so much so that I spent what little money I had on a volume about his life to enjoy when we got home.

But speaking about home, the day we arrived back at our little cottage overlooking Martindale Pond, I was in for a shock. I went to the backyard and, seated on the covered swing, asked Guy if he would collect the mail. He came back with the usual bills and a large brown envelope addressed to me. I took a look at the bills but was intrigued by the envelope. When I opened it a pile of clippings of my art columns fell into my lap. I picked one up, and then another, and another and each

one had the eyes of the head and shoulders photo (that was always used with the column) poked through with a red felt tip pen. In the borders were scribbled comments such as, "Why did you say that?", "That isn't right", and "You don't know what you're talking about!" Words likes "False!" "No!" "What?" and "Bad!" were sprinkled throughout. It was truly a heyday for exclamation points. I asked myself who hated me enough to skewer my eyeballs and spew venom over my work like so much Mexican hot sauce? I could think of only one person.

When I got back to work the next Monday, I took the envelope with its contents to the editor-in- chief to see what he thought. He asked me to check the handwriting with anything I had from Janet and it matched. We both agreed that she was disturbed, but my biggest fear was that if she'd do that to my newspaper columns, what might she do to me if she happened to see me crossing the street or trying to climb a curb or even just walking on the sidewalk? My walking was perilous and I could fall at any time but a slight push from behind or a car rushing towards me with no intention of stopping wouldn't see me run out of the way. I couldn't run, hell, I could barely walk. And might she throw something damaging at me while I was sitting at my desk? Everyone knew she worked there and nobody would say a word if she casually strolled into the office.

The police were consulted – we knew most of them and they knew us – and it was agreed that it would be kept as an internal matter. However, the company lawyer suggested that I take out a cease-and-desist order against her and they would mail it.

I don't think I ever saw her again but I did hear from one of our reporters, who went to the same church as she did, that she received the cease-and-desist order and it was my understanding that it was the same day she received a letter from the newspaper terminating her employment. Apparently she was quite ill and it wasn't too long after that episode that she died from a massive infection. I'll never know the entire story behind her illness and what prompted her to do what she did, but I know that as a columnist for the last 20 years I would want to be consulted if someone were allowed to take over what I do. She could've come back, resumed her job as a general reporter and taken the column back; but since no one could reach her to discuss her circumstances and she wasn't forthcoming, there remained many unanswered questions regarding the status of her health and what to do with the column. So I just carried on, and when she died, that was that.

**

When preparing the weekly art page, after I had laid out the articles and photos at hand on a layout sheet at my desk, I sent it downstairs where the newspaper was actually put together. It was customary for me to go down to the ground floor to see how it looked in type.

One morning at about 11:45, I carefully made my way down the metal stairs to the composing room where each page was laid out on a light table. Columns were stripped in and headings put on and screened photos placed above any advertising, which was usually at the bottom of the page.

On the day in question I happened to see something that I thought was out of place. I reached for the small knife used to move the pieces of waxed copy around, stuck the knife blade under a small piece of copy and the man beside me immediately threw up his hands and said, "Whoa!" After that, absolute chaos reigned and I had no idea why. As it turned out, no one, but no one, was supposed to touch the type except the workers in composing. That fellow had gone to the representative of the local of the International Typographical Union (ITU) at the paper, who immediately went to my boss. Members of the union had then threatened to walk out just when the first edition of the paper was supposed to go to press.

By the time I walked the length of the building on the ground floor, had taken the elevator up to editorial, and was back at my desk, everyone was in mid-negotiation. My boss immediately went to the publisher and both of them ended up downstairs in **composing, trying** to calm everyone in the ITU down. I had no idea what I'd done but it turned out I had committed the cardinal sin: I had touched type. I was called into the editor-in-chief's office and a stern talking to saw me red-faced and embarrassed.

I thought I was saving someone some trouble by moving the type and I laboured under the delusion that the fellows down in composing were my friends, as most of them would often wink at me and joke if they saw me coming. I soon learned that checking my page wasn't a smart move and I simply left well enough alone. If there was a problem after the pages were printed, so be it.

I always did my very best, checked all of my facts and was very detail oriented when laying out my pages. I liked to think that what I did meant something to somebody, so I hated to admit to myself that my mother was right in her reply to my worries over the content of an article or the look of a page, "It will be on the bottom of a birdcage tomorrow, don't let it bother you."

There's nothing more easily forgotten than old news but that didn't include typos. Just about everybody in the office read the

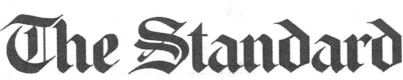

pc11.3

paper from start finish after the still press-warm copies were delivered to our desks. We'd often comment and chuckle at any typos we'd find and I still remember the ad for the humidifier that "shits off automatically."

Several years later the newspaper took a poll of their readers and asked them what they regularly read. Sports was at the top of the list and art was somewhere near the bottom. I'd had a good seven-year run and proved many times over that I could write, edit and set up a page. My art page, **however, was** cancelled.

***

One afternoon a woman in her 40s approached my desk and asked to see the editor-in-chief. I buzzed him and told him there was someone to see him and as she rounded the corner of my desk going towards his office she leaned over towards me and said, "I want your job." I looked at her and thought, fat chance lady, but in a matter of weeks I was asked if I would like to be the **assistant Family** page editor with a raise and a different start time. I was to be in around 6:30 in the morning and I could leave between 2:30 and 3:00. I gladly took the promotion even though I had no idea how I was going to make it in that early. My job was now based on a computer. The mainframe was so big it filled an entire room. My monitor was a big boxy thing. I had used one before when I set up my various columns, so it wasn't all new to me, but flying on my own and being responsible for the look of the Family section inside pages was a bit daunting.

Advertisements were always put in first, with direction from the advertising department downstairs, and they were always in the lower part of the page below the fold. Each morning it was my job to fill all the holes above the ads on the inside pages of the section with copy that came in from the various news services. First I would read what was available, then consider the length of each one and make sure they were appropriate for the pages; then cut, edit and paste them into the empty spaces and write a heading that fit above the article.

I really enjoyed the work and after the paper went to bed, around 11:30 a.m., I had all afternoon to interview anyone and write anything I wanted for the Family section. Everything from the stock market to tap dance lessons for tiny tots, the origin of Christmas cards and how to skin catfish was pounded out. I don't think I said no to any assignment and I came up with all kinds of ideas of my own. No one stopped me from writing whatever I wanted and I made sure there were photographs or illustrations to go with my articles. The Family editor and I didn't exactly get along so I tried to stay out of her way and was usually busy at my own work by the time she got to work in the morning. As long as I did my job she was happy and she usually did a good job of laying out my articles on the Family section front page.

***

The paper had given me the opportunity to let my talents develop, from using what I had learned in high school and working in the morgue at age 17, to writing thousands of obituaries, deciphering thousands of letters to the editor, working with the public, learning to write, edit and lay out pages; and we can't forget what I learned in the darkroom. The paper had been a long and, for the most part, happy learning opportunity for me and I soaked up every morsel of knowledge that was offered. Little did I know that everything I'd learned would see me go on to something that would touch the lives of thousands of people around the world.

12

Over and done with

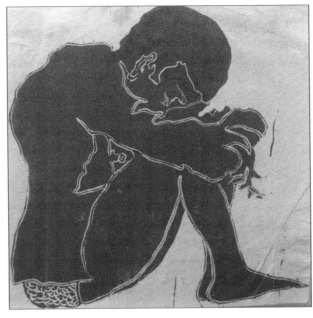

A linocut I did of how it felt to be me

To conclude the tale of our nine years of marriage, I can only say that Guy and I gave it the best we could, according to our abilities and expectations. I'm not sure what his were but mine were that we'd work together to build a secure and happy life for us both. That wasn't to be. His drinking finally got to the point where he'd get drunk on the job as a photographer.

One night after working at a large conference centre on the multi-laned Queen Elizabeth Highway, he pulled out onto the road, somehow managed to cross the grassy median and hit another car, which then flipped over and hit another car.

The result was a charge of driving while intoxicated and several other charges I can't recall but none were to be taken lightly. I think it was his second or third DWI. The car was a wreck but drivable. Guy wasn't really injured but the men in the car he hit, all bricklayers coming home from work, sued for a million dollars each and our car was in my name with my insurance. I couldn't let myself think about what that meant to my future. I was likely making less than $200 a week.

Thank heaven for a good insurance company. After months of lawyering and a few court appearances, none of which I had to attend, the suits were settled for far less than was asked because investigators proved that none of the bricklayers had anywhere near the injuries they claimed. I was so relieved when the verdict came down that I cried. And Guy hadn't had a driver's licence since the accident, so I could stop worrying about him drinking and driving.

95

Often Guy would come with me when I drove into work in the morning so he'd be downtown for the day. Those trips were so upsetting, so full of me wondering and asking why he wasn't looking for work instead of wandering around until noon when the bars opened so he could join his drinking buddies, and so full of me taking my sorrow and disgust out on him that I often couldn't remember driving to work. I was on autopilot, my mind totally preoccupied. It's a wonder I didn't have an accident. Come to think of it, I did have two. I slid into someone because I didn't stop on time but there was no damage to their car or mine, just a bump, but the fellow I hit got out of his car and came back to see why I had nudged him. I blamed it on my hand controls and that was that, but I'd really had too much to drink to judge my hand co-ordination on the controls.

I also backed into a car and took out its headlights, trying to get out of a parking spot at The Mansion House. Both times I was under the influence and both times absolutely mortified to think that if the police had been called I would have been hauled in on a DWI, becoming one more employee of The Standard with a drinking problem.

I remember Ma Paton, the paper's little old, but very tough, Irish cleaning lady, dragging a bag of clanking liquor bottles alongside a bag of paper garbage past me when I worked the odd evening. It was obvious that I wasn't the only one at The Standard who drank.

***

During our time together, I had my fallopian tubes tied so I could not conceive and eventually I had a hysterectomy because of problems with my monthly period. I don't know if it was my CMT or simply stress but it seemed as if I was either feeling down because it was impending, having incredibly painful cramps, or going through it. I had a great deal of trouble trying to manage pads and tampons with extremely weak fingers and no grip. There was one week a month when I felt okay. My gynecologist suggested a hysterectomy and I agreed.

One instance that has stayed with me occurred in hospital when I was having my tubes tied. The doctor actually took Guy aside and asked him if he approved of the operation. Guy came into my room and told me what the doctor had said. I think it made him feel important but it made me feel like chattel and demeaned. I was undergoing the operation because I realized I didn't want to have a child who would have an alcoholic father and a mother with CMT, and the child could very likely have CMT. Did Guy approve?! He hadn't a clue what a pregnancy could mean. I'd had many years to think about it since being pregnant as a teen. My future was sealed. I would have no children.

Money was a constant worry. There was never enough and it was always up to me to find it to pay the bills because it seemed I was the only one capable of holding down a full-time job. My artwork would sometimes bring in a few welcome extra dollars when anything sold but sales were far and few between. Trying to put together enough artwork for a one-woman show, I resorted to pen and ink drawings of myself sitting at the pine table pondering bills, Guy looking over my shoulder. I simply did not have the energy or desire to paint anything beautiful because life was pretty black-and-white at the time, mostly black. I did a pair of drawings like that and I think the gallery owner took pity on me because he bought them both. They weren't very happy drawings but, believe me, they came right from my soul. When I draw a person, I have a tendency to feel the body in my mind as I draw it and I think, because of that, my work sometimes hits a nerve with people.

Framing was always a huge problem because it was difficult to sell your work to the public unless it was framed and, if you couldn't do it yourself, it cost more than I could even consider at that time. I was fortunate that I was given Exhibition Assistance Grants from the Ontario Arts Council in 1976, '77 and '78 and it all went towards framing.

***

It was our habit to meet at The Mansion House after work on Thursdays and Fridays. I'd go over and Guy would arrive late, pretty well under the influence and very loud. After a draft or two, or more, with friends, we'd go home for supper.

Eventually when I told him I was going home to cook supper and asked if he was coming, he'd say no. I went home alone. It hurt but I was either going to stay and become an alcoholic or leave and get my life back. Eating alone became fine with me. Although I still cooked for two, the thought that, once again, he wasn't there to eat with me just confirmed what I already knew: our marriage was over.

The last straw saw us fighting in the kitchen. He'd just come home from an entire night out and I started at him. He'd slept at the Port Hotel with a waitress. Okay, I didn't really care who he slept with as long as it wasn't me but what did he think he was doing coming back?

I threw something at him and he threw something at me. One of us had a knife, I can't remember who but it was right there and then that I thought this was getting out of control. It was no longer just hurtful words; one of us could kill the other. I had often wondered if they'd put a person with a disability in jail. I couldn't plead physical cruelty. He'd never hit me. I'd tried many times to hit him, but he was so tall he could simply put one of his long arms out toward me and I'd be effectively swinging away at nothing. If I was going to get him out of my life I'd have to do it stealthily, from behind or in his sleep. Such horrible plans. But, as it worked out, I didn't need any of them. He left after that day of throwing things and didn't come back.

Slowly, day by day, I began to feel my life starting to right itself. I could rest without the fear of the police at the door or a call saying he was in jail. I'd stopped caring if he was in jail long ago, stopped waiting up at night, and stopped caring, period. I'd lost respect for the man I once loved so very much.

The following week back at work, I walked into Larry Smith's office, sat down and told him what had happened and that I needed a divorce lawyer but didn't know one. Everyone at work knew Guy, at least by sight, and I think everyone knew or could easily imagine our problems. Larry nodded in agreement and suggested I see the paper's lawyer. I called and made an appointment for that day during lunch hour.

When I told the lawyer I wanted a divorce, he suggested a trial separation. I said quite forcefully, no, a divorce, and that was that. He got the ball rolling. It was going to cost me $185.

Several months later I climbed the wide stone steps of our old courthouse, helped by our family friend Alice, who had replaced me in the paper's library when I left for my foot and ankle surgery and was a witness to Guy's considerable problems with drink. The divorce was granted and in 90 days we would no longer be married.

***

During the time it took for the divorce to go through, Guy and I went up to North Bay to visit Sandy and Dennis Geden, my artist friend from our Montreal school days and his wife, who both knew Guy well in his younger years. I was driving my first new car: a bright yellow Honda equipped with hand controls. Mimi, my epileptic miniature poodle, was also with us.

It was about 6:00 a.m., we had just filled up the gas tank and were on our way back home, heading south on the highway near Sundridge. There was no other traffic on the road. I can only tell you what I remember because some of it is pretty vague. All of a sudden I saw a black car coming over a hill toward us. That car shouldn't have been there as we were on the southbound lanes of a four-lane highway; or maybe *we* shouldn't have been there, that's what I still can't figure out.

In any case, in order to avoid the oncoming car, I pulled over onto the left side of the road and kept driving on the gravel. I also let off on the gas hand control and then pulled down on it very quickly. The result of that manoeuvre was like that squeeze acrobat toy you buy that has a little man on strings hanging between two sticks … when you squeeze the sticks, he flips. When I let go of the accelerator and then pushed it down quickly, I flipped the gas pedal attached to the hand control into full throttle and I couldn't change it. So there we were on the gravel shoulder with a 40-foot drop and only the tops of fir trees visible to our left and an oncoming car to our right. I was trying to control the car but it was going at full speed when Guy reached over and grabbed the steering wheel, pulling it to the right. The result of that saw the car flip into the air and land on its roof, circle across the median, and cross two more of what I thought were northbound lanes and then come to a rocking halt in a ditch.

When we realized we were both alive and began to take stock, we were hanging upside down from our seatbelts and covered with safety glass from the imploded windshield. The dog, her white fur covered with sparkling glass, was walking on the roof.

It wasn't long before we heard the whine of fire sirens and boots flying down the ditch to help. A fireman beside me said he was going to kick in my driver's side window. My face was right beside the window. I shouted, "NO!" He went around to the front of the car and, on his stomach, reached in through the windshield and undid my seatbelt. I slowly descended to the roof of the car.

Guy was bleeding. At 6'4", he sat so tall in the seat that as the car rolled onto its roof it crunched down on the top of his head.

In no time we were in an ambulance and then at Sundridge Hospital with several nurses picking glass out of our hair and skin. Mimi, tied to a stair rail outside, was having an epileptic seizure. I could see her from my perch on a gurney in the hall but dared not move for all the glass on me.

To say I was grateful to be alive is an understatement. I took a taxi all the way back to St. Catharines and left Guy to deal with the car and get back on his own steam. Callous, perhaps, but I was in shock and knew I needed to get where I was safe and could recover. I didn't feel safe with Guy and I knew he didn't have a driver's licence so he couldn't rent another car. My hand controls were in the wreck so driving for me was out of the question as well. I wrapped the dog up in towel, put her in my purse, and headed for home on my own.

Yes, seatbelts had saved our lives or was it something else? I thanked God for letting me live because that could easily have been the end of us.

What if we hadn't have had our seatbelts on? What if the gas tank had exploded as we swirled toward the ditch? What if, indeed!

Several weeks later, back at work at the paper with the huge purple bruise across my chest where the seat belt held me upside down beginning to fade, I wrote a column about the accident and how thankful I was to celebrate my 35th birthday.

Also during those 90 days, I gathered up all of Guy's belongings including his birth certificate and early one morning before work, before the bars opened, I left them in a green garbage bag in the middle of the big public parking lot beside The Mansion House. I figured it was the one place he'd most likely find it and I didn't want him to come up to the editorial department. I called the people at the Mansion and ask them to tell him where it was. I don't know if he found the bag or not but it was a way to get him and his things out of my life.

During those nine years I learned a lot about alcoholism. I saw a young man retreat into drink when he couldn't succeed. My attempts to pull him up failed. I gave it everything I had and I think he did as well. We can only give what we know and what we have in us to give. I also learned that, at least for me, when respect is lost, everything is lost. I didn't think I could not love him, but as the years wore on and wore us out, that's exactly what happened.

***

When Guy wasn't in my life neither was heavy drinking or smoking. I was healthier and happier living alone in the little house by the rowing course than I'd been in years. And I'm sure the neighbours were relieved that our frequent late-night all-out shouting and swearing matches had stopped.

We met briefly a couple of times after that but nothing had changed. I soon learned he had moved and was truly out of my life forever.

My lasting memory of those years is one of a half-consumed bottle of beer with a half-smoked cigarette floating in it – and I'd paid for both.

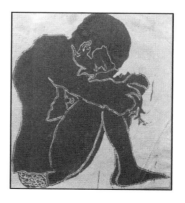

13

See who salutes

Even before my divorce became final, I knew I didn't want to live alone. It just wasn't me. Most of the time I appreciated the company of a man and enjoyed intimacy. I also wanted to share my life with someone.

Things had calmed down somewhat. The little old house on Canal Street was adequate but felt very empty, so I kept busy.

***

Writing my art column meant that I often interviewed artists in their studios. While visiting the exceptionally talented Dennis Lukas, at his home in Grimsby, I noticed that there was a huge pile of drawings amongst the layered carpets and pillows on the floor. May I take a look at them? "Of course." he said. "And they are for sale." How much? I asked. "Whatever you like." Knowing that I didn't have more $20 to my name, I offered him $15 for three that appealed to me. He just looked at me. "Why don't we say you paid $15 for one and I'll give you the other two?" It was never easy always being broke and continually confronted with some of the most beautiful artwork and handmade glass and pottery I'd ever seen. I often paid for a piece in installments.

Our conversation turned to his recent travels in Europe and he began to tell me about the guilds that were made up of skilled workers making everything from hats to cheese. I knew a great many talented craftspeople in the Niagara area because I'd interviewed them and loved going to local craft shows. Why couldn't we form a craft guild here in Niagara?

I drove home with a million ideas buzzing in my head. That evening I called artisans, Pat and Phil Waters. We talked about the concept and they agreed to call the craftspeople they knew to see if there was any interest. A great many of them were keen and before we knew it we had rented a room for our shop in a restored building in Old Port Dalhousie. The St. Catharines Craft Guild store opened its doors in 1976 and closed in 2008.

During those years the organization was run and the store solely manned by the craftspeople themselves. Thousands of dollars of juried local craftwork was sold. For several years, I sold batiked silk scarves, handmade cards and bead jewelry in the store.

I didn't really have a family to spend Christmas Eve with and remember working at the store, sitting beside the second-floor window in a yellow high-back chair, watching the snow fall on the sailboats tied up in the old Welland Canal lock across the road from the building. As the street lights began to slowly come on, I waited for locals doing some last-minute Christmas shopping to pop in... and they did.

I still have one of the drawings that I bought from Dennis back then. Unfortunately, he died suddenly, and far too young (age 56), but the entity that sprang from our meeting proudly served local craftspeople and the community for many years.

***

For many years at The Standard, part of my job was to take the obituaries from the undertakers each morning over the phone. I usually typed as I listened, my shoulder cradling the telephone receiver. Sometimes I took them down in my shaky scrawl by hand and then typed them. Once, while taking an obit, I actually typed my way right off the edge of my rolling office chair and ended up on the floor. Two reporters picked me up and, within a few minutes, I called the undertaker back to finish the job. It wasn't uncommon to have four or five obits to do in a given morning and after a three-day holiday they might run to a dozen or

more – all of them coming in within an hour and a half.

Several of the undertakers became friends and we'd chat for a minute before getting to work. The telephone console was usually blinking like mad with other undertakers waiting, so we got down to business quickly; but after talking to the same people five days a week for a number of years, you get to know them quite well. One in particular, Mary Darte, stood out. She was a common-sense woman and I felt close to her. We had met for lunch once and, upon meeting face-to-face, hit it off beautifully, just as I thought we would.

One morning when the obits were done and there were no others waiting, I told Mary that I was lonely but had no idea how I'd go about meeting someone. Her reply was, "For heaven's sake woman, you work for a newspaper. Run a personal ad up the pole and see who salutes."

Those were the days when there were no computer-based dating sites. The newspaper would include an entire column or section of personal ads. It was considered a bit risky to place one because you never knew who you'd meet, but people put themselves out there in print as there was no other way to meet someone unless you frequented the bars or were big on church. I was finished with bars and church wasn't an option.

I don't know why I hadn't thought of placing a personal but I hadn't. I think I was too caught up in the fact that I had a disability and how I'd tell anyone who answered. And I didn't think I could take face-to-face rejection after what I'd been through the past nine years. I hadn't truly known the definition of the word humiliation but I soon realized that I had been reduced from the daughter of a well-known and respected couple to the wife of a bumbling drunk. It wasn't easy to muster up enough courage to put myself out there again. My life had centred on trying to keep Guy sober and out of trouble for so long, I'd lost a part of myself. I'd look in a mirror and couldn't connect with the woman I saw there. I felt as if I didn't exist.

That afternoon I typed up an ad that appeared in the paper on Nov. 2, 1977:

Woman, divorced, mid-thirties, interested in art, antiques, nutrition, theatre and ballet, non-smoker, light drinker, would like to meet unattached gentleman 35 – 50 with similar interests for companionship. Please write Box 1116, The Standard, giving particulars, address and telephone number. Sincere and honest replies only please.

When I went downstairs to go home, I gave it to the girl in Classifieds. It was free and was to run for three days. Of course, everyone read it and the buzz that Crabtree was "looking for a man" was all over the building.

Trying to forget about the ad was near impossible and every now and then a surge of excitement would go through me. The suspense was electric. Who knows who would answer it? Would I meet someone who would accept me for what I was? A girl can dream.

At the end of the next week, after the ad had run for three days, I picked up the replies from the box assigned to me and went out to the parking lot where I sat behind the wheel trying to resist opening them. The need to know was overwhelming. Hope was still alive. I looked at them all, studying the writing or printing of the addresses, and decided on the thickest one.

After tearing open the envelope, I unrolled a length of yellow toilet-paper. The writer made reference as to what he was willing to do to me and signed it, "Banana Joe." I looked up at the brick wall opposite the windshield and thought, was this what it was going to be like? Was everyone who answered a personal ad a nut like this one? Was it all just a waste of time?

As I opened the next envelope, a photo dropped out on my lap. I picked it up and took a good look at the head and shoulders shot he'd enclosed. A nice face, light hair and, oh no, a shirt with roses on it. Flowers on a shirt suggested Western music to me. I called it "twang" and really didn't like it. But the letter was lovely. He spoke of that ineffable something between two people that makes all the difference in a relationship. His name was Graydon. His letter was a keeper.

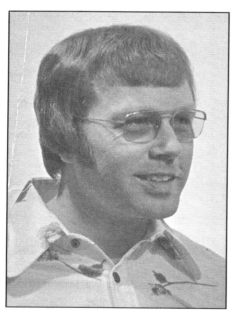

***My first glimpse of
Graydon R. Book***

When I got home I called him. I screwed up the courage to tell him that I had a disability and didn't walk very well. Better to put it out in front. He said he was okay with that as he was born with an eye condition that didn't impede his sight but made some things difficult for him. We made a date to meet the next Thursday night at the local Holiday Inn. The journey had begun. I was out there.

Pulling into a parking space in front of the hotel, the first thing I did was open the car door and lie sideways, my head out toward the asphalt to squirt decongestant spray up my nose so I could breathe. My allergies were so bad I was addicted to the spray that opened my nasal passages.

That done, I walked toward the entrance only to have to figure out how I was going to climb the one step to the door. Hanging onto the wall, I pulled myself up, hoping he hadn't seen me and run for the hills. Steps and curbs were still the most difficult things for me to navigate. With no push from my foot or lower leg, I had to pull with my arms, and without a railing it was darn near impossible.

Once in the lobby, I saw a good-looking man wearing a leather jacket sitting there. He stood up. Tall! He suggested coffee in the restaurant. Fine. We sat talking until the restaurant closed. When we parted, he said he'd call me again and he did.

In the midst of my personal ad project, I also joined a gym, Vic Tanny's. I'd go to the gym three afternoons after work during the week and work out on the machines. My upper body and back were strong, so a good 45-minute workout saw me begin to tone up the muscles that weren't affected by CMT and lose weight. My legs were pretty well useless and I had to be very careful with my wrists and hands because some of the machines could only be worked using your hands and I'd have trouble driving with my hand controls if I used my hands on the exercise equipment for any length of time.

Overworking muscles served by CMT-affected nerves can definitely slow down the nerves' ability to fire the muscle. In the case of my thumbs, the muscles had almost totally atrophied, as they barely moved. If I wasn't careful, I could lose the use of my hands completely. But I managed and loved feeling my body respond to all that activity. Yes, it tired me out, and I recall feeling shaky in the locker room when I was getting dressed after my shower but I had worked up a sweat, a welcome good sweat.

Working out in the gym was so different from anything I had done in the previous nine years that it was almost like going on vacation three times a week. There was nothing to worry about at the gym and, for me, time stood still while I slowly woke up muscles I hadn't used in almost a decade. I still can't hear the Bee Gees singing the music from Saturday Night Fever without wanting to throw my arms into the air to start my exercise routine, and it has been 40 years. I'd also drive home from the gym in my new little orange Honda with the windows down, singing to the pumped-up radio like a wild abandoned woman. For the first time in nine years I was free and truly happy.

Two more runs of the ad and more letters saw me having coffee with a fellow who turned out to be a hockey dad, when I expressly told him on the phone I wasn't into sports; and a date in the boiler room of the local hospital with a big, soft-hearted engineer because he worked shifts. As his story unfolded I learned that he had an eight-year-old daughter who badly needed a mother. I couldn't see myself taking on a child and housekeeping. It just wasn't me.

***

A couple of dates and a shower I'll never forget with a much older man who taught at the local university, didn't really go anywhere. And there were several fiery dates with a very interesting fellow, who I knew loved everything I did but I think my disability was the big elephant in the room. The sex was fantastic and I'd get weak all over every time he touched me but it just wasn't right for either of us. I could feel it and I'm sure he could as well. In fact, he told me that he felt he had to "perform" every time we got together and here I thought this was just his fantastically normal way of doing things. Silly me!

***

After our long conversation at the hotel, Graydon invited me for dinner at his apartment. He served Cornish game hen with a side salad and there was wine. Everything was lovely. The apartment was what you'd expect from a 40-year-old bachelor: not much furniture, but enough for one. A lone philodendron climbed up the wall and over the pass-through that looked into the kitchen. There was a small hibachi barbeque on the balcony.

As it turned out he wasn't into Western music at all. He had quite a collection of records that included the classics, jazz and the big bands. My father would have loved him. The rose-covered shirt, he explained, was an old one he had worn to wash his car when his best friend snapped his photo.

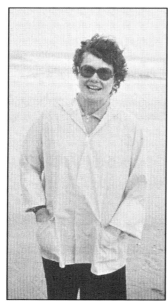

On the beach at Cape Cod

Not one to date a lot of men at the same time, not since my teens, I thought Graydon was the type of steady fellow I could settle down with. He drank moderately, smoked only after a meal and then only sometimes. He liked a pipe (especially the smell of the pipe tobacco) and we'd each light up a pipe and smoke it while doing the dishes together. Then that grew old. It wasn't healthy, why do it? We quit. He had a job

working payroll and accounting for a local company. He had a nice car and kept it spotless. He spoke well, he laughed at the same things I did and we grew to really like each other.

Trips to Toronto, restaurant meals, a bit of shopping, movies, long walks in the woods or driving around the back roads of rural West Lincoln (where he was raised on a farm in Silverdale and attended a one-room schoolhouse), even an evening at the National Ballet, all helped us to get to know each other.

A road trip to Cape Cod turned out rather

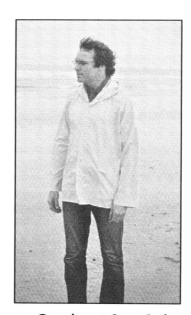

Graydon at Cape Cod

well although it rained most of the time we were there. We invested in bright yellow raincoats with hoods and carried on with our vacation, falling in love with a particular recipe for scrod (young whitefish) served at a seafood restaurant we found. We still talk about that scrod to this day.

We also took a farm vacation, spending a week on a dairy farm. Because I couldn't climb stairs, our bedroom was the glassed-in front porch and, much to my disappointment, Graydon would have no part in lovemaking with wall-to-wall windows all around. However, we did have one amusing incident. A woman from St. Catharines, Miriam, was also on vacation there with her young daughter. During a morning trip to the barn to see the "girls" after milking, one of them, who had her back to us, lifted her tail and proceeded to drop a pile of steaming manure. "Oh, no!" exclaimed Miriam's daughter. Of course, we all laughed and we've never forgotten that the highlight of our farm vacation was a natural bovine process of elimination and the disgust of a young child who had not too long ago learned to do just the opposite. Miriam became a friend and the young girl is now an executive in Toronto.

Only once did Graydon walk away from me. We were on our way to a movie theatre in a mall and he was walking ahead of me. I couldn't keep up but he didn't stop or slow down. That hurt more than a slap in the face. I told him that if he was going to treat me like that, we were finished. He never did it again.

I knew it was difficult for him to include someone else in his life. He'd lived alone for many years; gads, he was 40 when I met him. He could be cold and aloof. I was bouncy and liked big hugs. He admitted he'd gone on picnics by himself, made lovely dinners with wine for one and spent a great deal of his time, when he wasn't working, alone. I could tell he wanted someone in his life but it was a fight. He wasn't used to compromise, enjoyed his own company most of the time and sometimes he just needed space. On the other hand, I was lonely and loved to just be near him.

***

A carry-over from my marriage arrived daily with the postman. Graydon was a regular at my home now and on occasion he'd seen a pile of unopened mail on my kitchen buffet and wondered why it hadn't been taken care of. I told him I simply couldn't face it. The mail was mostly bills leftover from my marriage and since Guy was gone, I was responsible for everything. I'd been responsible for almost everything anyway, but having to pay after he'd left and after I had embarked on a new chapter of my life was like discovering a bag of stinking garbage in the trunk of a brand-new car.

Like a fool, I had signed a slip saying that I would be responsible to the company who advanced him the money he'd eventually get from his income tax return. He got both the advance and his refund from the government. I ended up paying back the people who prepared his income tax. I made so little at my job that I was barely making ends meet, but not facing my responsibilities wasn't the way to go forward. Graydon sat down with me and, together, we figured out how I was going to pay everything off. Together! How wonderful that concept was. Finally, there was someone in my life who respected me. I no longer felt like a meal ticket or simply a cigarette and beer provider.

***

Graydon's mother. Oh, his mother. When I first met Grace, I don't think she knew what to think of me. I was divorced ... almost. That wasn't exactly what she had in mind for her youngest. I worked at a newspaper and was worldly, you might say. The word "shit" and a few other choice

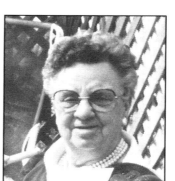

Grace Book

expletives were in my vocabulary but not used often. I was 35 years old, not a kid by any means. I had just been through the worst nine years of my life. And, obviously, had a physical disability.

She, on the other hand, reminded me so much of my father's mother, my Grandma Crabtree, that they could have been sisters. She laughed, talked up a storm, loved to play Scrabble, do crossword puzzles, knit and crochet, cook everything well-done, and make pies with crust so light you could barely see it. And Graydon cut her grass for her every Wednesday night after work. He'd pick me up and over we'd go. Grace and I got to know each other while we sat together and talked on the back patio, watching him push the lawnmower over what was a large double lot. Because it was a work night, we'd not spend too much time alone afterwards, but getting to know his mother, to see how he cared for and looked after her, made me think that he would do the same for me. I was right.

14

A new beginning … and end

Graydon and I were seeing each other on a steady basis now and beginning to really like each other ... a lot. And, we found something we both enjoyed: canoeing. Every Friday, immediately after work, I drove over to his place and we'd take his car out to Wellandport, a half-hour drive from St. Catharines, where we could rent a canoe. The Welland River meandered for miles through huge fields of corn and soybeans and by herds of cud-chewing Guernsey cows; it was quiet, calm and just what we both needed to deflate from the week's work. Paddling down the river and finally tying up to an overhanging branch and eating supper under a huge old willow was like heaven after five days of dealing with the public and trying to get things right.

Paddling wasn't easy for me but I soon learned to tie a shoelace to the end of the paddle and then around my wrist, so that when the water pulled the paddle out of my hand I could easily retrieve it. Graydon may

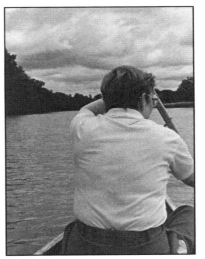

Canoeing on the Welland River

have done most of the paddling but I enjoyed the physical workout I got doing what I could.

Those days on the water were some of the best times we've ever had and I think they brought us together like nothing else could because it took two to move that canoe and, if nothing else, we learned to work together to get to where we wanted to be.

Don't forget this was back in the early '80s and alcohol was a pretty big part of people's lives. Graydon and I would have dinner and a few drinks or share a bottle of wine over a meal. I recall once getting very drunk, in fact both of us were quite drunk, and we promised we would stay together and in time adopt a little red-headed boy who wore glasses and was a nerd, definitely a nerd. That's about as far as we got that night except I got very sick to my stomach and Graydon cleaned up. He later remarked that you really don't know a person until you've cleaned up after them.

***

One day at work, my mother called me. It had to be important because she rarely rang me at work and this time she sounded excited and happy. Would I meet her after work at my place in Port Dalhousie? She had something to talk to me about and to show me. Curiosity killing me, I zoomed home and she was waiting. With both of us in her little brown Toyota, she drove two blocks north, turned the corner onto Bayview Drive and stopped. We were in front of a very old duplex. Two people were sitting on the front porch steps drinking beer. The grass hadn't been cut in I don't know how long and I found out later that there was a lawnmower somewhere on the lawn but the grass was so high you couldn't see it.

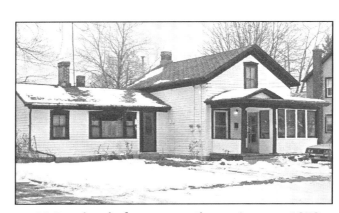

34 Bayview before renovations – January 1978

My mother was somewhat like me: if I'm hesitant to broach a subject, I sometimes compose a lead-in to what I have to say and then eventually get around to my point. However, Mom didn't have to do much talking for me to get the idea she'd come up with. There was a for sale sign tucked down in the grass so I got the drift of things pretty quickly: could we perhaps buy the house? I could live in the left one-storey addition and she could live in the original two-storey house right side. She wasn't getting along that well at #221 with my brother and his wife. She'd given him the house when our father died and I really think she was looking for a new lease on life with this house. What did I think?

Leaving all the memories of my life with Guy in the little house on Canal Street behind appealed to me and I told her to go ahead and contact the real estate lady named on the sign. The price was $29,500. It didn't quite back onto Lake Ontario as there was a small cottage between the lake and the house, but it was close enough so you could see and even smell the water and we'd have a bang-on view of the sunset every night.

The little house on Canal Street brought just enough money to buy the house on Bayview and Mom bartered the lawyer's fees with rare antique lighting pieces she'd collected over the years. Upon closer inspection of the house we found sagging ceilings, cracked walls, no insulation anywhere, and knob and tube wiring throughout. The floor on the right side living room sagged so much there was a small lake of smelly, yellow pee in the middle of it from the two cats left in the house when the former tenants moved out. I couldn't believe that people would move and leave their animals behind but they had. We called the humane society to come and pick up the cats and a flea-infested dog that was chained up outside the kitchen door. At least we gave them a chance, which was more than their owners had done.

Mom wasn't fazed by any of this. For decades she had been reading House Beautiful and any other magazines she could get her hands on that featured homes and home renovations. While Dad was away just about every Friday and Saturday night playing in the big bands, from the day they were married until the mid-'70s or so, she read house magazines in bed to keep her mind busy.

Being at work every day, it wasn't up to me to run the renovation, that was her job and she dove in headfirst. She hired a craftsman, Remi, who was experienced in many facets of home design; I mean, that fellow could make a grandfather clock from wood and the dang thing worked; and he was game to tackle pretty well anything and everything. He tore down plaster and lathe, ceilings came tumbling down, floors were torn up, and there was dust and dirt everywhere. One of the walls was a treasure trove of little items: an old

postcard, a shoe, pennies, razor blades, and a little round silver tin with "Three Merry Widows" embossed on the lid: a condom container from who knows how many amorous encounters in the upstairs bedroom.

I was trying to live in the house while all of the work went on around me. I'd come home at night and not know whether I'd have a bedroom, kitchen or even a roof over my head. The final straw, really two straws, happened when I tried to take a shower to get ready to go to The Standard Christmas party. I stepped into the shower, turned the faucet and nothing happened, but I could hear the water meter clicking away in the closet next to the bathroom. I got dressed and before heading out, climbed around the house in the snow to see a geyser of ice and water climbing up the clapboard siding. I had a broken water pipe.

Straw number two snapped when a couple of weeks later I climbed into bed with my two little poodles, praying that the fact there was no ceiling above me and I could see the raw beams and the underside of the roof didn't mean that there were a million bugs and maybe even bats up there. Silly me! When I woke up the next morning and looked down at my feet, the duvet was moving with spiders. I think if it had been one spider I probably would have screamed (I don't like spiders much), but there were maybe 50 of them (I may be exaggerating – slightly) and this wasn't a time for screaming; besides, who would hear me. It was a time for action. I slowly and very methodically moved the dogs out onto the floor and then I slid out, put on my slippers, and grabbed the end of the duvet flinging it off the bed and shaking off the spiders. That was it. Period. I was finished living in a house under construction.

I know Graydon could tell by my slightly hysterical tone of voice over the phone that things had to change and he suggested I come and live with him for the rest of the renovation. I accepted. But his apartment building was pet free. I couldn't bring my dogs.

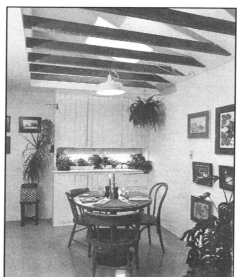
The pine table in the dining side of the new kitchen

Dogs? I know I haven't mentioned dogs, except for Mimi and Gus, but dogs have been a pretty important part of my life. I think they deserve a special place in this book so I'll tell you about them later.

That trip to Cape Cod where we fell in love with scrod prepared only as they can there, windblown walks on the beach, and depending on each other because we were in a strange environment, brought us even closer together. When the house was finally finished and it was time for me to move back home, I suggested that Graydon move back with me and he accepted.

***

Our home was beautiful. I had borrowed $50,000 from the credit union for renovations and once Remi and Mom had started tearing down and rebuilding, they didn't stop until my side had a lovely old pine buffet repurposed as a vanity in the bathroom and a beautiful white kitchen with a skylight over the round pine table from Canal Street; they'd even left the built-in hutch but put fluorescent lights in the back of it for my African violets.

One thing I didn't have halfway through the renovation was a living room and, again, fate stepped in when, Michael, my next-door neighbour, who wanted to build a large modern house on his lot but the city said he couldn't until he rid himself of two 16' x 22' summer cottages, said to me, "Linda, would you like a cottage?" That was the day my side of the house went from being fairly ordinary to fabulous. I found house movers in the Yellow Pages and within a couple of weeks they had put huge rollers under a cottage and rolled it across our lot line onto the cement block sill that Remi had built to hold it. Inside, a wide arch was cut through from the kitchen and a local bricklayer built a large fireplace on the wall next to the kitchen, featuring a hearth and a Heatilator that threw enough warmth to make a difference in that entire side of the house. The end of that room had a tall wall perfect for my artwork, as we had left beams exposed, and Remi had dry-walled the ceiling after putting in a large skylight.

Because the room had been an entire cottage, there were six windows facing the lake plus, and I loved this, a tiny mud room with a sliding panel in

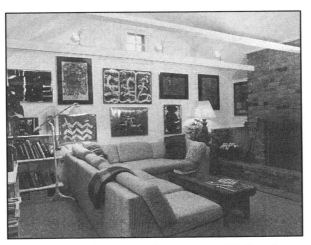

One end of the new living room with fireplace and my batik on rice paper art

the wall so that a mother could pass lunch or ice cream cones through to wet, sand-covered kids and not have them leaving tracks in the rest of the cottage. I left that slider in the wall to remind me where I was and what I was living in.

To say I was happy with the house and the renovation was an understatement. I never dreamed it would turn out so nice. And Mom? Her side of the house was just as gorgeous. What had been a screened-in porch at the front was glassed in and she filled it with beautiful tropical plants plus an old white Victorian wicker chair that she could sit in to read in the winter sun. Her kitchen featured a wall oven but her stovetop was set in a century-old oak counter from a grocery store, complete with bins with graphics showing what was inside. Her new back room had a large skylight in the ceiling, several comfy chairs, a long couch, a TV and beautiful watercolours she had bought from fellow artists on the walls. She had built a little two-piece washroom downstairs so there was no need to go upstairs until bedtime. Up there, under the eaves, she had her bed and a small kitchenette so she could stay up there, make a cup of tea and read at night just as she had most of her life. Mom and Remi had pulled it off and the three of us had a beautiful home.

Speaking of pulling, that reminds me, at one time during the renovation Remi noticed that the walls of the oldest part of the house, Mom's side, were starting to bow outward. Using a winch called a come-a-long, day by day the house was slowly pulled back into shape. I found out later that it had originally been the home of Port

Dalhousie's first butcher and was built in the late 1800s. I couldn't really believe that the house was in such dire straits and still standing, but Mom and that good man had all the faith in the world that it was going to be a safe and welcoming home again, and it was – thanks to them.

***

One afternoon while interviewing the wife of a high-ranking local military man for an article I was writing for the paper, she remarked that it didn't look good for someone like me to be "living with someone." I didn't really care what she thought but several days later after Graydon and I had come home from supper at his mother's place, I flopped on him on the couch and said, "Are you ever going to marry me?" He said, "Yes."

"When?"

"Soon."

"Really?"

"Yes."

"Really?"

"Yes"

"When?"

"I dunno, how about spring?"

"Okay. How about May?"

"Fine."

"Really?!"

He laughed.

And that was it. We were getting married on May 16, 1981, three years to the weekend we moved in together. It wasn't exactly a get-down-on-your knee proposal, more like an agreement of sorts, but then when did my life ever go according to convention? We decided that a very small family wedding on the banks of the Welland River would work and I began thinking about how we'd get everyone, including a minister, out there.

The next day I went into the office with a huge grin on my face. My friend, Andrea, asked me what I was so happy about and, unable to hold it in, I told her. "Hey, do you want to see Crabtree in love?" she said to anyone and everyone in the office at the time. Then, everyone knew.

Spring couldn't come fast enough. Literally. Always practical, Graydon decided that we'd both likely get an income tax rebate if we got married the last day of the year, so on December 31, 1980, the afternoon after an ice storm, with Graydon on one side of me and his mother on the other, I was almost carried up the slippery steps of our downtown police station. When I told the

114

woman at the reception desk we were to see Don Swift, Justice of the Peace, to get married at 3 p.m., she told us that everyone had gone home at noon. My heart sank. Then I asked her to call upstairs and, sure enough, he *had* sent everyone home at noon, but he was waiting for us. We were then told to be careful not to push the elevator's down button because that would take us to the cells in the basement. As we loaded onto the elevator, everyone watched as Graydon carefully pushed UP.

Outside the window, ice-covered tree branches sparkled in the sun as we were read the words and said our "I do's" that would join us as man and wife. My sister and my mother were there as well. A wedding photographer I knew from the paper had taken a portrait of us earlier that afternoon and a local florist had given me pink rose buds to wear on a lovely grey velvet jacket I'd bought for the occasion, which went with my grey satin blouse and new grey slacks. Graydon looked very smart in a tan corduroy jacket, dark

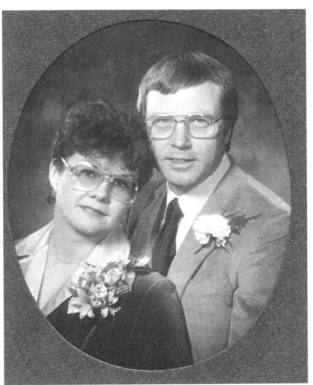

Linda Crabtree and Graydon Book
***Dec. 31, 1980** – pc14.1*

brown slacks, and a sparkling white shirt and brown tie topped off with a white carnation boutonniere. It certainly wasn't fancy but it was what suited us and what we could afford: the Justice of the Peace was given $15 for his time. We were happy it was over. We were married.

A reservation had been made for a wedding supper at our favourite Italian restaurant and sister Kathie had managed to drive a double-layered chocolate cake with green icing (her favourite colour) down there after the nuptials.

After a terrific meal with much laughter and kibitzing, Graydon's mother excused herself to go to the ladies' room and didn't come back. Kathie went to see how she was and then Mom went in and no one came back. The excitement had been just too much for Grace and she was quite sick. She wanted to go home. So Graydon paid the $114 bill and we had confetti thrown all over us as we exited the restaurant to return to our new, old home in Port Dalhousie. Grace was fine after some rest and we were back into our routine but as a married couple.

***

I loved putting a weekly art page together but when that reader survey revealed that sports was what our readers wanted, art was downsized to a column here and there when something was held locally. When you've edited a weekly page, written a great deal of it and set it up, and then you're suddenly hit and miss, the fun goes out of it. It did for me anyway, and I was ready to move over to the family department to see what I could do there.

regret throwing away) as well as thousands of obits, letters to the editor, public service pages and community listings. I had written about the things that interested me and actually developed a following. It was fun, I loved it, and thought I'd work at The Standard until I was too old to trundle in. Unfortunately, that wasn't to be.

Dealing in jewelry and smalls at Harbourfront in Toronto

Remember I spoke about fate when it came to the house? Well, fate stepped in again. You never know what's in store for you and I've learned that if I can go with the flow, I usually end up on top.

As I mentioned, the starting time was around 6:30 – 7 a.m. That's an ungodly time to have to start work and I found it difficult to get to sleep by 8 p.m., when people were taking their dog for the last walk of the day or watching the sunset go down over the lake. To do what I had to do in the morning, I had to get up at 5:30, or 6 at the latest.

I hung in there long enough to write many hundreds of articles (according to the scrapbooks I kept and, still to this day,

Graydon lost his job as an office manager soon after we moved into Bayview. We decided to try our hand at the antiques market at Harbourfront in Toronto, some 65 miles away. I was still at The Standard but went with him almost every Sunday to sell jewelry and smalls we'd bought locally. We sold my rusted out '76 orange Honda and his beautiful gold '78 Toyota for a long 1980 aqua Chevrolet Caprice station wagon bought from General Motors at an employee price, thanks to Mom, a GM widow, and really to Dad who had worked there for more than 30 years. That gorgeous car floated down the highway like a boat and when packed systematically by Graydon, held our entire stock, display cases, tables, everything. It was hell to park in the crowded Standard parking lot when I drove it to work in the early morning hours but I did it with nary a scratch.

***

One dark, snowy morning around 6:40, I pulled into the parking lot, opened the huge car door and actually fell out. I'm not sure why but I think I lost my balance and the car door being heavy helped to pull me sideways. Before I knew it, I was on the cement half-way under the car staring up at the exhaust system, and I couldn't get up.

Someone was shoveling snow in the bank's parking lot next door and heard my weak shouts for help. He took one look at me and summoned the paper-hatted, blue-shirted fellows busy at work in the pressroom next to the parking lot. Once they took a look at the situation a hospital-like triage began: one man was sent upstairs to tell my boss in editorial that I wouldn't be in and why, another was sent to call an ambulance and another stayed with me.

Ambulance personnel slowly extracted me from under the car and placed me on a stretcher. There was a storm drain under the car and cold water had run from the melting snow down my back and into the drain. I was soaking wet, shaking, shocked and didn't complain when I was bundled into an ambulance, and with sirens wailing, driven down our main street to the general hospital.

I was okay, just shaken up, but that experience and all the other problems I'd had trying to get there so early including very little sleep, my hair falling out in clumps and my hands going numb, made it quite clear that my body was trying to tell me something. I'd go out on an interview, thank the person I interviewed for their time, and fall down the stairs when I left — not exactly a great way to represent the newspaper. Because my hands were so weak from computing that morning, it was always a toss-up whether I'd be able to turn the key in the car's ignition when I left work or I'd have to wait until someone came out into the parking lot to ask them to turn on my car for me before I could head home.

Every couple of months I'd fall as I walked across the office, seemingly tripping over nothing. Craig Swayze, the city editor, picked me up once and said, "I thought we were through with all of this." I wasn't sure what he was referring to but if it was alcohol related he was right as far as work and alcohol went, but if he was referring to my CMT, I could only wish. Everything added up to the fact that I was having a really tough time coping, not only with the new job, but with the hours and, more poignantly, my CMT.

The managing editor, Murray Thomson, was very understanding and helpful as was the paper's publisher, Henry Burgoyne, and everyone else who understood my situation. Within eight months, and after being offered several other jobs at the paper, even my old job on the reception desk, and, following one incredible send-off party, I was retired on long-term disability. I'd been there 12 years, loved most of it, been treated exceptionally well and learned what I needed to get on with my life. Although, if you'd asked me at the time, I wouldn't have thought I had anything left to give.

***

I had always planned that whenever, and if ever, I left The Standard I would pursue my art full time. I had one-woman shows of my artwork confirmed for the Niagara Falls Library and Rodman Hall Arts Centre but knew the stress of putting them together and meeting exhibition deadlines would just about do me in. I canceled those as well. A one-woman show at Rodman Hall had been a dream of mine since I'd known what Rodman Hall was, and every time I covered a show there I could imagine my work on the walls, but I was so exhausted I knew that I simply had to divest myself of everything. I had to just stop. Everything. And see where I stood physically and emotionally.

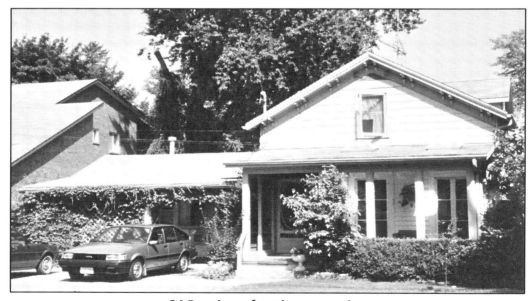

34 Bayview after the renovation

15

Depression and change

After leaving The Standard, I went into a deep depression.

Anyone looking at me would think I had everything to live for, but inside, I was lost.

Yes, I was newly married and had a husband who cared. Yes, I lived in a lovely old home by the lake we'd just spent $50,000 renovating and were putting $400 extra a month on the mortgage to get it paid off faster. Yes, I had a small pension to fall back on but I was only 41 years old and wasn't working. I needed a purpose.

To say I had loved my job at the paper was an understatement. There'd been one old fellow in accounting who was in his late '80s and still on the job. I'd hoped I'd be able to work there until I died or was too old to crawl in and reach the elevator button.

I enjoyed and cared for the people I worked with. I loved the work and had learned a great deal from my editor-in-chief and Craig Swayze, the city editor; even though the recent early starts got to me. The Burgoyne family, who ran the paper, had owned it for generations and they were generous, fair and fun. From the very beginning I was given an annual raise and everyone received a turkey and a bonus on their paycheque for Christmas. Our editorial department Christmas parties were outstanding and the lyrics to The Twelve Days of Christmas changed every year according to who or what had hit the fan during the year. The Standard was a family away from home.

Now, what was I to do?

I was angry and so depressed I wanted to die: just screw myself up into the heavens and disappear. Graydon knew I was in bad shape and so did my mother.

***

One day I decided that my hands were the cause of everything I was going through and I began bashing them against the plate glass mirrored doors of our bedroom closet. All I really accomplished was to severely bruise my fingers but that little episode told me that I needed to look for help.

I'm sitting outside on a beautiful sunny summer day, tears running down my face, saying goodbye to everything I loved including the trees, the flowers in my garden and our home. I was serious. I didn't want to live.

My mother sat down beside me and said she thought I needed to see someone about my depression. She rarely interfered in my life but knew I was struggling.

Taking her suggestion to heart, I asked my family doctor if he could refer me to someone. That someone turned out to be a top-notch psychiatrist and it was the best thing that could have happened at the time.

I was a bit hesitant at first. I knew I wasn't crazy. But, I'd just come off of 12 years of deadlines and productivity and couldn't see a useful future ahead. Trying to cope with the uncertainty of whether I'd ever find anything else I'd be able to do was deadly. As it happens, that's what depression can be all about. And this man was spot on with his diagnosis and treatment.

His office was north of Toronto about an hour and a half from us. Graydon said he'd drive.

After my initial appointment, it was suggested that I make double appointments so we didn't have to make as many trips and I'd be seeing the psychiatrist for 100 minutes each time.

Following each appointment I was totally

spent. I had cried, sometimes yelled, cursed, asked "why me?" more than once, and cried some more, but after five long sessions I was able to laugh and was starting to see the light. Truly. I know it's a cliché but I felt as though a dark cloud had passed and there was light beginning to creep into my soul.

I was on the mend and needn't come back unless I wanted to. I felt so much better that I didn't go back but I still didn't know what I was going to do with the rest of my life.

***

Again, my mother stepped in. She suggested I go back to school. I thought long and hard about this. I'd already put in three years of art school. What did I want to know? What could I learn that would help me get on with whatever was in store for me?

The answer was psychology and I decided to study death and dying because I'd come so close to being dead or at least wanting to be dead. And I wanted to know more about what had happened to me. What causes deep depression? Why was I so intent on leaving this earth behind when I had so much to live for?

An appointment with the registrar at the local university was fruitful. She didn't dismiss me, as I'd feared. Because I hadn't finished high school, I could attend as a

120

mature student. I certainly was, at 42. My three-year art school diploma gained me five credits. I only needed 10 more credits to complete my B.A. but I wasn't thinking that far ahead.

With that encouragement, I paid my tuition fee for one course, PSYCH 101, and became a student at Brock University.

But first things first.

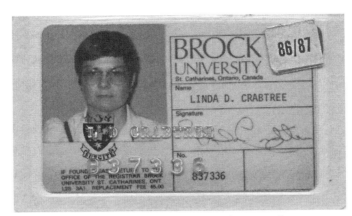

My Brock University student card

Parking was a huge concern. The campus stretched for what seemed miles and I had to park right near a door that had a ramp so I could walk up the ramp, open the door and get to class.

I was given a parking spot next to a door with a ramp.

I tried walking to class and figured out very quickly that I'd get knocked over if I didn't hug the walls. Students would walk four and five abreast, not giving a second thought to the woman they'd just breezed past who was trying to stay upright on the shining terrazzo floors. I felt like a frightened rat scurrying along the walls, trying to cross the hall when the way was clear. There had to

be a better way. I bought an electric scooter.

I was given the key to a utility closet where I could park my scooter and charge it while I wasn't there. As long as I could make the 20 yards to the closet from the exterior door, I was good to go.

To say I was nervous would be an understatement of the highest proportions. I was a wreck. Hundreds of students were taking the same course. It was held in a huge lecture hall with tiered seating for about 500 and the only way I could get in was to either park my scooter right at the very top or figure out an alternate way to get to the bottom on my scooter because there were steps all the way down.

The audio-visual department had access to all of the big lecture halls through a network of dark passageways behind the rooms so they could roll the projectors and other equipment the professors needed into the speaking area. I was given directions on where to go to get into these cement back entrances and who to ask for. Getting behind the action, so to speak, allowed me to sit on my scooter near the lecturer at the bottom of the hall. That way I could see what he or she was writing and hear every word. I used a tape recorder because writing notes was almost impossible, but soon figured out a shorthand style that only I could really read because listening to a taped lecture over and over was very time consuming.

The textbook was easy enough to read but "getting" the basics of psychology down took me some time. I finally twigged after a meeting at a seminar leader's home where we could ask questions and have the answers explained repeatedly until we got it. I recall feeling a lot lighter once I knew I had a working grasp of my subject. My "aha" moment came just in time for the Christmas exams.

There was no way I could actually write my exams. My hands were so weak, even back then, that holding a pen and writing for any longer than a few minutes was impossible. The pen would simply fall out of my fingers. I was given the okay to type my exam and an electric typewriter was put in a spare room used to store old desks and chairs.

Exam day came and Graydon drove me up to the university. I was too nervous to drive. On the way up – Brock is up on the Niagara escarpment – I told Graydon I felt as though I was going to an execution. Mine. Once there, I was ushered into the storage room, took my place behind the typewriter, and two-finger typed my answers for a couple of hours. To my great relief I was able to finish on time, although they had said I could take all the time I needed, and later found that I actually did okay. The same went for the final and by late April I had finished my first course at Brock. I didn't know it then but I was on my way to a whole new life.

16

Fifteen dollars and a few postage stamps

That spring of '84 I took a concentrated course at Brock and did well. There was nothing offered during summer evenings that interested me and I wanted to keep working and learning. I was so keen it was sickening and I was bored.

Sitting at my old cast-iron Underwood typewriter, a keepsake from my newspaper days, I mentioned to Graydon that I thought I'd try to find out more about this Charcot-Marie-Tooth disease that was slowly taking away my ability to walk and use my hands.

The first thing I did was put in a long-distance call to the Muscular Dystrophy Association of Canada in Toronto. I left a message, giving them my telephone number and home address. No

Do you have rare disease?

I am trying to locate people who have a rare form of muscular dystrophy, as I do, called Charcot Marie Tooth Syndrome or Peroneal Muscular Atrophy.

Because this disease is so rare, those with it don't often have anyone with which to share common symptoms, experiences, fears and triumphs, as do those with more common afflictions.

My goal is to set up a network across the country of CMT people, providing a much-needed line of communication and sharing, that we might not feel quite so alone with this progressively debilitating disease which leaves many of us wheelchair-bound in our later years.

Anyone with the disease who would care to share life experiences with others having the same disease is asked to please write to me.

Linda Crabtree
34-B Bayview Dr.
St. Catharines, Ont.
L2N 4Y6

Area woman has a rare disease

Linda Crabtree of St. Catharines shares a letter with her pet poodle, Siddeley. Crabtree, who suffers from Scharcot Marie Tooth syndrome, a rare form of muscular dystrophy, has spent the last few years reading medical texts trying to find out more about the disease. "What I'm trying to do is network people from all over and maybe together we can find something about this disease," she says.

From my archives: the letter that went out to many newspapers and a photo used on several articles. A woman called twice wanting to buy my dog, Sid. – pc16.1

one called back. I thought perhaps they'd send information in the mail. Nothing came. I called again. Still nothing. I couldn't quite figure out why they didn't respond, but no reply just meant I had to look elsewhere.

Then I hatched a plan. I had typed thousands of letters-to-the-editor when I worked at the paper. I had deciphered handwriting so bad it looked like another language and some of it involved translating sentences that were way beyond reason and shortening long verbal diatribes. I knew what editors would run.

A trip to the library saw me photocopying pages of Editor and Publisher, the worldwide compendium of all that is published. With $15 for paper and envelopes and a few postage stamps, I typed letters to editors of all of the newspapers in Canada, telling them that I had a rare disease with a strange name, knew no one else with it, and was looking for information and people to share our concerns and triumphs.

My letters were published in newspapers across the country and within a few weeks I had received so many letters from people also diagnosed with CMT, or suspecting they had it, and wanting information that I knew I was onto something.

My curiosity was piqued. How many people with CMT were out there? Now I had a real challenge. How many could I find? I went back to the library and photocopied all the addresses for the newspapers in the United States. Those letters went out and, before I knew it, I had more than 350 replies from people all wanting to know more.

Trouble was, I didn't have more to give

them. We'd have to learn from each other. And there was no way I could type 350 individual letters in reply. I had to figure out a way to answer them all at the same time. Personal computers were a rare commodity at that time.

The solution to my dilemma turned out to be a mass mailing and in the summer of 1984 the *CMT Newsletter* was born. It wasn't much – only eight pages, the columns typed, cut out and pasted down and then everything photocopied – but it was something.

Graydon and I had talked about wanting to find a way to make a living, something we could do together at home. Little did we know that our wish was being answered.

To make things easier, I asked IBM if they would donate an electric typewriter to the cause and a beautiful blue Selectric arrived not too long after.

That first little newsletter brought in more letters and I bought a filing cabinet to keep

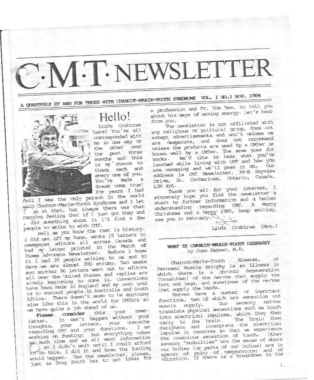

Our first CMT Newsletter November 1984

them in order. I moved my desk out of the tiny art studio, which doubled as a spillover for my clothes closet, into the living area where I could work beside tropical plants under a skylight. I also began to think that maybe we had something worth doing here.

Graydon began to think the same thing when he saw I was having trouble keeping track of the cheques that accompanied those letters. I'm the curious, artistic, photographer, writer, people-person in the family. He's the money, business, bookkeeper, taxes, quiet guy. We made a perfect team. But would he or could he work with me? We decided to give it a try.

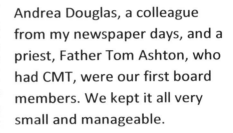

pc16.2

I knew how to get publicity and because we had begun in the summer and August is traditionally a slow month for news, the papers jumped on my story.

I had called our little publication the *CMT Newsletter* and that worked. But, if we were going to cash those cheques made out to me or to the CMT Newsletter, we had to open a bank account and we needed a business name. No one has ever accused me of thinking too small. We called it Charcot-Marie-Tooth Disease/Peroneal Muscular Atrophy International Association, Inc. (CMT International, for short.) Why not

shoot for the world!

It would be a federally registered Canadian charity so we could accept donations and issue income tax receipts to those who qualified. No one we knew had a background in charity law, but we found a lawyer in Toronto who helped us apply for charitable status.

Andrea Douglas, a colleague from my newspaper days, and a priest, Father Tom Ashton, who had CMT, were our first board members. We kept it all very small and manageable.

It took a while for CMT International to become a registered charity but by 1986 we had charitable status and began issuing tax receipts. We even kept track of and sent out receipts to those who had donated the years before, now that we were "legal." Anyone who donated got the *CMT Newsletter* every other month. A talented local graphic designer helped us out by designing a logo free of charge that we could use on everything: our letterhead, the CMT Newsletter, pins, and binders to hold the three-holed punched newsletters. All of these items were offered to help raise money to keep us going. Postage rates were high and printing wasn't cheap.

I found that if you ask people for a

donation, they give what they can. Some give $100, some $5 and a few, nothing. If you tell people what you want them to give, they will give you what you ask for, go below that or give nothing. By simply asking for a donation, we eventually received enough to pay for the newsletter to be typeset and printed and for Graydon to take a small salary. If someone asked, we suggested $35 a year but no one was ever turned away. There were always about 50 people on our mailing list who couldn't or wouldn't donate. The people who gave $50 and $100 a year easily closed the gap. We were pioneers in the CMT information field and it seemed we could do no wrong.

***

It was about this time that Graydon began using his middle name Ronald and preferred Ron. The name Graydon, it seemed, was a puzzle to many and he was often called Greg, Graham and one time Gaylord! Not that there's anything wrong with that but he sure didn't like it.

***

In 1985, we began talking about holding a convention in Toronto in July 1986. It would be the first ever and we were able to entice a full roster of physicians and researchers to come and speak. One hundred and forty

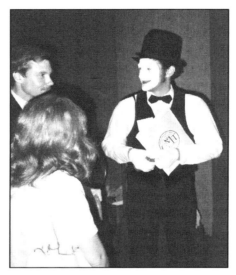

Steve Gulick, a mime with CMT, lightened the atmosphere during the first CMT International convention July, 1986

people with CMT attended. That number may seem insignificant now, but back then it was monumental. Just a year before, I'd never met another person with CMT. We began CMT International on $15. Our food bill at the convention was $12,000.

We'd never run anything like a convention before and I was as nervous as a kitten up there introducing speakers and people I'd only admired from afar. The thirst for answers was so great that women were even asking me questions when I was sitting on the toilet. Stall to stall we'd discuss high arches, foot drop and hands that were weak or always cold.

Everything went smoothly and we believed it was well worth it, except for my complete exhaustion when I got back home. I was horizontal for a week and unable to move anything much but my eyeballs. Slowly my strength returned and away I went again. Letters were piling up and we had a newsletter to get out. We also set a date for the next convention, July 1988, again in Toronto.

***

That same year, we outgrew our side of the

duplex. Mom agreed to move upstairs and let us have the entire bottom floor of her side for an office. It wasn't long after her move that doctors Rebecca (Gabi) and Victor Ionasescu visited from Iowa. Both were dedicated physicians and researchers in the field of neuromuscular disease and Gabi, in particular, had an interest in Charcot-Marie-Tooth disease.

After a tour of the house, and a long discussion about CMT International, the conversation turned to my CMT and how I possibly came to have it. Victor asked about my mother and when I told him that she was in her apartment upstairs, he asked if she would come down. I called up the stairs and Mom said she was still in her housecoat and didn't want to meet anyone but I knew instinctively that was an excuse. She had always denied the fact that she might possibly have passed anything on to me or that there was anything wrong with her. I finally begged her come down five or six steps, just far enough so that we could see her feet through the bannisters. When she did, Victor took one look at her tiny, high-arched feet with cocked toes and said, "Textbook CMT feet."

I hated to call Mom out on this. She was in her 70s, there was nothing that could be

My graduation photo
pc16.3

done and I didn't want her to feel bad about anything that neither of us could do anything about. However, it was nice to have confirmation that I, indeed, had inherited CMT from my mother's side of the family and that I was not a de novo or original case.

***

At university, I had turned a corner. Learning came easily to me and as I began taking third- and a few fourth-year courses, my focus became more on sex and disability rather than the death and dying I thought I'd major in when I signed up in 1984. CMT International had given me something exciting to live for: the digging for information and the gutsy wonderful people always steadily moving forward; it was all good. I was no longer depressed. Every day brought something new, someone to help, a reason to be alive.

On the day I graduated from Brock, in June 1987, I put on a black gown like all the other graduates and rode my scooter into the huge university gym. I was with 300 other students graduating but, unlike them, I couldn't climb the steps to the stage. Arrangements had been made for me to receive my degree down in the first row and when my name was called, I moved forward and a hood was placed over my head, my degree handed to me and they shook my hand. I noticed people began to stand and applaud. I thought perhaps someone really important had entered the gym and I was blocking their way. Then I looked back and realized that the standing ovation was for me. Wow! How did they know this day was huge for me, that I had worked my heart out toward it, that I had pushed the university to recognize the problems students with mobility impairment had trying to attend lectures and to take part in events? I don't know. How did they know that my years at Brock had changed my life and taught me how to work smarter and think more productively? They didn't. They just saw a woman obviously disabled and wanted to give her a hand. But behind it, only I knew there was so much more. I had always wondered what went on behind the walls of our university. Now, I knew, and it had changed me. I had done something I once thought impossible. Wow, indeed!

***

People with CMT in the UK were beginning to organize. In order to publicize a disease most people had never heard of, it was thought that it would help to have a speaking tour arranged for me there. A Canadian woman with a disability, pushing a rare disease, was mildly newsworthy, just a few notches above a Brit pushing a rare disease. I wanted to go. I'd been talking to the people who were attempting to get things going over there and wanted to meet them and see how it was all being handled.

Did we have funds to fly me to the UK? No. I'm not sure how we did it, but funding was found. However, there was one huge concern: I couldn't go alone. I needed help getting in and out of a bathtub, couldn't drive without hand controls, and I needed someone to push a wheelchair as I couldn't rely on there always being curb cuts in the UK; my scooter would be a liability.

An acquaintance volunteered her newly married daughter, Ann, a nurse. I couldn't see how she could bear to pull herself away from her husband but Ann agreed and on July 3, 1987 we set off on our journey: two strangers to a strange country. I really disliked giving my independence over to someone and I imagine she wasn't thrilled about pushing me everywhere either but we certainly managed.

We flew all night and arrived in London sometime very early in the morning. Once at our hotel, The Tara, which was booked for us by the London Club for the Disabled, we were told our rooms weren't ready. I thought I'd die in the hotel lobby, trying to sit up while every bone in my body ached and all I wanted to do was sleep. Please,

God, let me sleep.

Finally, our room was ready and a bath seemed the right thing to soothe frayed nerves and overall jet lag. The tub in our tiny cement-block-walled room was so big and so deep there was no way on earth I could get into it, much less out, even with help. I cried out of sheer desperation. A sponge bath would have to do. The room wasn't air-conditioned and there wasn't a window that opened. For lack of space, my wheelchair had to sit in the hall. And this was THE hotel deemed accessible in London?

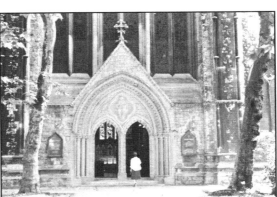

Entrance to St. Mary Abbots Anglican Church in Kensington, London

Sweat-soaked, we woke up after suppertime and headed out for a meal. Trying to find out what had gone wrong with our accommodations, I contacted management and learned that it had been assumed we were travelling on the cheap. It took two more rooms before we found one where we could manage.

London was magnificent. We toured Kensington several times, went to church (St. Mary Abbots where I received communion for the first time on 30 years), took a cruise on the Thames, saw Buckingham Palace and even stayed at Westminster Abbey long enough to hear an organ recital.

Without my pusher, Ann, I wouldn't have done half of that. London is such an old city that the sidewalks weren't ramped. She must've pulled and pushed me up hundreds of curbs. We spent half a day shopping in Harrods, a huge upscale department store. I think it was the best shopping trip I've ever had.

We found the pubs and pub lunches. I didn't drink alcohol then and I don't now, but I found Kaliber non-alcoholic beer brewed by Guinness and it became my beverage of choice for the trip.

While in London, Ivor Dartnall-Smith, our national coordinator in England, his wife Mavis, and my companion and I visited P.K. Thomas, said to be the top neurologist in the country. I remember sitting in his office, feeling as if I was in the presence of God, the all-knowing. I asked him about pain and he told us there is no pain associated with CMT. I told him about the many letters we had received from people with CMT who experienced pain and of the research that Dr. Hardy of Liverpool had done through our organization and the resulting article recognizing pain as a secondary condition resulting from CMT. Mr. Thomas dismissed it all as something else, perhaps aggravated by the CMT.

No one spoke as we left his office in utter dismay at the arrogance and lack of compassion and empathy this man had shown to the obvious plight of those with our disease. Unfortunately, this attitude can still be found among some, but not all, professionals practicing today.

That same day, I spoke on the London BBC about CMT, then we headed out for Enfield with the Dartnall-Smiths to visit Kathie and Ray Boreham. Kathie had one artificial leg due to a birth defect and wore a brace on the other thanks to her CMT. Our visit called for a special dinner, typically English: roast beef, potatoes, veggies and Yorkshire pudding – all delicious. Then off to Upavon and through Windsor where I took a picture of the contrast of a newly cleaned building's facade after it had been divested of 200 years of coal soot next to a building that badly needed cleaning. We got used to seeing buildings all over England with their facades hung with scaffolding as they were being cleaned from top to bottom. The result was a beautiful bright facelift.

Once in Upavon, a tiny village featuring thatched roofed homes, the lovely clean air and roses that Ivor grew revived us and we finally got some real sleep. We also rented a car and managed to make side trips to Bristol, where Ivor and I spoke on the BBC, and to Wales where we tried to look up one of the driving forces behind CMT UK, but it was a weekday and she was likely at work. We also visited Stonehenge and because I was in my wheelchair, we were allowed to go in under the ropes and actually feel

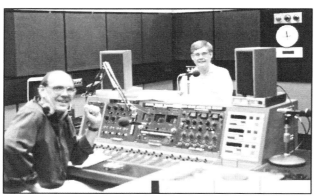

Taping an interview about CMT for the BBC in Bristol

those magnificent stones. Then it was onto Bath, Cleverly, Blenheim Palace and Stow-on-the-Wold, as well as many side trips in between.

In fact, I think the most fun we had was when we got lost. Whenever we saw an interesting back road, Ann and I took it. We really had no time limits as long as we got to our destinations in time to check in and "get lost time" was factored into our schedule. A caravan of gypsies rattled down the main road in Pewsey and I watched as their dogs stayed perfectly in step with the small shadow of the back of the caravan.

130

Every back road, every hedgerow, every stable we found by mistake was an added bonus.

One of our most enjoyable finds was Bowood, a beautiful huge old estate near Calne, where I climbed three flights of stairs and almost did myself in. And in looking for the Etherington Park Hotel, we ended up in the stables out back, talking to a Mr. Stewart and his Beddlington terrier, Joseph, who looked very much like a lamb. When we finally got around to the front, the place was magnificent but it is the terrier Joseph who has stayed with me all these years.

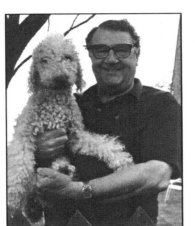

Mr. Stewart and Joseph

On another venture, we were looking for an old abbey but again our traveler's luck held and, as usual, we pulled up lost somewhere in the back of someplace. There we witnessed a touching scene: the Earl of the Sandbourne had been married that afternoon and he and his bride had just returned from the church at Pewsey. She had given her bouquet of Shasta daisies to someone else and the household staff of about 20 people circled around them as they arrived back from the church to the huge back courtyard. The dog, a big black lab, had a wrapped gift for the newlyweds in his mouth. At first he wouldn't come out to give it to them, so they carried it out, but then he caught on

and went from person to person showing them how terrific he was, present in mouth. The Duke put the Mercedes away and everyone went in the house, if you can call it a house: it was one huge estate. I can't imagine how much it costs in money, management and staff to keep it going.

In about two days Ann had learned to drive confidently on the left-hand side of the road, and we stopped ducking and sucking in our breath after three days. She had mastered the traffic roundabouts as well and sometimes we'd just go roundabout for the fun of it.

***

Sunday, July 12, was a very special day. A large meeting had been arranged at Wednesfield and every person with CMT in the UK that the coordinator was aware of had been invited. After the business part of the meeting was over and tea had been served all around, I spoke a little while and then asked if people wouldn't mind my taking some photographs of CMT hands and feet, outdoors on the patio. Of course, we all did more sharing out there and I was held by the waist by someone's husband, so I could get close up photos of the feet and not fall flat on my face. The day ended with cake and ice cream and I met more CMT people that day than since the convention the year before.

From the meeting, we drove directly to Brigg in Yorkshire to stay with Richard and Susan Lund. Richard was the CMT representative there. The next day was Monday and, after several newspaper interviews and photographs, I was asked to speak before the Brigg Rotary club.

From our lodgings at the Lund's, we managed Stratford-on-Avon, Beverley, Oxford and York: where we toured the Jorvik Viking Centre, way down under York. I actually reached out and touched charred wood from a Viking hut burned some 1,000 years ago.

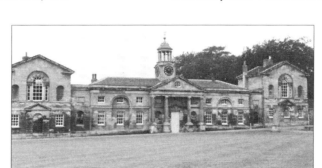

Bocliffe Hall – We picked peacock feathers off the lawn

I was introduced to one of the most fascinating people I've ever met while at Richard's. Dorothy Hilton, a quadriplegic, lived in a little house not far from the Lunds, all on her own, running the household with the help of a POSSUM computer and some visiting outside help. Dorothy was in bed most of the time and I remember pink linens, long wavy red hair splayed out over her pillow, a small white face and huge blue eyes behind great, round glasses. There was a fishpond within view from her bed and her computer was on an arm that came out in front of her so she could turn on the fishpond fountain and pretty well everything else in the house. She could also answer the door, unlatch it and lock it when you left. She very patiently wrote letters, articles and dissertations for school: as a scan of the alphabet passed by her eyes and she picked the letter she needed, only to repeat the alphabet again, and again pick the letter she needed.

Dorothy and I wrote back and forth for years until she finally passed away, having earned a degree and travelled to several conferences. I can only imagine what getting out was like for her.

You might think that people who have severe disabilities are inspirations only to people who do not have disabilities - but, in fact, Dorothy was a huge inspiration to me. I have never forgotten her. It's not so much about the disability, it's about the spirit that drives the person and how they make a life for themselves. Dorothy shone.

As we left Brigg, we managed to find several beautiful old estates, namely Bocliffe Hall and Bramham Park. I'll never forget the misty quiet, sheep grazing under huge dripping trees and the cry of the peacocks on the lawn and rooftops; the only constant was the sound of our tires crunching the gravel as we drove around the circular driveway of Bramham Park. We were too early for the tour but got more out of the 20 minutes we spent there than we ever could have on a tour. If I had energy enough to get out of the car, Ann would push me anywhere we could go as not everything was wheelchair accessible. We got used to seeing what we could, when we could, and that was good enough for us. It had to be. We savoured everything we did like a chef over his favourite dish.

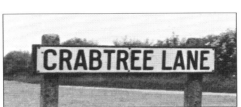

On our way to the English Lake District, we toured a beautiful old estate called Harewood House and even found a Crabtree Lane near Keswick.

We stayed at Bowness-on-Windermere in the Lake District and I bought a mohair throw at a spinning mill near there that kept me warm throughout the rest of the tour. Feeling slightly damp all the time made my muscles ache, so I wrapped myself up in that beautiful mo and relaxed in the luxury of it all. I still have it.

As we headed north toward Eskdalemuir to visit a doctor we had met on the plane over, we saw fabulous scenery. I thought to myself that England had left me with an overwhelming sense of green, chimney pots and pink roses; and Scotland felt deep green, rich brown and deep purple dotted

with white. Indeed, the first time I was actually out in the country, I looked at the hillside and remarked to myself how many white rocks there were, until the rocks started moving and I realized they were sheep. Where I come from, a flock of sheep on a hillside is a rarity.

At Pitlochry, Scotland, we stayed at the Atholl Palace Hotel, a huge old place with high ceiling bedrooms and a view, through cleaning scaffolding, of miles of hills and dales. The next day we were off to Carnoustie to see Lillian Fyfe, our chapter coordinator in Scotland. I stayed wrapped up in my mohair throw, as it was still cold and damp.

Lillian had a tiny home with a long, broken-up backyard. In the house, two large tortoises, a dog named Ben, a black cat and a huge tank of tropical fish all lived with Lillian, her husband and their son: who played the guitar upstairs while we visited. Lillian was very friendly and outgoing but in a great deal of pain and you could see muscles constantly twitching in her thighs. She was also very weak but very healthy looking. No wonder she was frustrated. She said the pain played havoc with her sex life and she felt like she'd been hit by a truck afterwards. This is something I heard from quite a few women over the years.

Following a tearful goodbye, we headed for St. Andrews and a retail shop, the Woollen Mill. Shopping wasn't as much fun there because I felt really weak, likely from all the talking, so we found a beautiful beach and took pictures of low tide and all the old ruins. St. Andrews is famous for its golf course and I thought of my father and how much he'd have loved to have played a round there.

Scotland has some of the most beautiful country I've ever seen: clouds reached down like fingers touching the tops of huge humps of mountains - green in patches then brown rock and green trees. The heather was just starting to bloom and all the shades of green, brown and purple were sharply vibrant and vivid because it had rained for three days. We grabbed a bun and beer and carrot cake at a pub and ate while on the road. I had never seen such huge foxgloves. They were everywhere, tall and healthy (I thought), majestic and very purple. I asked Ann to stop and I pulled one into the car, only to find it was absolutely covered with little black aphids. Oops!

At 6:30 that night we pulled into Oban to find the Great Western Hotel – a huge old lady overlooking the water. The entrance to the hotel was majestic, to say the least. Some 25 wide steps led up to the front door and I looked at the place with a huge sigh: more stairs. I didn't know if I could manage more stairs. Ann went in to talk to the people at the front desk. Yes, the hotel was accessible, inside. The lift was so small there wasn't room for me in my wheelchair and Ann as well, so they offered me the back entrance where they take delivery of the beer barrels. There were only three steps there. If memory serves me right, there was also a very shiny metal chute that they slid the beer barrels down. We all joked about that chute and my possible use of it but for me it wasn't really a joke because, if I had to, I could very easily see myself sliding down to gain entrance to the hotel and my blessed bed.

From my bed that night I could see miles of open water and a huge old house in the trees on the far shore and, beyond that, another lake and more mountains with clouds climbing over their tops. The sun was trying to come out from behind the clouds and it was 9:25 p.m. Because we were so far north it got dark very late in July: much like home.

From there it was down to Ayr and then Prestwick and then our flight home. During our 16 days in the UK, we had met some wonderful people with CMT and many others who didn't have it, but all were kind and helped us on our trip. After that I knew CMT UK was in good hands and it has been ever since.

17

One hot summer

For three years Ron and I had put out the newsletter, answered letters and spread the word. Fund-raising projects were springing up everywhere to help us continue. Members ran pub nights, walkathons and yard sales. We were even given a large collection of vintage cookie jars that were sold at auction. We never knew when a cheque would arrive or from where. People with CMT simply just took it upon themselves to do what they could to promote the flow of information. A one-day conference was put together by Sammie Hammon in Seattle, Washington, for people living out there. I decided to go and got to meet some terrific people with CMT that I'd only corresponded with by letter. The city was beautiful. A group in British Columbia also began to meet.

A yard sale at 34 Bayview – the public donated items and we brought in $1000.

***

In March I decided to do something about my allergies. My nose was always stuffed and I was addicted to the inhaler that shrinks the swelling. Cryosurgery to take away some of the tissue in my nasal passages was suggested and I went for it.

No one thought my CMT might affect the healing or even be part of it all, but it was. No one told me that my nose would be totally plugged with dying tissue for ten days either, but it was.

I'd been to see Dr. Charlie Chan, a pulmonary specialist in Toronto, and he did extensive tests on my breathing. The result was that my diaphragm was weak, mainly on the left side, and when lying down I was unable to breathe out well because I didn't have the benefit of gravity while prone. Not breathing out well enough meant I was retaining CO_2 and the result was a hangover-type headache that woke me up every morning.

With my nose plugged, if I tried to swallow with my mouth closed I felt as if my ears were going to implode. My weak diaphragm didn't help the situation. After the surgery I struggled to eat or drink, and sleep was a horror show. I'd wake up in a panic; I was suffocating. I had to sit up. I moved out of the bedroom so Ron could get some sleep and set up the pull-out couch in the living room.

My mother came to stay with me night after night. We watched TV into the wee hours, the only thing on was a loop taken by a cameraman as he drove the highways around Toronto. As I began to fall asleep and awaken with a start because I couldn't breathe again, Mom would rock with me as the panic attack subsided and together we'd chant over and over: "It's okay. Everything is going to be alright." I was 45, she was 72. Mother and daughter.

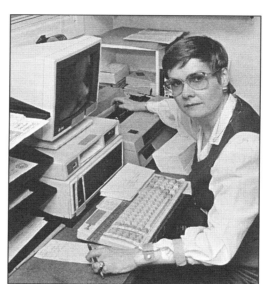

One of our three computers – note wrist brace and pencil to stiffen typing finger

pc17.1

On the ninth day I was looking in the bathroom mirror and I saw what looked like white tissue in my nostril. I pulled at it with tweezers and it came away. Hallelujah! Air flooded into my nostril and my brain settled down. I could breathe through my nose. The other nostril cleared the next day and my ordeal was over. But it had brought

home just how weak my diaphragm was and how easy it was to upset the delicate balance my body had taken on to keep me going.

***

I also received a letter from my former managing editor, Larry Smith, telling me how much he admired the fact that I hadn't just given up when I left the paper. He'd read about me in the media and I'd been on TV quite a bit. That letter meant a great deal to me because, I think, part of me still felt that if I'd just tried harder I could have kept working there. And Andrea Douglas, my friend from the paper who served on our board, had nominated me for the Ontario Medal for Citizenship. In June of 1987 Ron and I went to Toronto where I received the medal and could use O.M.C. after my name. I didn't know the honour existed and was overwhelmed.

***

Computers were just coming in as glorified word processors. We tried several and were really underwhelmed by their lack of precision and constant breakdowns. I plugged away on my IBM before finding one I liked. I had used a computer for years at the paper where the main frame was big enough to fill an entire room. I expected the ones that we could afford for the office to work as well but none did. The Maycourt Club, a local women's group, funded the very first of our three computers.

***

Then the summer of 1988 hit us. It was one of those Canadian summers that are so hot you really don't want to go out. That July we held our second CMT International Convention in Toronto. This time around we had specialists on board, who we'd been working with for several years, as guest speakers and four of them agreed to hold

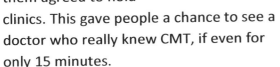

Rest and good fun with Karen Roth in Texas

clinics. This gave people a chance to see a doctor who really knew CMT, if even for only 15 minutes.

Andrea Douglas, arranged more than 300 appointments over three days and no one I know of got their times crossed, although doctors were always running late because no one wanted to leave without having their questions answered. To see a sweaty, exhausted doctor falling into a seat in the hotel coffee shop at 10 p.m. wasn't out of the ordinary. He'd been at it since early morning. One doctor told me he'd seen more people with CMT in three days than

he'd seen in three years in his regular practice.

Following the convention I was so burned-out I couldn't say CMT without feeling sick so I headed for Texas to rest, staying with Karen Roth and her family. I had met her at the convention when she asked if she could play a piece on the piano for me. I looked at her hands, so weak I didn't think she could play anything, but play she did and it brought me to tears. We became fast friends and remained so until she died in 2015.

It was just as hot in Texas as it was back home and we spent a good part of my stay in the Roth's swimming pool or on the road in her air-conditioned van to Carlsbad Caverns and the salt flats in New Mexico. She drove with hand controls from her electric wheelchair. It was during that trip that I learned you could become dehydrated from air-conditioning blowing on you for hours. At one time I was ready to pass out and after that kept sipping from an extra-large cup of water in the holder on the dash.

***

Back home, trying to work in the office, saw sweat running down our faces and dripping from our noses and chins onto our work. It was an unbearable situation and I was exhausted trying to keep up. We couldn't air-condition the old house because it had three add-ons and two furnaces plus no basement under most of it, just a crawlspace. And the old floors were so slanted, I'd be chugging up to the living room and running down from the bedroom. How many times I lost my balance on those uneven floors I can't say but they were a problem. We could see no financially reasonable way to change things.

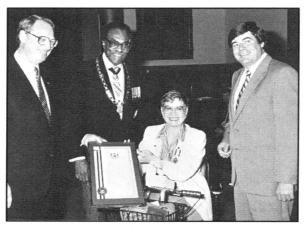

Robert Nixon, Member of Provincial Parliament; Lincoln Alexander, Lieutenant Governor of Ontario and Peter Partington, local MPP, at the 1987 Ontario Medal for Citizenship ceremony – pc17.2

We talked and the upshot was two-fold: for the present, we'd put an ad in the paper and see if we could hire someone part-time to do the typing and filing for me. And, we'd put the old house up for sale and see what happened.

***

In the meantime, Howard S., a scientist interested in CMT, had gotten in touch with us from the United States. He was doing CMT research, had started a group, and asked if we would like to join him, as in become part of his group.

He also invited Ron and me down to Maryland to visit some researchers at the National Institutes of Health (NIH). He was keen on his CMT work using gas mass spectrometry and was trying to find funding to do more. We went and came home even more confused by what happened down there. After Howard's presentation, we were all told that the powers that be at the NIH didn't see any funding forthcoming in the future for his work. We saw no benefit to us or the people we served by linking up with those in the USA, and said no to a collaboration, although we corresponded when needed. I don't know if he was in competition with us. How can you be competing for peoples' lives and their health, both physically and psychologically? You can't. I went forward with the firm intention to simply keep my head down, work smart at what I was doing and stay focused on getting the very best information out to our readers.

It seemed that everything that had come before was coming together as I did this work: my art school training, my newspaper experience with layout and design, my joy of writing and photography, my interest in people, and my ability to draw out bits and pieces during an interview that they didn't think they'd ever tell anyone. The many psychology courses I'd taken at Brock certainly didn't hurt either. The *CMT Newsletter* was a success.

***

Speaking of psychology courses, one of my professors at Brock asked me if I would give a lecture on what it's like to live with a disability. I could think of no better way than to use myself and my life as an example. I probably talked far too long but no one in the tiered seating in front of me moved, so I kept talking and as I did, worked up the courage to include my teenage pregnancy. When I finished to a round of applause, the teacher said, "Well, I hope you found that cathartic." I respected this woman and we both laughed.

As the applause died down and some of the students began to leave, I noticed that some of the young women were staying behind and slowly four or five made their way down to me. "I am so glad I was here today," one of them said, and all of the others said something similar. Some had tears in their eyes. "The same thing happened to me and I've never been able to talk about it." When I left the lecture hall that day I felt a lot better about myself and I also hoped that I had done the same for those burdened young women.

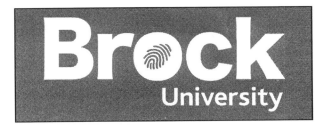

pc17.3

***

I went through several people who answered our ad for clerical help pretty fast. Not being able to spell wasn't an option. Neither was an inability to type a decent looking letter. After two or three false starts, Dorothy, an experienced secretary well-versed in typing from dictation, filing and pretty well anything else clerical, was asked to join us part-time. That took the pressure from me to answer the many letters that came in every week. She typed what I dictated and we answered those letters, all of them. I knew how gut-wrenching it felt to pour your heart out to someone while searching for answers and not even get an "I don't know" back.

***

The problem with air-conditioning was solved when we photocopied a handmade "House for Sale" sign, stuck it on a post in the front lawn, and put a small ad in the Globe and Mail in Toronto. A woman who lived just around the corner from us saw the ad in the Globe and asked to see the house. After several visits, accompanied by friends, she said, "I like your house and would like to buy it." We were in shock.

The house had sold so fast, we weren't prepared for what was to come. Our asking price was met, less what we would have paid to a realtor. The one stipulation was that we had to be out in three months. It was late fall. Winter in Canada is not a great time to start looking for a place to live. Ron and I were working hard to keep CMT International going, I was looking at graduate school, and now we had to figure out whether we were going to buy another house or build, and if we were going to build, where? Huge changes were in the offing.

18

Our new home

Designing a house wasn't something I'd ever actually done. I'd drawn rough plans of my dream home for years but to sit down and plot out rooms for a place that we would actually live in wasn't something I ever thought I'd do. I mean, this was real!

And where would we build it? We didn't have a lot.

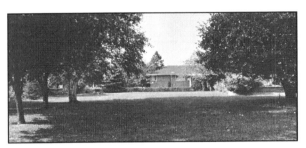

A perfect 60 x 120 foot lot

I searched all the real estate pages in the newspaper for building lots and called several agents but there was nothing much available. On our Sunday country drives, I spotted a few beautiful pieces of property that would make wonderful places to live but all of them were too far from civilization and neither Ron nor I knew how long we would be able to drive. We opted for property in the city.

Our search took us to four city lots that were for sale. We had just about given up, as the first three were tiny pieces of land subdivided from the owner's home and no

bigger than a long garage. That wasn't at all what we were looking for. The fourth lot was in a subdivision that had been built in the 1950s on an apple orchard. The property in question was a corner lot that had been kept as a small park for 35 years. Now it was up for sale. As we drove down a tree-lined street and I read out the house numbers, I could barely contain myself. This lot was perfect. It was close to Mom and Kathie, within walking distance of downtown, and backed onto a private school. Ours would be the newest house in an established neighbourhood featuring middle-income homes very much like the ones in the area where I grew up.

A phone call to the owners who lived next door to the lot, a meeting over our kitchen table, a survey, some lawyering, a cheque, a bill of sale and that 60' x 120' lot was ours.

Now to choose a builder: I called five or six, and three returned my call. One said the project wasn't "high end" enough for him, another couldn't start until spring, and the third was interested. His father had been in the construction business for years and had a good name. I figured I couldn't go too wrong with him. His name was David.

My drawings, as finished as my knowledge of housing design could make them, were sent off to an architectural draftsman to be translated into plans a builder could read. The draftsman kept adding features like fancy tray ceilings and recessed lighting that I didn't want. I kept sending them back for revisions. Every time he revised, he charged. I finally told him that I wasn't paying anymore and he stopped revising.

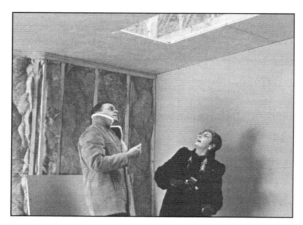

The walls were all pink with insulation and the skylights deep into the pitched roof

What I did want was no steps or stairs anywhere, no basement, 5' wide halls, 36" doorways and pocket doors wherever possible so I wouldn't have to go around doors if I was using a wheelchair or scooter. I wanted every room to have two entrances to allow me to go from one to another without backing up or having to make a four or five-point turn. The kitchen had to have low drawers because I couldn't reach up and grab without dropping things and I needed to be able to slide pots from the stove to the sink and beyond, and food from the refrigerator to the counter, sink and stove, without lifting because I simply didn't, and still don't, have the hand strength to lift. For me having that "slide factor" included was huge. It meant I could function independently in my own kitchen. Electrical outlets throughout the house had to be high enough to allow me to plug something in without falling over. Light switches had to be low and easy; I loved dimmer switches. And most of all, I wanted a bright, welcoming house. To that end, I drew in 14 skylights. Fourteen! Was I nuts? I couldn't get out easily, so my idea was to bring as much of the outdoors in and to my way of thinking that meant light.

The foundation was dug for the concrete slab the house was to be built on, just before Christmas in 1988, and the house began to take shape. Our address was to be One Springbank Drive. David had said it would take three months and a bit, and it did.

I remember walking around in it with Ron on February days so cold our breath hung in the air. But it was ours and it was wonderful. Two-by-six interior and exterior framed walls were soon packed with what seemed like miles of pink fibreglass insulation. For a while the entire house was bubblegum pink. Then that gave way to off-white dry wall and the rooms I'd drawn began to slowly take shape.

It was important to get the roof on and the house closed up. I'd wanted a flat roof, but considering our snow loads in winter, that wasn't something David recommended. So to speed things up, I okayed trusses for a peaked roof. That meant every skylight had to have a tunnel built from the roof down to the interior ceiling. We visited the site regularly and one day while stopped to watch workers on the roof, one man shouted at me: "Too many skylights!" I had no idea what was involved constructing skylights in a peaked roof, only a flat one. I think if I had, I would have reconsidered or at least cut the numbers down, but David didn't say a thing. He just kept building. Now, those skylights brighten the house beautifully, but in winter the heat rises into them and the house can be colder than I'd like. I sacrificed heat for light.

We moved in through the Ridley Heights

In the jetted tub with a raised surround to sit on and swing your legs in – beveled mirror backsplash

Drive carport door on April 6, 1989, as the carpet layers worked their way out the front door on Springbank Drive. It was that tight. I had chosen to have the entire house done, excluding the kitchen, in sand-coloured low-pile industrial carpet. It lasted through my scooter, two dogs and 26 years, although we soon installed non-slip vinyl in the bathroom, and tile in the utility room and guest washroom. The popular wall colour in the late '80s was peach so our large family/dining room, what I called the Jacuzzi room, the kitchen and everything but the entrance hallway and the offices were painted peach.

There was a small angular room just off the family room, where I had a large jetted Jacuzzi-style tub installed with a beveled mirror backsplash above it. It looked ever so elegant but I soon found that the tub wasn't deep enough to keep my knees warm and I had a terrible time getting in and out of it. Sometimes my ideas didn't pan out as well as I hoped they would.

I had included a small private yard off the main family room with a pond and waterfall. Just down the highway, Ron found about a dozen huge granite boulders that had been cleared out of a vineyard. We paid the farmer $100 for them and on the morning of my 47th birthday, I looked out the kitchen window to see a huge rock-covered flatbed truck pull up to the curb. The neighbours must have thought we were nuts because we'd already spread tons of Lake Erie beach stone all over our corner lot so there wouldn't be so much grass to cut.

Dogwood, pines, cedars, hemlock and ornamental shrubs went in that spring. My mother had told me not to wait to landscape. "A good yard takes several years to look established," she said. "Plant as soon as you possibly can." Greg Pillitteri, who had just graduated from the Niagara Parks School of Horticulture, took on the job and set about sculpting the yard with a small front-end loader. He moved those boulders to form a waterfall with a pond and then fenced in our pocket-sized, very private backyard. It promised to be quite beautiful.

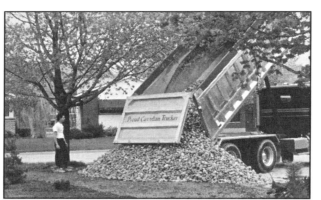

Greg supervising the dumping of one of four truckloads of stone spread around the property

Indoors, two rooms were devoted to CMT International: one had space for our secretary and Ron, who looked after everything from the banking and books to membership and mailings ... everything I couldn't do. The room behind that was my office with my computer, desk, a bank of file cabinets that held every letter we'd received since 1984 and our *CMT Newsletter* production board, where we mapped out the pages several issues in advance as information, stories and photos came in. I got to know many of the physicians who were doing work on CMT and could look to them to vet everything that I wasn't sure about for the newsletter. I believe all of them wrote articles for us.

My plate was full answering letters, taking phone calls, writing articles and putting the newsletter together. It was routine to spend six or seven hours in the office during the day and then another two or three at night. If I could get my feet on the floor, I could get my body up and into work. As a rule, I did. Most weekends were no different except we'd go out for breakfast at Betty's restaurant in Niagara Falls on Sunday mornings.

That fall I had begun classes at the State University of New York (SUNY) at Buffalo. The plan was for me to eventually do rehabilitation counselling. I would work on my own as a private counsellor in the

144

afternoons when not busy with CMT concerns. The house was designed with solid core doors for counselling privacy and had a large entrance hall that would double as a waiting room. There was also a two-piece washroom for guests or clients. I'd tried to think of everything.

***

The government was paying my way, for my books, and even for a driver to take me to Buffalo, some 50 miles away across the international border, two and sometimes three times a week. Art, my driver, a retired gentleman of about 70, would regale me with tales of his home life as he drove. I still remember the time he told me about his wife kicking him out of bed because he farted. I mean, what was the man supposed to do?

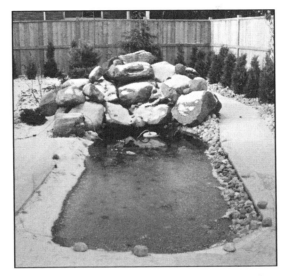

A fence, 50 cedars, a small hemlock and two dogwoods plus a granite boulder waterfall and a shallow pond with a concrete rollway surround made up our private pocket-sized backyard

I loved class, was miles ahead of the young kids just out of university, and felt like the den mother. Not only did we have class but seminars and a practicum. Mine was at the Erie County General Hospital. These were above and beyond my regular everyday work. And when I got home, I had chapters to read, papers to write and notes to transcribe because I had to tape a lot of lectures due to not being able to hold a pen for any length of time. I hung in there until just before Christmas exams. I was working all hours of the night trying to study and keep up with the demands of CMT International. I'd dictate letters to CMT people, work on the newsletter, read a couple of chapters for school, transcribe the notes of the day and fall into bed exhausted around midnight or later. Eventually I began to realize that I wasn't going to be able to keep up the pace. Something had to give. I was exhausted.

A visit to my doctor told me that I was in pretty bad shape. I had begun using a cane, sometimes two, for balance when I wasn't on my scooter, was rundown and not getting enough sleep. He said I might graduate if my current pace didn't kill me first. I listened. Should I give up my dream of being a rehab counsellor with a master's degree in science or should I give up CMT International? It was a terribly hard decision to make.

I thought long and hard. Ron worked for CMT International, my secretary relied on us for her salary, the house was perfect for CMT work, I knew what I was doing and I loved it. And we were educating and helping thousands who knew nothing about their CMT.

School was a maybe. I loved it but would I get work as a private rehab counsellor? When all was said and done and I'd graduated, would I like it?

I had to admit I already had a CMT tiger by the tail. After what had been a five-year journey of regaining confidence, doing very hard work, learning to love to learn, and learning to dig, build, plan and dream for my future, I quit school. It almost killed me to admit I couldn't physically do it all, but I quit.

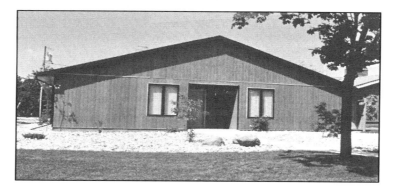

Exterior of our home 1990 (above) and 2017 (below) – that's a pink Dogwood on the left and a Japanese Maple on the right. Brown canvas awnings over doorway and windows.

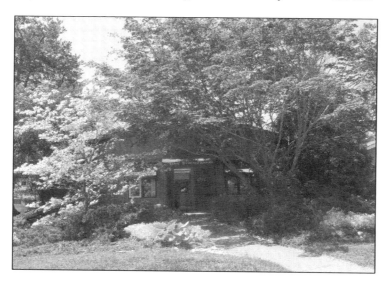

146

19

How to get back to England

There was definitely life after academia. Without the pressures of school, I could launch my energies fully into CMT work and enjoy it without worrying that I was neglecting my studies.

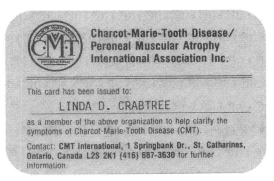

The CMT ID card (front) introduced in 1989 to help people explain their condition

In 1989 we also introduced an annual index to the *CMT Newsletter*, so people could find what they were looking for in back issues, and a laminated registration card that said they had CMT. Too many people told us that because of an awkward and often off-balance walk, they'd been mistaken for being drunk or, because CMT doesn't show unless you have trouble walking or your hands are affected, not disabled at all. They wanted proof that they had a debilitating condition. Those cards were a huge success.

I replaced a time-worn paragraph vaguely explaining CMT, I'd photocopied out of a book in the library and carried in my wallet for years, with one of our cards myself.

Charcot-Marie-Tooth disease is named after three doctors. It has nothing to do with the teeth and is also known as Peroneal Muscular Atrophy. It is one of many disorders classified under Hereditary Muscle and Sensory Neuropathy. This genetically inherited, progressively debilitating, neuro-muscular disorder affects the peripheral nerves and their insulation. The messages from the brain through the nerves to the muscles are slowed. Healthy muscles can therefore weaken and atrophy. Loss of feeling and/or movement **may** result. Hands, feet and lower legs are usually affected. Arms and thighs are usually spared however they may be affected in later stages. Breathing **may** also be affected. Loss of balance and fatigue are common symptoms. Certain drugs can make CMT worse. Test lungs BEFORE administering anesthetics. Life span is usually normal.

A brief explanation on the back

CMT breathing problems, pain, orthotics, hip dysplasia, scoliosis, and grieving for lost movement and abilities was discussed in the newsletter. Articles were written by doctors, some who had CMT themselves. Everything was in layman's terms.

***

That year I received the Canada Volunteer Award, "In recognition of outstanding voluntary service in improving the health and well-being of Canadians." I was flown to Ottawa in a small commuter plane out of

Hamilton. No one had thought to find out if I was able to climb steps and there was no way into the plane except steps. I turned around, sat on the second from the bottom step and, using my arms, pulled myself into the plane, one gritty step at a time. My travelling companion took several photos that I used to enlighten the powers that be in Ottawa upon our return. A couple of steps weren't going to stop me from making an appearance. Good thing I always wore slacks.

Boarding the plane the hard way

I was also given the YWCA Woman of Distinction Award. I was in hospital recovering from a kidney attack (maybe just sheer exhaustion) days after we'd moved into the new house when, after lights out, I heard high heels clicking down the terrazzo corridor. "You got it, you won," Andrea and Denise Archer leaned over the bed rail and whispered so as not to wake my room-mate. Being acknowledged for my work by my peers meant a lot to me then and it still does.

In 1990 our new home won a Premier's Award for Accessibility honourable mention. The competition was only open to architects but I thought, why? Why couldn't people with disabilities take charge of their living conditions and, if capable and given the chance, design what works for their lifestyle? I don't think my entry was too welcome but they couldn't very well kick me out, could they? I was delighted with an honourable mention. It was a step forward for all people with disabilities. I thought the phrase "Nothing about us without us," referring to no policies or decisions made about the disabled (or any) community without the involvement of that group, very much applied here. That's why I entered the competition. One of the judges said he only voted for my design because he liked the "pocket" backyard. Whatever the reason, Ron and I gladly accepted the award from Premier David Peterson, who coincidentally was using a cane at the time due to a skiing accident, while the builder and his wife looked on.

***

CMT UK was growing beautifully and we were hearing from people in other countries who wanted to start a CMT International branch or separate entity in their country. We gladly suggested how they might begin and helped in any way we could. Because getting the word out via the press and radio to find people with CMT was so important, having a free and accommodating social network in any country truly helped.

148

Also in 1990 we held another convention but this time in Niagara Falls. Instead of individual appointments, we organized workshops where a group of people with CMT could watch and listen to a demonstration or talk and then ask questions. That format seemed to work well as those running the sessions often used the people with CMT, who were asking the questions, as examples to illustrate what they were talking about. The physicians had real-life case examples of CMT right there in front of them.

CMT UK announced that they would hold the 1992 CMT Convention at Stoke-on-Trent and I was delighted to know that things were progressing as they should. I wanted to be present but our funds didn't allow for international travel and I didn't want to go alone. Ron preferred to stay at home and run things but gave me his blessing to make the trip. It was awhile off but I began planning to get there, one way or the other.

Government had given us a little funding, but when we asked for continual funding, we were told that because we were international and not just concerned with people who had CMT in Canada or Ontario, we didn't qualify. Go figure? We were disqualified because we included everyone.

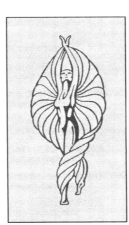

YWCA Award to Women gold pendant design

CMT doesn't respect borders, why should we? That was my take on it. We'd just have to work a little harder to get the funds we needed.

Sophie Abarbanel, a librarian in Ottawa, funded a scholarship we put together in her name. In 1990 the first winner of the Sophie Abaranel Educational Assistance Award of $1,000 was a young man in Mississippi who had been accepted at Duke University. He had been a student at the Mississippi School for Mathematics and Science, was president of a fraternity and was involved in many other academic pursuits. He hoped to major in political science. His family didn't know CMT existed when he was born but, in looking back, the signs were there. From an early age, his sport was swimming and he took the positive energy from his successes in the pool to his academic pursuits. To find out what you can do and do it well when you are young, makes all the difference when you have CMT. The disease may limit your mobility but it doesn't limit your ability to use the good mind you were born with. Today he is working in government, just as he said he would.

Dr. Joseph Antognini did work on anesthetics and suggested that succinylcholine might not be a drug we'd want used on us, as it is used to relax the muscles during surgery and the muscles release potassium. In people with CMT too much potassium can be released, causing heart malfunction. Dr. Antognini also sent out a questionnaire through us to find out more about anesthetics and how we react to them.

Dr. Simone Blajan-Marcus, in France, became our resident psychologist and answered questions far too complicated for a lowly psychology major like me.

A youth column was established to address the particular concerns of those coming to grips with adolescence and CMT.

We also set out to find answers from professionals in Australia, New Zealand, France, the United States, Canada and the UK for an assortment of questions of interest to our readers.

We had great interest from Western Canada, particularly from a retired gentleman, Bill Neily, who set out to find everyone he could who had CMT in British Columbia and personally visit them all. We also planned a trip across the country to attend a one-day seminar in Burnaby, B.C. Ron and I flew to Calgary, Alberta, where Lynn Parmenter, my old friend from my YWCA days in Montreal, drove us up to Banff for supper and the next day I had a meeting with Albertans who had CMT. The Calgary Herald announced our visit and wrote about the meeting. Then we climbed aboard the Canadian National (CN) railway for a trip through the Rocky Mountains to BC. I'll never forget lying in my window berth as our train snaked through the mountains under a full moon.

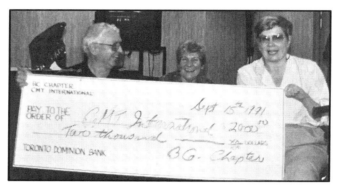

Norm and Gladys Schmidt presenting the $2,000 cheque

The meeting in Burnaby saw Dr. Robert Sampson, an orthopedic surgeon who has CMT, hold two two-hour workshops for 77 people and then come back to give a talk on feet, balance and bracing. Dr. Stuart Patterson, yet another orthopedic surgeon, along with occupational therapist Dorcas Beaton, were there to look at hands.

Dr. Patterson and Dorcas worked into the wee hours of the morning, seeing 50 people in 15-minute one-on-one appointments. Hands weren't the main concern of most doctors because CMT usually affects the feet first, but when you lose your hand function you very quickly learn that you can't do much without them. To those 50 people, that appointment was likely the first time someone really took an interest in their CMT hands.

Gladys and Norm Schmidt had arranged the conference for us and, in spite of dealing with colon cancer, Gladys did a terrific job of pulling everything together and then, at the end of the event, the couple presented us with a $2,000 cheque.

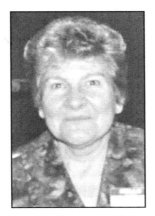

Gladys Schmidt

Someone remarked that they could feel the love and caring in the room. It was always like that when we had a CMT International meeting. No one was selling anything, no one asked for money, no one was neglected or told it was all in their head. As for me, I floated on that warm fuzzy love for about three days and then we flew home, where I hunkered down for a week to recover. But it wasn't long before I found myself revisiting the question of how I was going to get to England for the next convention.

20

Supersonic

The last time I travelled to England, the all-night flight from Toronto to London almost did me in. I arrived absolutely exhausted. My knees had been bent so long and my legs hurt so bad that I learned the true meaning of the word agony.

Dare I think Concorde? That beautiful plane would get me there in half the time. However, the airfare was not going to be cheap, and we were in a recession; lesser challenges had come my way and been dealt with. The question was, how? If you are not familiar with the Concorde, according to Wikipedia, it was "a British-French turbojet-powered supersonic passenger jet airline that was operated until 2003. It had a maximum speed of over twice the speed of sound at Mach 2.04 (1,354 mph or 2,180 km/h at cruise altitude), with seating for 92 to 228 passengers."

A few phone calls and I was in touch with a travel agent in Toronto. It was October 1991. There could be some seats available,

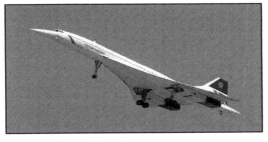

The British Concorde – pc20.1

please call back in November. How much? One way: $4,500. I thought deep and hard and everyone agreed I shouldn't travel alone, not in my condition, so that meant $9,000 for two. Gads! No way. I thought about the QE2; too long a trip and I'd never sailed. What happened if I was seasick all the way over? No, it was Concorde or nothing.

After several false starts, I finally got a price of $2,615 per person one-way or $5,230 for two. It was still a huge amount for a tiny charity to come up with but a little more reasonable. We would take a regular flight home.

The money? Well, after much letter writing, explaining that the founder and head of a Canadian-based organization that worked with people all over the world couldn't attend the overseas convention of her own organization by regular air because of her health and that special plane fare was required, two branches of Health and Welfare Canada (International Affairs and

Health Services and Promotion) together arranged to donate $5,000. That worked wonders. CMT International put in a considerable amount and CMT UK paid for a room and meals while at the meeting. With four entities working together, my niece Samantha and I were away on the Concorde on August 13, 1992, from Toronto Pearson International Airport's Terminal Three. Ordinarily the Concorde didn't fly from Toronto. It normally flew from New York to London, but a group of seniors had chartered the 100-seat plane to fly from Toronto and there happened to be a few seats not booked.

We left home that morning at 7:30 a.m. and arrived at the airport around 9 a.m. The plane was to leave at 11:30 a.m. As we inched our way up the line, praying our luggage wouldn't be overweight as they DID care how much you took on the plane. We overheard that there was going to be a three-hour delay; something had gone wrong with the plane. What was three hours after all those months of planning and waiting? We just hoped we'd be in England before the day was out.

Directions were given for us to wait at Swissôtel, where everything in the cafe was complimentary. The airline also made arrangements to call someone at our destination to tell them we would be late. Eventually we were back in the lounge at the airport.

I made three observations during that three-hour wait. People who could afford to fly the Concorde seemed to be middle-aged or older, and may have filled out, if you get my drift. Some of them seemed to feel they had no one to consider in this world but themselves. They smoked openly in the no-smoking section of the lounge and they constantly ran into my wheelchair. I can't suck my wheelchair in to let people pass; I wish I could. I can't tell you how many times I was banged, jostled, hooked onto and pushed. Put it down to poor eyesight and poor coordination on their part. I hope so. The smoking business was just plain lack of consideration. I breathe so shallowly that I'm hardly here in the first place, and they sat talking, drinking and laughing, while I fanned the air and tried not to faint.

The third observation was that the bathroom to the VIP lounge was so tiny you couldn't get a wheelchair into it. The accessible one is "only down one floor," to quote the hostess. I hung onto my niece, stood up, and managed the tiny one. Not a lot of thought went into that waiting area. With 100 people waiting in that VIP lounge, there wasn't much room for wheelchairs and I think there were four of us. Scrimping here made the place look and feel cheap. Most of these people could afford to fly the best, recession or not. Why not give them some space and luxury?

Finally the plane arrived and shortly

afterwards was ready for us to board. In return for our boarding passes, we were each given a little model of the airplane – a nice surprise.

Next to the door of the plane, I stepped out of my wheelchair and hanging onto the plane, with the help of a hostess and my niece, I made it to my seat. The wheelchair was whisked away to the baggage compartment. Manual wheelchairs, electric wheelchairs and scooters with dry cell batteries travelled free of charge. They were classed as part of us, as well they should be, and not as luggage.

Weeks before I had the forethought to arrange for a bulkhead seat through a note to the airline from my doctor so I would have as much legroom as possible on the plane. This really helped because I'd been sitting with my knees bent for almost seven hours before we boarded the plane.

Once on board everything was handled so professionally, we felt that we were in very capable hands. I was surprised at the closeness in the cabin and the amount of gum on the carpets, but I guess it is inevitable. Why should I expect perfection!

Our plane was *Alpha Charlie*, one of the older Concordes, built in 1976. There were 20 and British Airlines flew seven. Alpha Charlie was sleek, white and beautiful on the outside and all done up in shades of grey leather and carpet on the inside. There were two double rows of 25 seats each. The plane carried 100 passengers plus a crew of three and three or four flight attendants.

The seats were comfortable but there wasn't a great deal of legroom or even head room. In the centre aisle of most large planes there is room for the beverage or food cart and you can pass if you turn sideways. In this Concorde there was no way on earth you could do that. It was all very tight and passing meant someone had to go up to an open space and pull in while the other person passed. It's awkward but for four hours everyone got along fine.

I tried to take pictures but it wasn't easy. They wanted us seated with our seatbelt on and when the plane's engines were on, there was a constant vibration. I have a few blurry testimonials to that and I was shooting with a fast speed film.

Each cabin section had a digital computer with bright green letters mounted in the bulkhead wall to keep you informed. Ours was right in front of our seats and it showed the plane's altitude and speed. I took notes.

There wasn't a sound from the passengers on takeoff but the plane made a mighty roar. The captain told us we'd be going 184 miles per hour on takeoff, 212 mph on liftoff and 240 mph leaving the runway. To reheat the after-burners, the speed goes up to 300 mph. They run the engines particularly fast after takeoff to cool them down, as they don't cool down evenly. This means we are going 300 mph with 38,000 pounds of thrust.

We could feel the surge forward from the four Rolls-Royce Olympus turbo jets. It forced us back into our seats. I sat there as we ascended on a very real slant, watching the curtains begin to hang away from the doorframe in front of me. Afraid? Not really. What will be, will be, and on a Concorde plane, going that fast, there wouldn't be much chance for survival anyway. Not with 25,000 gallons of fuel around us. We'd be dust!

Once up, the captain continued his banter about the plane and hot, damp, lemon-scented hand towels were passed around to help us refresh ourselves. Then came the menu for the on-board meal. We were told we would be supersonic in 45 minutes, we were heading for a corridor to Labrador, and we'd be in England in three hours and 40 minutes where it was 60°F and partly cloudy.

Now to settle down with a good book. I'm kidding, of course. A trip on a Concorde plane was a happening (as they used to say in the '60s.) There wasn't a dull moment.

The menu wound its way through canapés of smoked salmon garnished with dill, deep black caviar and foie gras mousse with apple, along with spikes of lobster with green mango and papaya relish. For a main course, we had a choice of fillet of beef with wild mushrooms, shallots and parsley served with grilled tomato, French green beans, carrots and jetee promenade potatoes; or baked fresh salmon with cracked pepper, tomato, corn and coriander salsa, asparagus, baby carrots and parsley potatoes; or steamed breast of chicken with julienne of root patty pans (cute little orange baby squash, as far as I could tell.) Delicious decisions!

At 8,000 feet we cleared the clouds and were headed straight for Labrador, where we would be going 760 mph depending on the temperature. The captain compared our passage in the airways to the wake of a ship creating a sonic boom 35 miles wide. It was allowed only over uninhabited land and over the water. Champagne was served in miniature crystal stemmed flutes. I didn't drink. I kept watch on the computer: Mach .61 – 10,000 feet up: Mach .63 – 10,500 feet up and on and on. We were climbing 500 feet every 10 seconds.

The canapés arrived on a china plate with a silver underplate. Each one looked like a miniature gourmet meal and tasted delicious. The sun was out; we had left the rain and the clouds below. The low hum of the engines, the rushing sound of the plane, that nice feeling of luxury and everything running smoothly and getting even smoother as you realize you are definitely getting the very best, pervades everything.

The salad course: first a crisp white linen tablecloth on your foldout tray. We noticed the chatter of people anticipating good things, the clinking of crystal glassware and silver cutlery.

Looking outside it felt that the plane was standing still, but we were almost going the speed of sound; the computer says .94 — almost Mach 1.

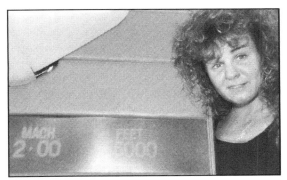

Samantha, my niece, beside the digital screen that told us how fast and high we were flying. Everything vibrated.

The linen napkin came next and it actually had a buttonhole in it to help us hold it up. Thoughtful! It was 3 p.m. Canada time. The salad was full of pine nuts, orange, yellow and pink flower petals, and about a dozen different kinds of greens.

The captain was talking about the winds and said we were seven minutes from supersonic acceleration.

I was in the middle of a forkful of fiddlehead ferns when the plane surged forward. Now THAT was acceleration. A few seconds later, just as I was about to bite into a perfect piece of lobster, the computer screen in front of me flashed Mach 1. Everyone around me clapped and cheered. I smiled to myself: Wow! I'm going the speed of sound and I can barely walk; isn't life something!

At Mach 1.14 everything was on a slant. I was holding myself forward to eat. My choice for the entree was the chicken and it was excellent, right down to the spinach.

The food was picture perfect and tasted as good as it looked. This meal proved to me that, indeed, on-board food can be good if enough money and care is spent on it.

I looked out the window. It was triple thick and smaller than an average plane window by about half and it radiated heat like a small furnace. I felt as though a little fireplace was burning near the left side of my face. It was the heat from the plane going so fast. The plane actually stretched 7½ inches in flight because of it. We were Mach 1.90 and 48,000 feet up. There was a low engine hum and a constant deep vibration but we could hear each other. It was very bright outside, considering we were flying into night. We left at 2 p.m. and would get in by 11 p.m., as there was a five-hour time difference.

Mach 2 at 55,000 feet and 860 mph.

Another round of applause. The captain announced birthdays and a wedding anniversary; another round of applause. He said it was 21:24 in the UK. Let's see, that's 9:24 p.m. It took me two minutes, considering my weak fingers, to set the hands on my watch to the new time.

During the flight I had been noticing a packet tucked in the pocket in front of me that held instructions and magazines. It was a gift for all of the passengers and on opening it, I found a lovely little writing case with a silver pen that had the Concorde name on it and the plane's logo on the tip of it, in blue and white. There were postcards, information on Concorde, writing paper and envelopes. What a nice touch. We were getting spoiled!

Some items from the Concorde flight including a model and a silver pen – the dark squares are chocolates

As I started to think washroom, there were 99 other people on the plane all thinking the same thing. I decided to watch the red and pink sunset over my left shoulder. Finally, the trail to the washroom slowed and I ventured forth. Most people wouldn't even mention the washroom when writing about an airplane trip, but for people with disabilities, especially those travelling alone, the washroom can be a very real obstacle. This washroom was very small and very messy. The constant vibration of the plane and I think the age and physical condition of most of the passengers, led to a sloppy mess that I wanted to get out of quickly. I cannot squat: I'm either up or down. I cleaned the area as much as possible and then did my best to stay away from the mess. My silk-lined slacks fell to the ground. I sat in the mess and then couldn't get up. There was no room. I couldn't bend over and I couldn't spread my arms enough to push up. I had to call for Sam to get my slacks up and me out of there. I'm very glad I wasn't alone and the trip was short.

Everyone was invited to visit the front cabin and have a certificate signed saying we flew supersonic from Toronto to London. Plenty of people went forward and eventually Sam and I did too. The cockpit was a tiny area: all a-dazzle with lights and switches, with three very competent men squeezed in to make it all happen.

The bulk of the trip behind us, the passengers became quite active. The excellent food, good company, the champagne and wine, and cameras flashing as people took turns standing beside the computer readout saying Mach 2; all made the mood quite festive. And then the captain was talking about Bristol. The sunset was behind us in a dark rainbow of colour. Sam saw lights below. It was 10:25 p.m. and we felt it. We were travelling at Mach 1.91 and 55,500 feet up, then Mach 1.88 and someone put on the brakes. We were staying up but we weren't going as fast. There were foam wedges under our feet. I was getting very uncomfortable because I couldn't get up and walk around. I needed to badly.

We were subsonic now, Mach 1 at 40,000 feet, and we could hear a lot better. We could also see city lights. Sam said they looked like rivers of lava. She was right and we were going down. The plane descended just as it ascended: 500 feet every 10 seconds. The no-smoking light was on and jackets and coats were being passed out.

We were given landing cards for customs. Eight miles out, the landing gear came down and the computer lights went out. That huge nose that makes the Concorde look different was coming down for landing. The ride was a bit rough compared to the calm when we were really up there. At 1,000 feet up, we were 2.8 miles from touchdown. It was 10:55 p.m. We held on as the plane stopped with a mighty roar. We had made it!

We had been going 175 mph at touchdown. The flight took four hours and 10 minutes. We had flown Mach 2 for two hours and 20 minutes, and Mach 1 for one hour and 15 minutes; the rest of the time was in takeoff, landing and getting to the supersonic corridors.

Everyone had a good stretch. We collected our carry-on luggage that was still there after 98 people had disembarked. There was a wheelchair waiting for me at the door of this sleek white old beauty. My personal wheelchair was with our luggage at the baggage carousel.

We arrived in London bright and fairly energetic considering we'd been up, way up, for hours. What a ride!

The Concorde-type of plane was retired in 2003, after the crash of Air France Flight 4590, in which all passengers and crew were killed.

We stayed with Don and Cherrie Gilliland. Our gracious hosts were Canadian: Cherrie had CMT and Don was with the military. They lived in a huge third-floor apartment in an old six-storey red brick townhouse on Palace Gate; Kensington Park was at the top of their street. I rented a scooter and had it delivered so that I would have a way to get around on my own steam.

Speaking of the scooter, that townhouse had about a dozen stone steps up the front to the entrance. One day, on our way out, Sam and I had gone down to the entrance before everyone else. I had my raincoat on and it had large loose sleeves. I pushed open the front door with my scooter and the sleeve of my raincoat caught on the tiller that I pushed to accelerate the scooter. The scooter took off towards the steps. Sam quickly saw what was happening and grabbed the back of the scooter seat, while she still had her hand on the front door handle to anchor herself. There she was, splayed out between me - just about ready to plunge down the stone steps to God knows what kind of damage - and an open door. Could she hang on? Seconds later, a son of the family arrived and quickly sized up the situation. He held the door open so that Sam could grab the scooter with both hands. By that time I had figured out what had happened with my scooter and unhooked the tiller from my cuff. Sam grabbed the scooter with both hands, tilted it up, and pulled it back. We just looked at

each other. Tumbling down a dozen stone steps with a metal electric scooter on top of me would have certainly ended my trip or worse. Sam saved my bacon. I still can't help wondering "what if," but we soon recovered and carried on. Later that day, shopping in Harrod's, I caught the tiller in my cuff again in a washroom and the scooter smacked into a wall. I'd had whiplash before from hitting a wall on my scooter and I didn't want to spend the rest of my vacation in a neck brace. The jacket was retired for the duration of the trip.

***

This time around I wanted to see London, as I didn't have a lot to do at the meeting except give an address to the gathering, take in the presentations, talk to everyone and enjoy myself. What a change that was from all the worry and stress of running conventions with my crew in Canada. This time other people had done all the work and they had done it beautifully. I could relax. I can't remember much about the meeting except remarking that so many people in the UK had amputated toes. Instead of surgeons pinning them to stop them from curling or becoming otherwise deformed, they were cut off.

Several wonderful concerts at Royal Albert Hall and the stage production of *Cats* were enjoyed by all of us. Royal Albert Hall was close enough that we could walk/roll to it. Sam and I also visited the Tower of London. Everything went smoothly until our group was led up a flight of steps and we were left behind. We'd seen the Crown Jewels and the ravens, so that would have to do. It was going to make us late for supper but we decided to enjoy the beautiful weather. We took a boat from the Tower of London but were still 2.5 km from home. It was decided that Sam would jog back to the flat while pushing me in my wheelchair that I'd used for that outing because a wheelchair was easier to get into taxis and boats. We jogged past dogs, squirrels, a million pigeons, ducks of all kinds, men, women, children, horses, cabbies, cars and lorries, flowers, fountains, statues, Royal Albert Hall, and churches. We went down underpasses, over bridges, around lakes, across roads until, finally, we were home.

All of that time I had clutched the money in my hand for a phone call to Cherrie to tell her not to hold dinner, but we didn't see a phone box anywhere and no one carried a cell phone back then. We were more than an hour late. Selfish, I know, but that glorious trip home through all those beautiful green spaces in the middle of one the world's oldest and largest cities is a memory that has stayed with me all these years.

It was when we were out in the older area of London, where we were antique hunting, that I felt my age. Usually I got the whistles from the construction workers but now I was on a scooter and the fellows were whistling at Sam as she jogged beside me. Middle age and my CMT had finally caught up with me and no one whistles at a woman who has a disability. It was Sam's turn to feel special.

21

A new voice

By the early 1990s the *CMT Newsletter* was 12 pages long and we had space for a series of articles on some of the lesser discussed, but nevertheless important, side effects of CMT. Heart and lung specialist Dr. Charles Chan wrote an article on breathing and sleep, and we also talked about vocal cord and diaphragm paralysis. We made sure to tell people to never chalk up their symptoms as simply part of their CMT, because what was ailing them could be caused by a number of things and CMT was just one possibility. We did an update on bracing and burning feet and even how to tie shoes to make your feet feel sturdier. We talked about relationships between parents and children, marriage and having children, and sex and disability. We also looked at the Passy-Muir trach speaking valve that lets you speak while on a respirator.

Some of our readers simply couldn't bear to hear about the downside of CMT and I was chastised for always writing about the problems we faced with the disease and how to cope with them. The truth, as far as I could see it, was that our newsletter was about putting the problems that we found trying to deal with our disease out front and having them solved or, at least explained, by specialists or, as it happened many times, by other readers. I did my very best to make the newsletter a mix of ups and downs and I think succeeded, but to some readers any mention of a problem was too much. Denial anyone?

***

In my work for CMT International, I shared start-up experiences with several women, including Betty Bednar who founded About Face as well as Elizabeth (Liz) McHenry in Quebec who founded the Canadian Marfan Association (now the Aortic Disorders Association of Canada) and Maureen Gaetz-Faubert in Alberta. Maureen, like me, saw the need for a Canadian Organization for Rare Diseases. There was the National Organization for Rare Diseases in the US. Why not here? When I found out that Maureen and I had been working on the initiative at the same time, I gave her the logo I'd had designed and she incorporated the charity in 1995. I've learned that it

CORD

CANADIAN ORGANIZATION FOR RARE DISORDERS

doesn't matter who does what or gets credit for what, it's that it gets done. And, that you should pick your battles wisely because some things are better off left in others' hands. Sharing with Betty, Liz, and Maureen gave me comrades-in-arms, so to speak, as we travelled the founding and funding of a new charity together.

***

I had begun painting again in 1991 and thought one of my paintings, a large poinsettia, would make a nice Christmas card. We sold hundreds of dozens of those to raise money and I went on to do several more paintings for Christmas cards and hasty notes.

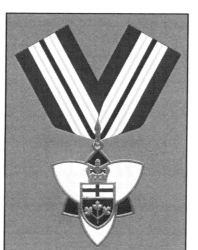

The Order of Ontario insignia

pc21.1

Meanwhile Ron and I were not getting along. He was distant and, I think, worried about what the future held for him. Perhaps the possible severity of CMT had dawned on him. To give him some space, my niece Sam and I headed for Florida, where we visited Busch Gardens and Epcot Center and did some shopping. When we got back, Ron told me I was to receive the Order of Ontario, a high recognition indeed from our province. My sister Kathie had nominated me and 14 people had supported the nomination. I would like to thank them all but you don't often get to know who your supporters are when someone nominates

you for something.

That October, in my wheelchair at a reception at Queen's Park in Toronto, I received the Order of Ontario from The Hon. Henry N. R. Jackman, Lieutenant-Governor. While we were waiting for everyone to assemble, we got to meet other recipients. No one even thought to squat or sit down so they'd be on my level. I can't recall what Pierre Burton said to me, but I'll never forget looking straight up into his white nose hair. I also talked to a lot of belt buckles that afternoon. Lincoln Alexander really impressed me as a likable fellow and I also met the renowned Canadian pianist, Oscar Peterson, and the fabulous Shakespearean actor, William Hutt. I was in good company, indeed. I could also use the initials "O.Ont." after my name if I wished.

I was also invited to a theatrical presentation of Canadian talent put on for people who had the Order of Canada or the Order of Ontario, or both. After the theatre, we were all treated to dinner at Ed's Warehouse, a fairly upscale restaurant – with steps at the entrance. My dear friend, Beryl Potter, a triple amputee with only one arm, and I sat on the sidewalk and watched stage and screen stars, politicians, writers and other recipients of the Orders and their spouses file past us into the restaurant. Very few even looked our way or, if they did, they looked at us then looked down, choosing not to get involved. Finally, Norm Howe, husband of local recipient, Margherita Howe, came rushing over to us, said he was disgusted by our situation, and he would find a way for us to get in. Apparently no one in the awards department had even thought about the fact that the recipients in wheelchairs couldn't climb the restaurant steps. I allowed myself to be carried, wheelchair and all, but Beryl, who was in a large, heavy electric wheelchair and weighed quite a bit herself, went home. I was so disappointed I wrote about it in what has become a regular column on disability issues for the St. Catharines Standard for the last 21 years.

At dinner I met actor Gordon Pinsent and architect Eb Ziedler, who was at that time designing an addition for The Hospital for Sick Children in Toronto. His addition would be built around an atrium so patients could see green growing plants. He was a huge proponent of trees and of nature as a part of the healing process. I had always felt the same way. Remember when I had a plant in my room during my hospital stays? To me a live plant is a constant healing presence and Eb was obviously a kindred spirit.

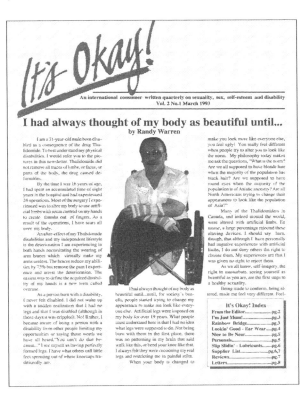

Soon the *CMT Newsletter* expanded to 24 pages and we began planning for the next convention in July 1994. Articles in that newsletter focused on pregnancy and the plantar fascia release that could be done to let down high CMT arches, plus the genetic cause of CMT1B was found. I also began writing a column for the newsletter called *From the Heart* that let me talk about personal issues I thought might be relevant to readers. Ron and I had been married for 12 years and we were coping, but it wasn't easy.

***

Using the experience and resources I'd gleaned from publishing the *CMT Newsletter*, I decided to start a small magazine called *It's Okay!*, on sexuality, sex and disability. There was nothing like it anywhere and the topic was taboo. I mean everyone knew people with disabilities weren't interested in sex, were they? After all, we were too taken up with our conditions and trying to cope, why would we be interested in sex and who would want us even if we were?

The little magazine received very good reviews and even some interest from the press and TV. Suddenly I became an advocate for sex and disability issues. I was part of a panel on a series of shows on sex and disability, produced by TVO, and it was there that I met Dr. Rob Buckman and Dr. John Lamont, who were both very outspoken on the topic. I was also invited to be a guest on the *Sex with Sue* radio show that was tittering on everyone's lips.

A woman who looked as if she could be a grandmother but was the proprietor of an adult sex shop in Toronto that featured all manner of films, books and toys, suggested I make a visit and take what I wanted. I did and it was an education, I'll tell you. I'd never heard of butt plugs, cock rings, or dildos with little fingers on the end and rough nubbins on the sides. I was invited to speak about sex to a gathering of people with disabilities in Kitchener, Ontario, and I took my toys with me. The

press covered the meeting and, wouldn't you know it, my demonstration to the audience of how to put a condom on your lover without the use of your hands made the newspapers. Just in case you're curious, I used a banana, and the condom was purple and tasted like grapes.

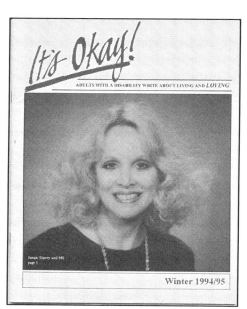

A later, more sophisticated, cover of It's Okay! featuring Susan Tipery and her journey with MS

Light adult erotica drifted my way via the mail and I even had a series of videos on female masturbation and how to reach an epic height, shot by a group of women all masturbating in a circle, sent to me. I considered it all fun stuff, devoted to letting people with disabilities experience what those who didn't have a disability often took for granted.

I also learned a lot from people with disabilities who agreed to put themselves out there and wrote very personal and, may I add, very beautiful and heartfelt articles for the magazine. A man with spina bifida, another who was born with tiny limbs thanks to thalidomide, a woman who had lost her sight, a lesbian who was disabled, to name just a few, all gave of themselves to help others feel not quite so alone. The magazine went to 36 pages, included ads and even a colour on the glossy cover, but after eight issues and two years, I concluded that paid subscriptions and advertising simply weren't enough to keep it going and I didn't have the time to give it what it needed to grow. I gave it away but, like many things that only survive because of that something special only the originator can provide, it eventually died. Now, with the internet, there is everything you can think of out there, but I hope my little effort gave a tiny push to the "Yes, we are disabled, and yes, we have sex, so get used to it" movement.

***

An old friend, Susan Wheeler, nominated me for the Toronto Sun newspaper's Woman on the Move award, which I received at a reception in Toronto that *was* accessible. Several years later I nominated her and she received the award as well. And my mother, my wonderfully supportive mother, received the Canada 125 Medal for her work raising $20,000 back in the '70s to save the gorgeous old Looff carousel that has been on the beach in Port Dalhousie, now a part of St. Catharines, since the 1910s. Her one condition, when she presented it to the City of St. Catharines, was that the cost of a ride remains at five cents, and it still is.

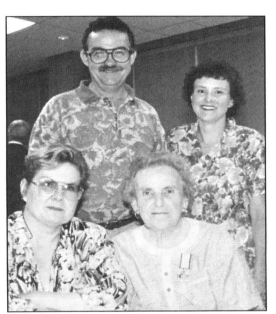

Mom wearing the Canada 125 Medal for saving the carousel at Port Dalhousie. Front: me and Mom. Back: brother Ronald and sister Kathie

One morning, still in bed and not feeling too happy about my world, the back doorbell rang. Probably someone selling something; they usually came to the back door. Ron answered it and came back to me, holding a registered letter in my name. I was to receive the Order of Canada, the highest form of recognition my country can give. Holy cow! Talk about how to wake a girl up! I was thrilled but wasn't supposed to say anything about it until it happened. Are you kidding? How are you supposed to keep something like that from escaping your bubbling-over-with-news-and-excitement lips?

To this day, I'm still not sure who nominated me for the Order of Canada. My guess is Rosalie Floyd from British Columbia, who was the inventor of the Jiffy female urinal. Rosalie was a devoted fan of the *CMT Newsletter* and called me often, first from her home, and then from her room in long-term care before she died. At one time she told me that she was going to give me the patent for her urinal. I declined but I should've taken it, as the Jiffy is the best female urinal I've ever used and still use to this day. To my knowledge the manufacture of these urinals stopped when Rosalie retired, but she was another obviously very talented person with CMT, one of many that I heard from while publishing the newsletter. Whoever nominated me, I thank them.

It is not an easy thing to nominate someone for something like the Order of Canada or the Order of Ontario. I have nominated people for both and it requires months of background work and searching out people to support your nomination. These things are not done easily nor taken lightly.

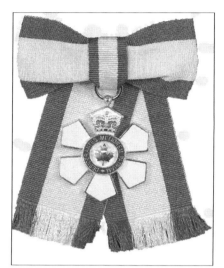

The Order of Canada Member Insignia – pc21.2

Joe West, a long-time local advocate for people with disabilities and a polio survivor, was my nominee for the Order of Canada. He died before the recipients' names were publicized, but I am confident he was on the awards list. I did, however, upon knowing that Joe was in bad shape, give him my copies of the support letters I received to accompany his nomination. I was told he read them in his hospital bed and I hope they warmed his heart.

My nomination for the Order of Ontario

was David Lepofsky, a Toronto advocate for those who are blind, and really, everyone else with a disability. His energy and ability to persuade with incredible logic and unfathomable memory still leaves me in awe. My nomination was successful. David already had the Order of Canada.

***

I mentioned vocal cord paralysis at the beginning of this chapter because it was something I experienced personally, but it was rarely ever thought of as possibly being part of CMT. It all began while on a trip to Florida with a woman I met at a conference. We had rented a red convertible and one day threw abandon to the wind, put down the top, hiked up the volume on the radio and, singing at top of our lungs, drove like a couple of maniacs down Alligator Alley to Miami.

My voice was a bit rough from then on but, after my flight home, I noticed at the airport that I could no longer hear and I really couldn't speak; there simply wasn't anything coming out when I tried. My limousine driver explained to the customs official at the border that I had laryngitis and we whizzed through. I figured this was temporary and, like every other time, a few good swallows and my hearing would pop back and I'd probably regain my voice in a day or two. But it wasn't to be. My hearing came back but my voice didn't. I went to my doctor and then to two or three ear, nose and throat specialists. One told me that I'd never learned to speak correctly and another told me I had a bad case of "Canadian Crud," whatever that was. He was from another country and thought that, due to our climate, the whole Canadian population had postnasal drip or worse.

When I spoke, I sounded as if I had two voices, one overlapping the other, and it wasn't very strong. Trying to live with it, I stopped using my hands-free telephone because projecting my voice simply made it worse. Then one day, after coping like that for almost two years, I just happen to read an article in the Mayo Clinic Health Newsletter on vocal cord paralysis and procedures that could be done to fix it. This could be the answer for me, I thought, but first I had to find a doctor who did throat surgery. After calling around, I managed to find one in Toronto and made an appointment. I was assured, after an examination that threaded an endoscope (a thin tube with a light and camera on the end that allows the doctor to see down your throat or up other orifices) up my nose and down my throat, that I did indeed have a paralyzed left vocal cord. The newsletter talked about silicone injections or the Isshiki laryngoplasty and it was decided the latter would be the best way to go.

I had to be awake throughout the operation so the doctor could hear my voice as he inserted a small battleship-shaped wedge, made from a silicone-like material, from the outside of my neck to the inside, up against the paralyzed vocal cord or fold. The wedge would push the paralyzed cord over next to the working one, so they would touch and I could produce a single sound. The operation wasn't painful or all that difficult and I had my voice back after everything healed. It wasn't as strong as it had been but was no longer double and it took a lot less energy to speak than it had when I was blowing a great deal of hot air just trying to make a sound.

That was July 1993. On June 3, 1996, Ron and I were out dining with Dave and Annette Masser, who were visiting from England. Annette has CMT and is a delightfully funny woman so our visits are always enjoyable, but this time I had such a stabbing pain in my throat that my eyes teared up every time I swallowed. Something was very wrong. After our meal, I asked Ron to take me to the emergency department of our local hospital: it was that bad.

Several doctors took a look but could see nothing. It was suggested that I be examined using an endoscope. The only problem was the endoscope was in Niagara Falls and wouldn't be back to St. Catharines until the next day. I was amazed that there wasn't one for each hospital. I could drive to Niagara Falls if I wanted to be examined there.

Emergency room visits are notoriously tedious and long in our part of the country and I was exhausted. I told Ron I just wanted to go home to bed. However, once in bed there was no way I could sleep so I sat up the entire night trying to watch television, falling asleep from time to time but then waking up again with a start every time I swallowed. Somewhere around 5 in the morning, I fell asleep through sheer exhaustion. When the early morning news awakened me, I felt the need to clear my throat. I can still recall

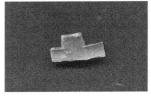

The wedge, about a half inch long

how frightening that was because it wasn't just a simple clearing of the throat and I knew that if I didn't take a big enough breath to get whatever it was down there up, I might never get it up. One large try and I coughed up a mucus covered wedge; the same one that had been placed from the outside beside my vocal cord three years before. The relief was palpable and like magic I no longer had a sore throat. A few hours later, when I thought the doctor might be at the hospital, I called his office. "Didn't I tell you that could happen?" he said, "If it had come out any lower you probably would have choked to death." Thanks for telling me doc, thanks a lot. The good news was I still had a voice ... and do to this day.

170

22

It's all good

In the spring of 1994 a chauffeured limousine took me and my friend Sandra to Ottawa, where I received the Order of Canada from the Right Honourable Ray Hnatyshyn, then Governor General of Canada and representative of Queen Elizabeth II.

The presentations take place at Rideau Hall, the official residence and workplace of every governor general since 1867. This beautifully maintained national historic site, on 79 lush acres, has been made accessible and everything was programmed like clockwork. The ceremony went off without a hitch; Sandra pushed me to the front of the room in my wheelchair, where the medal was clipped onto a little receiver that had been pinned on me prior to the ceremony. I shook the governor general's hand, had a picture taken with him, signed a book and then retreated back into the audience. All of this may sound like

On April 13, 1994, I was invested Member of the Order of Canada by former Governor General Ramon Hnatyshyn — pc22.1

it was very easy, but it took months for me to figure out what to wear and have it made, to get permission and funding to hire a limousine, and to find someone to help me shower, get dressed and to push my wheelchair. My brother offered but I could only take one person with me and I needed a woman. I'm not sure why I opted for the wheelchair, but I think it was because my scooter wouldn't fit in the trunk of the limousine and there wasn't room in the back of car for it and us as well.

The dark brown silk velvet ensemble, I had made, still smelled a bit like smoke from the dressmaker. When I went to put it on before the ceremony, I realized that she had sewn the bottom of the skirt together, perhaps in retaliation for me giving her hell for smoking while she was sewing. Thanks to Sandra, the skirt was opened in record time.

I had always worried about shaking hands with people because my fingers won't uncurl and some people might think is very strange to be offered a hand with closed fingers. Now that I've been around a few more years, I realize that people with important positions, like governor general, get used to all kinds of different handshakes and mine was just one of many.

After the medals ceremony, we were all treated to a fabulous sit-down dinner that topped anything else I have yet to experience. Huge centerpiece flower arrangements on round tables greeted us as we filed in. Beautiful blue gold-rimmed plates, various-sized crystal stemware and so many heavy silver eating utensils just boggled the mind. A lavish, gourmet buffet was set up in the large, high ceiling, chandeliered room where dinner was served. Fortunately, I had a military aide de camp seated next to me and it was his job to make sure that I could manage and that I got everything I wanted. He was a lovely man, very kind and patient, and that dinner was one I'll never forget. Not only was the food excellent but the service, company and entire ambience was perfect. Did I mention we were serenaded by a string quartet throughout the meal?

Having the Order of Canada meant I could use the initials C.M. after my name. When we got back home I was interviewed by the newspaper and received flowers, cards and

a ton of emails congratulating me. Nice.

Experiences like that were a little bit of heaven away from the office and my day after day, night after night, CMT International work getting the newsletter out and answering letters. When I was through attempting to sort out other peoples' CMT in the office for the day, I would close the office door and go into the other part of the house to look after my own CMT. I never got away from it and, you might say, my life was steeped in CMT. But I had asked for it and I had received it, so plentifully that it almost felt like a miracle. Realistically, though, I think it was because we were a first with a newsletter offering information and empathy that had never been out there before, thus the incredible interest we experienced and the rush of people connecting with us.

Most of my trips away mixed CMT and a bit of R&R and involved a conference or at least one meeting. I recall a meeting in Florida where I spoke and answered questions for five hours. After everyone had hugged me goodbye, my travelling companion and I went out to the back of the hotel and, drink in hand (you can get a virgin anything if you ask), watched the sun set over the Gulf of Mexico. The meeting had begun at 10 a.m. and ended around 6:30 p.m. I was exhausted but it was a good exhaustion and I felt like I had done what I was supposed to be doing in this world. And what a strange world it was, away from the newspaper, away from university. Who knew my life would turn out like this? Who, indeed? Certainly not me.

One day, during the summer of 1994, I looked at Ron and said, "Sometimes I feel as though I ducked into my office in 1984 to begin a small journey into my disease and looked up 10 years later only to find myself fat, wrinkled, stiff, tired, feeling old and using a walker to move around the house." His reply was, "I'm 10 years older, too. How do you think I feel?" We had been publishing the *CMT Newsletter* for 10 years and nothing had slowed down, except we weren't going to have another convention. This time, registration was slow and my heart simply wasn't in another meeting with all the incredible detail involved, but that was just a little blip; we carried on.

Because of my experience with vocal cord paralysis, we published explanations and diagrams about vocal cord issues and CMT, as well as the swallowing problems and the frightening episodes of choking some of us experience. Dr. Philip Chance and Dr. James Lupski, both with CMT, wrote about their research on the disease for us and we also put out an issue regarding a person's choice to remain childfree. We also did articles on abortion; male impotence, as CMT can affect the pudendal nerves; and erectile difficulties, which had really upset some of our male subscribers. Some women with

CMT also have difficulty reaching orgasm and some never do. Personally, I have never reached an orgasm during intercourse but have experienced some wonderful orgasms, thanks to my dreams. During times of extreme stress, I find that I wake up having the most delicious orgasm and I'm able to carry on dealing with whatever is plaguing me. Strange, perhaps, but true.

Speaking of the bedroom, I had moved out of the large master bedroom into the smaller spa room that featured a large jetted bathtub. Ron and I weren't getting enough rest trying to adjust to each other's sleep patterns and not getting along most of the time. A good night's sleep and I could concentrate on my work. I was much better off on my own and he seemed happier alone.

There were so many good articles in back issues of the newsletter that I was able to put together separate publications dedicated to specific topics, such as *Toileting, Exercise, What happens when you fall, How to travel when you have CMT, How to talk to your doctor, CMT from birth to age 21*, and *CMT and keeping well*. We also published a list of more than 100 journal articles on CMT and continued putting out a CMT identification card, so the people who were stopped by police and asked to walk a straight line but couldn't, could produce it to back up their claim that they were, indeed, sober and living with a progressive

173

neuromuscular disease that affected their ability to walk and, most of all, to balance. Every year we offered hasty notes, Christmas cards, and a full index of everything that was published in the newsletter that year so people could find what they were looking for and – *ta-da!* – we also introduced colour to the newsletter. It was just one colour, but it made a big difference to how the newsletter looked. I loved messing around with screens behind the text until several of our readers told me they couldn't read text with coloured screens behind it. That limited my newsletter layout fun, but it still looked better than it ever had.

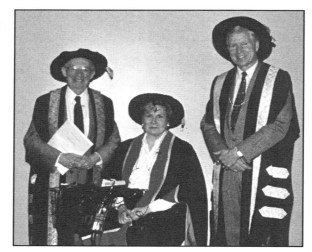

With Robert Welch (left), Chancellor of Brock University and Terrence White, President of Brock at the conferring of my honourary doctorate (LL.D.) in April 1994

Probably because I was also writing a newspaper column about disability issues and people felt that I had empathy toward anyone who is different, I received a phone call one day. The man on the other end told me he was gay, was having a tough time, and thought perhaps he could help people with disabilities as he was pretty handy with tools. There was something about his voice and the fact that he was baring his soul to a complete stranger over the phone made me feel that I wanted to meet this man. I suggested a visit that afternoon and we spent several hours together. He had left a marriage, certainly wasn't afraid to tell anyone that he was gay, and wanted a new start in life working for himself. The outcome was that he began doing renovations for people with disabilities: building beautiful ramps for those who had lost their ability to walk and were using wheelchairs and scooters, renovating bathrooms and kitchens, putting in elevators and building additions, and eventually an entirely accessible home.

When I received an honorary doctorate from Brock University, I had a red gay pride ribbon on my purse as I gave the convocation address to more than 2,000

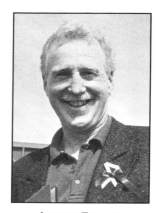

Jasper Zwarts

graduates and their families. Jasper was in the audience looking up at me. Now, many years later, coming out as gay isn't looked

174

upon as it was back then. Today Jasper is retired and a grandfather, and we are still friends. It's out-of-the-blue meetings like this that can change your life and add someone quite wonderful to it.

This was a busy time in my life, busy but fulfilling. Sometimes I felt like I was just being carried along on the current and I didn't really have any say in what happened; I just went with it. In 1994 I also received the YMCA Peace Medal. I wrote this in my journal: *I'm lucky because I'm being used or, in the words of Marjorie Williams, the author of The Velveteen Rabbit: "I'm becoming real, and that's the most satisfying feeling in the world. When I go, there'll be virtually nothing left of me. Everything will have been used up." What a wonderful way to go.*

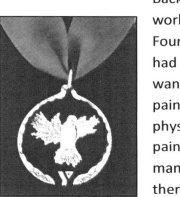

YMCA Peace Medal

***

The next year we did an issue on pain and also featured letters on suicide, as the pain comments came rolling in. Some people understood but some were appalled that we would even touch on the subject of suicide. The indirect push was: God gives us life and only God can take it away. Sorry, but I don't believe that and sometimes the knowledge that we can take our own life can be the only thing we have to hang onto, because it's the only thing we can control. More letters came in and people really

started talking about pain and how it affected their lives. Because many had no means to control their own pain, suicide wasn't far from their thoughts and, to add insult to injury, many doctors still believed that there was no connection between pain and CMT and that the person complaining of pain was simply drug-seeking.

Back in 1987 Dr. Paul Hardy, who worked at the Pain Relief Foundation in Liverpool, England, had gotten in touch with us. He wanted to do some research on pain and CMT. Since many physicians had said there was no pain associated with CMT and many of us knew firsthand that there was, we worked together on a pain questionnaire that included the McGill pain survey and sent it out to 1,750 CMT International members. The results were interesting in that only 205 replies came back, but in those 205 there was everything we see today associated with CMT pain: cramping, throbbing, burning, tingling, sharp and/or shooting pains. Having had CMT pain for more than two decades now, I know that Dr. Hardy's work was groundbreaking. I can't fathom being told that my pain is imaginary. I think by now, with so much anguish over unrelenting burning pain, I'd not feel too kindly toward anyone who still suggested I couldn't possibly be in pain because of my CMT.

Because the newsletter had spread worldwide, I was getting queries from Australia and one man in particular would call me around 3 a.m., my time, on Sunday mornings almost begging me for answers. He was an independent miner at the Coober Pedy opal mines and loved what he was doing but his CMT was making it very difficult for him to shuffle around on his stomach and use his hands in the slender tunnels. I could feel his frustration on the phone and no matter how tired I was, he never failed to make me wish I could sit with him, look straight into his eyes, and tell him there was life after opal mining. I don't know whether my approach would've done any good though because he was talking suicide. There wasn't very much I could do about it from Canada to Australia but I did make a few telephone calls to see if there was any kind of outreach where he worked. There wasn't.

When his calls stopped coming and our request to renew the newsletter went unanswered, I feared the worst. A year or so later, I received a call from his sister telling me he had indeed taken his own life. I held one of the beautiful opal pins he had sent me in my hand and prayed he was in a better place than one of those skinny dark tunnels that had held such a fascination for him.

Speaking of empathy, when I talked to people on the phone who were in pain or read their letters, I often wished that I could experience what they felt because I didn't have pain. Be careful what you wish for. I had been experiencing a burning pain in the back of my right thigh, had gone to a chiropractor, and the pain had disappeared. But now it was back and, wouldn't you know, nothing the chiropractor could do would take it away. My wish had been granted: I now had chronic neuropathic pain and it is still with me to this day.

***

Sometimes people who received the newsletter stopped by our office. One case in point is Ethel and Howard Seagraves from Jennings, Louisiana. We had a lovely visit and before they left they asked me if there was anything they could do. I told them straight up that I would like to visit Louisiana as I really needed to get away during February or March. The darkness and cold Canadian winters really made it difficult for me to keep my spirits up and if I had something to look forward to, I was a different woman.

A year later, in March, I got off an airplane in New Orleans and the humidity hit me like a brick wall. I've never experienced anything like it. Howard and Ethel were wonderful hosts and Howard showed me all over the Jennings area in his big floaty car. When she wasn't working, Ethel accompanied us. My vacation ended with several days in New Orleans, just after

Mardi Gras, when there was still a sad afterglow in the air … a morning-after hangover. The ornate wrought-iron balconies, out-of-the-way alleys with ivy growing on the brick walls, a lacey black table and chair set up for anyone to use, and the jazz, all gave the city a dusting of rotting, rusting melancholy that suited me perfectly. I could live there.

What I saw, what I felt, was too strong to ignore. I wrote this sitting in bed in a gorgeous room in Le Pavillon Hotel:

New Orleans – Two days after Mardi Gras

Big city, very old
Skyscrapers, very cold
Dirty beyond belief

Two days after the big celebration of the end of nothing and the beginning of something

Vagrants, grey all over with one exception: ropes of purple, gold and green beads gleaned from garbage bins knocking belly- buttoned beer guts

An already immaculate postage-stamp park sits ready for tourists in the grey morning cold

A lone mockingbird sits in a bare-bones tree giving us all his wide repertoire

No one lives here but Stonewall Jackson on his black iron horse in a bed of perfectly groomed blue pansies

No littering, loitering, skating, dogs, spitting - no living allowed

Life is on the steps that lead to the Mississippi boardwalk where grey all over, shaven-headed, gold-studded kids offer hair wrapping and body piercing, "Anything you want

pierced lady? Anything?"

Beside their squatting spots are smudges of white on the concrete

I guess you could call it some kind of baby powder, not made for babies

Shutters everywhere, balconies festooned with glittering purple, green and gold leftovers

Bits of strings of beads on lamp posts, hydro wires, mixed with leaves, in flower planters, hiding in garbage and floating in gutters

A small white harlequin face looks up at me as my wheelchair slides down a 200-year-old curb

Hot Cajun gumbo that makes you wonder what you really ate and how to make the burn go away

Hot seems to be my only food sensation in Louisiana

Alligator hot, crawfish hot, crab hot, catfish hot, water chlorine

My gut feels dry and bleached

A prostitute on 5-inch heels, red hair longer than her skirt, talks to an open car window for a few minutes and then speeds off

Bass guitar drones from a dark corner bar warming up stiff cold fingers after a day of purge

Lent is here – it's back to the business of hawking your soul and gaudy T-shirts

Cheap glitter, masks, good music, bad music, soul and Cajun music, fancy curly-cue wrought-iron balconies, old sounds, old smells meld

New Orleans – two days after Mardi Gras

***

Now, back to reality and life at the office. For years I'd had the vision of a resort for people with disabilities that could be built in Niagara Falls. During one of my more productive times, I even put together a board of directors and a local firm of architects drew up a beautiful set of drawings depicting my ideas for a fully accessible resort that I called Trillium Forest. I worked with a doctoral student to pull together a business plan, but when estimates came in at more than $50 million for the infrastructure alone, I saw the light. This wasn't something I could bring to fruition. I had to quit wasting time, but how many nights, before sleep came, would I wander through the pathways connecting the ponds and the glass walkways from pod to pod, thinking how wonderful it would have been to be able to take an accessible vacation in Niagara. I still think it would be a good idea to have a resort for the thousands of people with disabilities who visit Niagara Falls every year. Their vacation should be about having fun not about whether they can find an accessible hotel room or how to rent a wheelchair.

I was asked to be part of a university-level credit course radio series on the contemporary issues of human sexuality.

That little *It's Okay!* magazine had made quite an impression and I remember Peter Gzowski laughing on air, when I was on his CBC morning show, as he said something like, "Who knew I'd get up this morning and be talking Canada-wide about oral sex." I think I countered with something like: "Whatever it takes Peter, whatever it takes."

That year I also became an international honorary member of Beta Sigma Phi. It was ironic really, because when I was in high school I was never one of the girls asked to join sororities. Now I was welcomed with a ceremony and everything that went with it. I think I told you, I'm not a team player: I was curious to find out how sororities operated but as for becoming active, I was, and am still, a self-starter. I'm sure they knew that going in. When I wear my sorority pin, I'm still amazed at the number of women who recognize it and come up to say hello.

If it sounds like awards, medals and honours came my way left, right and centre, you'd be right. It was an amazing time in my life. I mean, Reader's Digest even gave us a free one-page ad. Can you imagine how many people saw that?

23

CMT International just keeps growing

Even When it Rains

The doctor says that laughing helps …
so much better than if you cried.
For crying dampens the spirit but,
laughing's like jogging inside.

by Ann Gasser

The mid- to late '90s saw us steady the course. Donations remained constant and information flooded in, from people with CMT and doctors, like welcome flotsam on waves after each newsletter. I never had to worry about not having enough good copy to fill newsletters and we usually worked two, sometimes three, newsletters ahead. We covered areas such as alternate therapies, aging and CMT, what smoking and cancer drugs do to us, driving with CMT and using hand controls, exercise and how we cope with anxiety and stress, and foot and ankle surgery.

Some of our members were interested in learning about amputation and we heard from several who had their feet amputated. It was comforting to know that they did better without their CMT-affected feet than they had done with them. Losing part of your body is always a traumatic experience but when that part of your body stops you from living a full life, in my opinion, it's better gone. Why hang onto something if it isn't working for you just because you were born with it?

Speaking of surgery, we surveyed our people and found that many of them were absolutely exhausted after surgery. So, we queried some of our consultants. I believe it was Dr. Greg Carter who said it was very important that operating room staff know that people with CMT should be kept warm before, during and after surgery. Simply trying to keep our bodies warm in a cold operating theater actually wore us out and when we came to after the anesthetic, we didn't have the strength to recover the way other people do. There was also some question as to whether the anesthetic succinylcholine was appropriate to use on us. A spinal or regional anesthetic is best, as we tend to recover quickly. We also made sure that our readers knew that their anesthetist should have information on the fact that they have CMT, so they could be looked after properly during surgery.

Working with our local college, I put together a short video that explained Charcot-Marie-Tooth disease in a way that it could be used in hospitals for teaching purposes and also for people with CMT to slip into their VCR player and show their family what CMT was and how it affected them. Quite a few people bought that tape, as they finally had something solid they could take out and say, "See? This is me. This is what we've got in the family!"

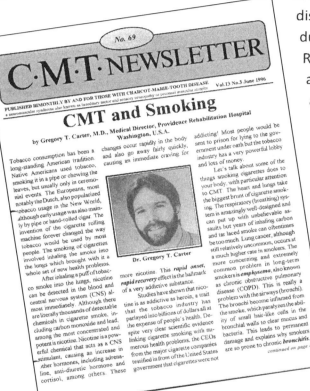

To keep things light, or at least as light as possible, the delightful poetry of Ann Gasser was sprinkled throughout the newsletters. And the newsletter was going out with 32 pages several times a year, always three-hole punched (they called it being drilled at the printers) so people could easily keep it in a binder. Many people kept every issue and I believe our annual cumulative indexes helped them find topics they were looking for.

In the office we had a disaster to contend with: during a memory backup, Ron's computer crashed and took 4,700 names and addresses of our member-donors with CMT and advisors with it. Those names and addresses were why we existed and to lose them was to lose our reason for being. We tried everything and finally ended up sending the hard drive over to computer specialists in Toronto, but in spite of the hefty bill, they couldn't recover anything we could use. We had to rebuild from scratch or almost scratch.

Ron got up very early every morning, for I don't know how long, and went through the files, copying down every address of every person who had ever written us and adding it to the *new* mailing list. I sent the next newsletter out to all of them asking them to please fill in a form for us, so we could rebuild our mailing list and asked them to talk to anyone they knew who had CMT and might be receiving the *CMT Newsletter* to tell them what had happened. I also wrote to newspapers and, because we were online now with a membership group (CMTIlist) and a webpage, I was able to get the message onto that as well. After four months or so, we had more members than we had when we'd lost everything. Our push to get everyone back had found most of our original members and a great many more people living with CMT.

The question of whether to tell or not to tell a person who might become your spouse was discussed in the newsletter at length and the upshot was that it was far better to come clean and deal with the reaction and feelings that ensued than to try to keep something hidden that was eventually bound to come out anyway. We also talked about how and when to tell a child they have CMT. Science had come up with preimplantation genetic diagnosis (PGD), which meant that a couple didn't have to have a child with CMT if they had the money and time to have the testing and procedures done. I know that parents love their children, CMT or not, but I had heard from women who had five or six children, maybe more, many with CMT. What would they have done with the knowledge that, with planning, they might've stopped CMT permanently in their family? Makes one wonder, doesn't it?

Personally, at this point, I had to have cataract surgery on both eyes; I was seeing a halo around everything at night and during the day everything had a lovely golden glow to it that I knew wasn't right, even though it made my surroundings a nicer place to live. I was a bit young for that at 57, the eye surgeon said, but he thought perhaps the drug, theophylline, that I had been on for years for my breathing, had affected my eyes. That drug may have been the only thing there was at the time back in the early '80s when I started taking it, but it made me nauseous every day at 3 p.m. The nausea would go away in about an hour, but what a reminder that I was taking a potent drug for my breathing.

When I found a local pulmonologist, he switched me over to Symbicort and there were no side effects. Since the cataract surgery, my eyesight has been excellent; in fact, I sometimes joke that the lens in my left eye is so good that I see like a hawk. Optic atrophy can be part of the type of CMT I have, 2A2, so my ophthalmologist checks me for that every time I see him, but so far I only have a tiny bit on the edge of the right side. I'm doing fine vision-wise.

As far as walking went, I wasn't doing much and was using a manual wheelchair for restaurants and meetings, an electric scooter outdoors and a walker inside to get me from room to room. One afternoon when I was using my walker and, as usual,

181

rushing to the washroom, I stumbled and fell. On my way down, I managed to push the walker away so I wouldn't hit myself on it, but ended up on my knees with my head in a corner. My kneecaps had floated somewhere else many years before and being on my knees was like torture, but I couldn't fall to the left or the right because I would break my neck. All I could do was shout into the carpet for Ron to come and lift me up and out of the corner.

Considering what the outcome could have been from that fall, we decided there and then that a small scooter was likely advisable for me to use indoors. Why a scooter? Why not an electric wheelchair? I had tried one and found the footrests that stuck out in front were continually in the way of my getting close to the sink, into the fridge, and just about anywhere there was something they could block. I would have to renovate the entire house, take out cupboards under all of the sinks and lower most of the counters. A scooter, on the other hand, saw me sit higher, and it would let me drive up parallel to a sink or counter and turn my seat sideways, so I only had my knees and my little size five feet to contend with. Because I had designed the house with wide doors

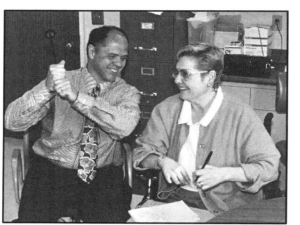

With Dr. Michael Shy at his clinic

(most rooms have two doors so you never have to back up and turn around), wide halls and absolutely no steps, I have been able to use an electric scooter in the house ever since.

I've only had one horrendous fall since then and that was when I slid off a slippery shower seat, my feet under my torso, and pulled every muscle and tendon I owned so badly I spent almost six weeks recovering. The company that makes those commode seats has now put a texture on them so you can't slide off of them as easily but it was too late for me, the damage had been done. I learned my lesson, though, that it's very difficult to fall when you're sitting and your feet are up, so now when I'm sitting in the shower my feet are up on a small shower stool and I feel safe.

I also visited Dr. Michael Shy and his group of doctors at the CMT medical clinic at Wayne State University in Detroit, Michigan. (Dr. Shy is now a professor in the Department of Neurology for the University of Iowa Health Care and practices medicine in the Charcot-Marie-Tooth Clinic there.) They did a lot of poking and prodding and I contributed a little bit to their research but that was about it. I'm glad I went, as I was able to write several interesting articles for the *CMT Newsletter* about the clinic, but nothing really came of it for me. I had looked after just about everything I could by myself and most things they could suggest had already been done.

There are some things that I just can't accept for myself and one of them is rigid bracing for hands at night. Sleep is one of the few things that I cherish. When I'm asleep, I dream and I have no pain in those dreams. Put my hands in bracing and chances are very good I would wake myself up several times a night hitting myself with the braces. I sleep with my hands curled and that's the way it has been most of my life. Unless my wrists need some kind of stabilizing while I sleep, and that's a definite possibility, I choose not to use hand braces.

When I was a little kid, before I was diagnosed with CMT at age 12, at bedtime my legs were strapped into huge padded braces that we're supposed to stretch my Achilles tendons because the doctors thought that was why I had foot drop. Those braces were hot and heavy and smacked into each other every time I tried to roll over. I couldn't move in them and felt violated when I had to wear them. Even though I was too young to recognize that feeling of violation, I knew way deep down in my soul that I didn't like them. I feel the

same way about rigid hand braces.

Dorothy Gosling, a retired nurse, took it upon herself to decipher a great many journal articles for the newsletter, so people that didn't have a medical background could understand what was being written by researchers about CMT.

Someone said I was like a beacon in the fog. I liked that comparison. I found myself included in the *Who's Who of Canadian Women*, and was made a Paul Harris Fellow by Rotary International, thanks to my longtime dentist, Dr. Matthew Taylor. A founding member, The St. Catharines Craft Guild invited me to their 20th anniversary dinner. And, I was one of many… people invited to meet the Queen at a reception in Ottawa, but I had no way to get there, and they weren't offering free limousine service.

One of the little sayings we threw into the newsletter as a space filler was: "Don't let yourself get too hungry, angry, lonely or tired." I think that goes for everyone but it is especially true for people with CMT. There is also a graphic online that shows what looks like a little thermometer: first thing in the morning it gives us four green degrees, we're stoked, we've got a bit of energy; then getting ready to go out takes away one of those degrees, travelling takes away two more and we're more into the orange; two to three hours at an event takes away another degree; and then all we have left is a red one. By the time we get home, we are down to nothing; we are absolutely depleted. That sums it up for many of us.

***

During the CMT International years I was exhausted a great deal of the time but there was work to be done and schedules to keep, with deadlines just like I had at the paper although, thank heaven, they weren't daily deadlines. One example of this devastating fatigue was when I flew down to Plano, Texas, again to visit with my old friend Karen. If you recall, I met Karen at one of our first conventions and she played the piano like an angel. My reason for this visit was that her husband had left her and she was in a bit of a state. We had messaged back and forth via email for months while she watched her marriage dissolve.

Once there, Karen and I packed up her van and headed for Branson, Missouri, driving through Oklahoma. I had no idea how long the trip would be. When we finally got to Branson, I hurt so much and was so exhausted that I couldn't get off the bed. Karen had energy because she was on a BiPAP machine all night that did her breathing for her and she didn't have neuropathic pain. Me? Well, I struggled along breathing on my own and woke up already into the orange. We didn't take in any of the concerts and didn't really do much while we were there because I was so exhausted. I also dreaded the drive back

because I knew I'd be in so much pain, but we both made it in fairly decent shape.

When I went to Plano, Karen always loaned me one of her Jiffy electric wheelchairs and she and I would take to the streets and shops together: two shopping divas in our chairs, side-by-side.

***

By 1998 CMT International was in its 15th year and we were getting email from Zimbabwe, Ukraine, Columbia, Russia, Pakistan, India and Hungary. Our website, CMTINT.org, featured a great deal of the information that we published in the newsletter and many people found us through it. Ron said we were sending our information out to 44 countries and people far away were asking how to start a CMT organization in their country. I was always willing to help and learned quite quickly that not all countries have freedom of information. It wasn't easy for some to find others with CMT and in some countries being disabled meant you were shunned, expected to stay behind closed doors, and were definitely looked upon as a second class citizen, which made it even more difficult to find people with CMT and get information out to them.

Dr. Greg Carter in Washington State had always been interested in CMT and neuropathic pain, but every time we mentioned it we were reminded by various physicians that there couldn't be any pain with CMT. The survey we'd done with Dr. Hardy from Liverpool, years before, told us that indeed people with CMT did experience pain and Dr. Carter wrote a paper on the topic: *Neuropathic pain and Charcot-Marie-Tooth disease,* which was published in the December 1998 issue of the Archives of Physical Medicine Rehabilitation. After that there wasn't much denial regarding CMT pain. We had validation.

***

In 2000 the part-time secretary who had been with us since the house by the lake, left. However, I was very lucky to find Eileen who had begun her newspaper career when she was young, just as I had. She had worked as a writer and proofer for many years and could spell, type and file. Best of all, she had previously worked on a magazine, could contribute ideas and proof everything we both wrote. We got along like gangbusters.

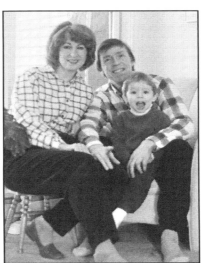

Artist, Doreen Benenati, her husband and son, Claude and Stuart Larochelle

Eileen was what kept me going that year. My brother Ronald had a major stroke, we faced a human rights suit, and my very good friend, artist Doreen Benenati, whom I loved and had corresponded with since our art school days in the '60s, died of leukemia.

The newsletter, at that time, featured articles on meeting people and marriage, and we looked at achievers: people with CMT who had risen to heights in their work life when no one expected much of them at all. We talked about assisted breathing and the BiPAP and CPAP machines that some of us used to help us breathe at night. I reviewed the best book I've ever read on living with pain and chronic disability: *Full Catastrophe Living: Using the Wisdom of Your Body and Mind to Face Stress, Pain, and Illness* by Jon Kabat-Zinn, PhD. Something he wrote has stayed with me for years, and I paraphrase: If your pain has you at the breaking point and you don't think you can take any more, ask yourself if you can bear it another 5 minutes, then 10 and 15? The answer for me is always yes, and somehow the pain doesn't seem as bad after that. I'd diffused the thoughts that I had been in pain too long, that it was unbearable. Now, the pain was just there, one minute at a time; I was living in the moment and not looking back at the painful hours I'd already been through. Kabat-Zinn remains involved with stress reduction and can be found on Google.

We also looked at creative CMT people who made clothing, quilted, wrote poetry, designed websites, made really spiffy canes, and painted up a storm. Then we got serious about raising children with CMT, pointing them in the right direction at home and in the school system.

Hands were another topic: some people experienced numb extremities instead of overly sensitive or paralyzed ones. Numb hands were a real problem. You could cut or burn yourself and you'd never know it and you couldn't feel if you had a grip on anything. CMT hands could be big, small, gnarled, large knuckled, stubby, rough or smooth, and lovely: just like everyone else's hands. Some beautiful hands simply didn't work at all. Others worked but looked like the person had arthritis: large knuckles and little muscle in between. Hands became clawed when the tendons pulled the fingers up, but made it difficult to make a fist and could become a distraction. I experienced this when I spoke during board meetings and found people watching my hands rather than absorbing the gist of my message. I think Ron and I were both feeling our years and that prompted me to write about aging and CMT. The year had been extremely stressful. I put together an ethical living will. We were both feeling old.

24

One ends, one begins

In 2001 Ron and I began to look at retirement. He'd soon be 65 and had been working since he was 17, and I'd be 60. To be totally candid, I was burned out and so was he. We had run CMT International for almost 18 years. It had grown to 2,500 members and we'd heard from more than 10,000 people in 44 countries. I was working two or three newsletters ahead and every day our mail would come with a great thump in the corner of our porch, which we'd made into a receptacle beside the front door.

I was beginning to lose the thrill I'd long felt when I heard that thump: the excitement of hearing from new people, learning about their lives, and how I might be able to help. The curiosity about what would be in today's mail was waning. And, the most difficult thing of all, because it took away my ability to do my job properly, I was beginning to not care.

I couldn't get away from CMT. I felt buried in it. Five days a week I'd work in the office as much as I could. When the pain got too bad, I'd take letters out to the back patio and dictate on the lounge. Weekends I'd work, if need be, and I remember getting up from the couch most evenings after supper to put in a few hours before bed. If I could get up enough energy to swing my feet down onto the floor, the rest of me would soon follow.

When I did have downtime, I had my own CMT to contend with. I had stopped walking altogether and could only stand to transfer to the bed, couch, toilet and driver's or passenger seat in the van. As I mentioned, I used a small scooter in the house now and we had our Chrysler van converted into an Entervan with a lift, so I could drive the scooter onto the lift, push a lever, be lifted up to the van, and drive in;

C·M·T· NEWSLETTER

No. 102

Coping with retirement and CMT

the lift would automatically fold up against the door. I could stand up well enough to hang onto the two front seats and step between them to either be a passenger or drive using my hand controls. With that arrangement I was independent and could go wherever I liked. My life was not only my own CMT but 2,500 other families' CMT as well. It was CMT 24/7 and 100 proof.

We published our 100th *CMT Newsletter* in August of 2001 and I began hearing from members who had been with us for 10, sometimes 15 years. In December 2001 my front page article was on coping with retirement and I'm sure it got some of our readers thinking the same thing we were thinking: it was time to say goodbye.

But how do you retire a charity that individuals donate to at different times of the year for a newsletter that goes out to them on a regular basis? We knew it wouldn't be easy and it wasn't. We looked for someone to take the newsletter over because we knew the written information was what people would miss the most.

The charity had to be dissolved according to

our Canadian federal government laws. Ron worked tirelessly on the final audit for our auditors, who were given six months to get our final papers filed with the government before we closed up shop. Because we were a registered charity, any funds we had left had to go to a Canadian charity. They went to Dr. Mark Tarnopolsky at McMaster Medical Centre in Hamilton, Ontario. He was, at the time, one of the leading authorities on CMT in Canada.

The newsletter was taken over but, unfortunately, it didn't last. Some of our readers were very disappointed and some who had made a recent donation to continue receiving the newsletter were upset, but there was no other way. I felt terrible letting some of our readers down; I'd had such personal relationships with so many, for so long, and they felt like family.

The one thing we did do was put the best information from all of the 103 *CMT Newsletters* on a website called CMTNEWS.com, where it stayed for many years. Now this information is on my personal website at lindacrabtree.com. It's an archive. The data is dated, yes, and some of the links have been lost, but people still read it so I'm leaving it there. So much has happened since 2002 in the field of CMT research and awareness that it makes my head spin, but some people just need to begin with the basics and a lot of what is there is just that.

During the final weeks of CMT International, with the last *CMT Newsletter* under our belt, I spent hours every day going through 20 file drawers of letters, cards and journal articles, remembering the terrific people who had written and called and been such a huge part of my life for the last 18 years. I lost 10 pounds doing it. A huge white van pulled up to our front door and Ron carted out box after box of documents, letters and emails to be shredded right at the curb where we could see it actually being done. Ron told me that 10,200 people had contacted us in those 18 years.

Our timing was right. Everything was switching from snail mail to email and there was nothing really tangible anymore. If we were going to do more newsletters they would likely have to be done online and at that time it was very difficult to bring in any money for anything online. As well, we had already put so much on the CMT website that I felt we'd brought CMT International to a fair and decent close.

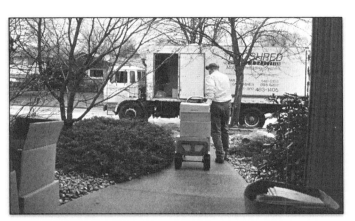

Thousands of letters and hundreds of files being shredded at curbside - Feb. 2002

Cards, letter and phone calls from members telling me how much they appreciated our work over the years poured in and softened the realization that it was over. Dave Fielden of Silvis, Illinois, wrote: "You have helped in ways you may never know." I liked that. Others wrote to say they had saved all of their newsletters and that information had saved them many doctors' visits. Knowing what were common CMT symptoms and what weren't had really helped. Knowing what drugs not to take had also helped. The cards and letters spoke of gratitude and love. They made me feel as if many of the people that inspired what I'd done through the last 18 years felt the same way about me as I did about them. Now there were no more newsletters to get out, no more phone calls asking for help: no more.

But that's not actually accurate. I've remained online since, to talk to anyone who has CMT and through several forums, including one I run. I talk to people with CMT all the time but only on my own time, when I have the energy.

In 2002 I received the Golden Jubilee Medal, marking Queen Elizabeth's sixty years on the throne. It seems everyone with the Order of Canada got one.

***

As always, after a long successful run at something had finished, I was really down. I'd learned to recognize the symptoms and knew if I wanted to be reasonably happy again I had to find something to do that excited me.

I'd always wanted to sculpt so I tried my hand at that but found that the wet clay made my hands ache and I wasn't really very good at it. I joined the local aquarium club as I had always had an interest in tropical fish and got quite involved but it eventually became too much for me and I gave my tanks away. I bought a sewing machine: one of those tricky ones for quilting that will do your initials and all kinds of fancy stitching. Trying to hold fabric was very difficult but I managed to make a pair of long embroidered spaghetti bibs before I called it quits. I loved the machine but didn't like the frustration I experienced trying to handle fabric with no use of my thumbs. I call them my $400 spaghetti bibs.

I also signed up for a course in writing erotica. It's not quite as sleazy as pornography; it lets your imagination do all the dirty work. The day Ron and I went over to the local shopping plaza, to pick up some men's magazines that feature some of the work freelancers can do writing erotica, convinced me that I'd wasted my money on the course. Erotica was easy to write but to what end? To get some guy off? I really didn't want to be part of it and considered it then, and still considerate it, a waste of my time. But, when you look at the success of erotic fantasy novels and the huge demand for them, I sometimes wonder if I quit too soon. I was at a crossroads in my life and I could either turn towards writing erotica or toward people with disabilities. I took the only direction my conscience could live with, and I know I was right, but I'm still curious as to what may have happened if I'd gone the other way.

Years before, one idea I developed while running CMT International was a website called AccessibleNiagara.com to help people who are disabled, wanting to come to Niagara as tourists, have a barrier-free holiday. My thinking has always been that if you see a need and can fill it, it's your responsibility to do just that.

After developing the website, I found that my work with CMT International and trying to do AccessibleNiagara.com was too much, so I gave it away to the Niagara Centre for

Independent Living. They, in turn, obtained a government grant to update it and keep it going, but when the grant money ran out the site was no longer updated.

Later, I was looking for something to do. By chance, I took a look at the website and saw that it was sorely out of date and the domain name was in limbo. Without a second thought, I bought the domain back and it was like bringing home a child I thought I'd lost. I was excited about life again and couldn't wait to get it updated, new venues audited and added, and improvements made.

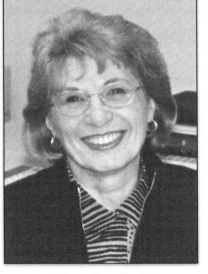

Eileen Zarafonitis

As usual, Ron was the voice of reason. I needed money to go running around auditing places and I shouldn't be doing it on my own. The March of Dimes agreed to be the lead applicant on an Ontario Trillium Foundation grant to allow me to set up the site, as it should be, and eventually I had enough money to afford to put gas in the van to go to Niagara Falls to do top-to-bottom audits of hotels and to journey out in the boonies of Niagara to wineries tucked into hillsides and hidden behind acres of rolling vineyards.

Eileen, who had worked with me so well for several years before CMT International

closed down, was also good to go with me. We had a lot in common and about 100 years of writing, proofing, editing and publishing between us. We could do this.

I had always been interested in the concept of universal design and took an online course on it. I also live in a world where barriers are commonplace. You don't have to tell me how bad things can be. I experience it every time I go out.

An auditing checklist was made up and away we went. Soon the site grew to include 40 hotels, 20 wineries (there are now more than 80 in Niagara), all of the accessible venues run by the Niagara Parks Commission in Niagara Falls plus some others, and all kinds of information a tourist with mobility impairment would need when travelling to Niagara.

In 2003 we put out 20,000 copies of a 32-page printed directory we called *Accessible Niagara: Opening Niagara to people with disabilities*. I managed to raise $20,000 from sponsors to do that. It was always free to the traveler. Again, in 2005, we put out 50,000 copies of a 40-page one. In 2011 we raised $12,000 and went to a huge foldout map format featuring more than 170 accessible venues. We had 40,000 of those printed and when the printer delivered them, they were so dark you couldn't make out the photographs. I refused to accept the delivery, even though they were piled up at our front door, so they were printed yet again. I had put these together, Eileen proofed them, and we went over and over them until they were good to go.

Finding the money for printing was almost more difficult than doing the actual work on the mock-up. Asking people who aren't disabled to fund something for people who are, often gets you a lot of blank stares. They have to compute why this is needed. They don't think twice about walking into a hotel or booking a room, parking, or if they can get on a bus or see an attraction. They don't have to. We do.

Distributing the guides was something we hadn't thought would be difficult, but I found out it would cost a great deal of money to get them to where they should

be, if we left it up to the local distribution company. So, Eileen and I began what we eventually called our *Thelma & Louise* runs.

I'd first make up a list of the hotels in geographic sequence and how many guides would go to each. With that list and boxes

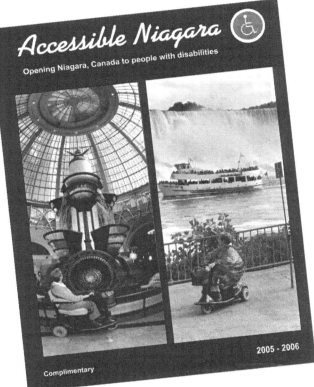

of guides in the back of the van, we'd head out, me using hand controls at the wheel and Eileen with her runners on, ready to hit the pavement as soon as I pulled up under the lobby entrance of a hotel. I'd keep the motor running and she'd be into the hotel with the bundles in her arms and back in the van in under three minutes. Once, she opened the door of another van. I can only imagine what that driver thought was about to happen.

We had a good laugh every time we did something nutty. We were also exhausted by the time we'd put in four hours and delivered guides to 10 or 15 hotels. We did that twice but exhaustion didn't stop us. We are tough old girls. We did the same thing with a list of wineries: first, we delivered west of St. Catharines into Jordan and Vineland, and then east into Niagara-on-the-Lake, where most of them are located.

When the magazine-sized guides became too expensive to print, we went to the foldout guide like a map that I've mentioned. Again, we did our *Thelma & Louise* runs.

When the maps ran out several years later and a new company took over the boat trip into the base of the Horseshoe Falls, making our guide truly out of date, it was suggested that the AccessibleNiagara.com website be updated to make it accessible to people who have vision impairment and easier to navigate for everyone. That sounded like an excellent plan but a great deal of work and I didn't have a clue where to begin. I tucked it away in my mind vowing to tackle it in the future.

***

Personally, things were not going well between Ron and me. When the newsletter ended, he told me that he wanted to leave. I was trying to find myself after 18 years of knowing exactly what I would do each day

and for how many hours, and I think he'd just had enough of everything including the house, yard work and looking after the dog plus cooking. As he said, "I've just realized that I'm going to have to look after you for The. Rest. Of. My. Life." For months that stretched into years, I felt an aura of resentment around everything I did, everything I asked him to help me with, and if I wanted to do something for fun I felt terrible asking him for help because it was just one … more … thing. And there was no sex and no intimacy; consequently, I began to feel terribly lonely. Ron may not have moved out physically but emotionally he had left the marriage. Trying to talk it out usually ended up with him disappearing into another room and me sitting at my computer, neither of us talking.

Sex can be a delicate subject even between two people who love each other. For me, sex is something that gave me great pleasure and it was something I could actually do. You don't have to have legs to have sex. I was only 60 and had hoped that I would be sexually active until I was an old lady but when one half of the partnership is not willing, things don't go very far. A friend of mine drove me over to Dr. John Lamont in Hamilton, who specializes in sex counselling, and I spoke to him about my problem. He told me that without Ron's cooperation, there was very little I could do about it. (Why did I always call it sex and not making love? Perhaps because it never felt that way but I still glowed after each rare encounter.) Ron, like many men, said that he had peaked in his teens and just wasn't interested.

To say I was twisting at the end of my rope pretty well describes how I felt. I mourned the loss of intimacy and possibly the end of our marriage. After such a long run and working so well together and, I thought, enjoying it, why this reaction? Then I had second thoughts. Perhaps he didn't like working for CMT International. I had never been a boss per se; I thought we were working as partners. Maybe he saw it differently. I didn't know where we were going. All the things I wanted for our retirement weren't what he wanted. I thought perhaps we'd be able to travel a little, that we would become closer and enjoy more things together and that because we had more time and less stress with no deadlines, there would be more intimacy. I was wrong.

25

Confronting the elephants

Ron didn't leave. He said he had no place to go. I thought to myself that if he really wanted to go, he would find another place to live. So, we carried on, not speaking much, not touching except for the help I needed, living in a house that seemed to have clouds of resentment and sadness drifting from room to room, as we went about our daily chores.

Ron had told me that he would never lie to me. I believed him. Sometimes the air was so thick with tension that I'd start an argument just for some relief. We'd talk, I'd end up shaken and in tears and he'd end up in his bedroom with the door closed. One day when we were standing at the kitchen sink, I asked him if he loved me. He said he didn't. I asked him why he was still here and he said, "Have you ever heard of loyalty?" I just about sank to the floor. I was married to someone who openly admitted he didn't love me but was going to stay with me out of loyalty. Thank you very much, but that isn't what I had in mind for the rest of my life.

When we were out in public, everything seemed fine. When we were with family, everything seemed fine, except Ron was very rarely out with me or with my family. Our imploding relationship was like the elephant in the room. We knew it was there but carried on in spite of it because it hurt too much to discuss.

***

Sometimes things happen that make you realize how much you really do care for someone and I think Ron gained a new appreciation for me, as I did for him, in December 2005. This is what I wrote in my journal on Wednesday, December 14th of that year:

Hearing Ron in the kitchen, I wake up slowly, lifting my head to see what time it is on the VCR at the end of my bed. It glows 8:55. Head back down, thinking how warm the bed is, I take mental stock of the day ahead. I have to get ready for a meeting of the Mayor's Accessibility Advisory Committee scheduled for 12:30 and make up my mind about going to Buffalo the next day for a meeting with architectural students at the State University of New York at Buffalo who are designing Heartland Forest, an accessible resort in Niagara Falls. The weatherman is predicting a major snowstorm and anyone living in southern Ontario knows that Buffalo, New York, always gets the brunt of it all. I'd have had a meeting the day before as well and I can tell if my body is tired when I try to move. If it hurts to stretch then I'm not in good shape. Every meeting takes its toll and every day I work outside of the house adds onto the next day and by the end of the week, I'm totally exhausted. It takes two days to get over one meeting. Three meetings in a row, like this week, and it takes a full week to recover. The last thing I needed was to get stranded in Buffalo and end up trying to cope by myself in a strange hotel room.

After hauling my legs over the side of the bed with my arms and putting on my slippers so I can stand, I swiveled my body around and sat on my electric scooter, pushed in the key to get moving, flipped on the lights over the bookcase greenhouse full of violets besides my bed and headed out into the living room, down the hall and into the master bath. I had to pee.

While sitting there, Ron came into the doorway and said, "When you're finished, there is something I want you to see." Now Ron isn't that kind of man. He isn't secretive, or at least I don't think he is, and we talk openly about many things ... and he isn't into suspense. Right now, he has my full attention ... something's up.

"Show me, now," I said, "I may be awhile."

He left and came back in five seconds holding a small, clear plastic bottle. "That's my pee." It was as red as pomegranate juice.

"God, how long has it been like that?" I gasped.

"I've been noticing it getting darker for three weeks but it has only been like this for two days."

"You've got to do something about it, now."

"I'll call the doctor's office this morning," He said looking down at the ominous dark liquid that had us both frightened.

It was okay to be peeved at our relationship but when it came right down to it, and things got serious, we were both on the same page. We cared and we knew it.

I'd wondered why the water in the toilet bowl have been purple for the last little while and meant to ask him as he was the designated toilet bowl tender but figured maybe he was using a new cleanser. Usually, it's a turquoise blue. We are "If it's brown, flush it down, If it's yellow, let it mellow" people and sometimes I see what's in the bowl before I sit. Sounds strange, I know, but being artistically inclined the colour is always of interest to me. Turquoise bowl cleaner and yellow urine makes the water green but turquoise bowl cleaner and red blood make purple.

First, he called the provincial medical hotline. The nurse on the other end told Ron that they considered blood in the urine a medical emergency and he should go to the emergency department of his local hospital immediately; it was life-threatening. This really frightened us but we calmed down enough to think that the government has to cover its tail against lawsuits and they were going to tell anyone with anything that seemed remotely serious to go to emergency. We knew that we'd likely wait six to eight hours to see a doctor and the thought of the hospital frightened Ron just as much or more than the thought of going to the doctor.

I asked him why he waited so long. Why he was so afraid to see a doctor. We've been together 28 years and he's been to the doctor three times: twice for a flu shot and once to have his blood pressure and cholesterol checked.

"When I was a kid living on the farm, the only time we saw the doctor was when there was something really seriously wrong or someone died. I think of doctors and death together," he said. "I have an irrational fear of doctors. I know that and I admit it."

I just prayed to God that his irrational fear wasn't going to kill him.

Ron called Dr. Chan, our general practitioner's office, and told them what the nurse on the government hotline had said. They agreed and when they asked some more questions including how long his urine had been like that, the secretary said she'd ask the doctor what he thought and call back. Ron told me she had exclaimed, "Three weeks!" and had asked, "Why did you wait so long?"

"I thought it would go away," he answered. "I had it for a short time last year and before I decided to call you, it had gone way. I thought it would likely go away again."

But it hadn't gone away; in fact, it was getting worse.

While waiting for the doctor to call back, we took stock of Ron's nightwear just in case he really did have to go to the hospital. One pair of pretty worn PJs, house slippers in decent shape and a camel-coloured, polar fleece housecoat I bought years ago and had only worn once. It fit him because the cuffs on the sleeves could be turned down to cover his long arms and I always buy housecoats for comfort rather than looks. I told him what he needed to take with him as he'd never stayed in hospital before. As it turned out the doctors said something like, "If it's been three weeks, what's two more days." Ron wasn't sent to the hospital, an appointment was made with the doctor for

Friday at 2:40 p.m. In the meantime, we searched the internet for blood in urine. There were a lot of reasons for it and all suggested that a doctor be seen as soon as possible.

That Friday morning Ron left a small bottle of urine on top of my jewel box in the bathroom. I noticed that as it sat and settled, there was a definite very clear, light top section and then a cloudy reddish white bottom section. There was obviously a lot of sediment in it and something was really not right.

That evening, we made a list of things Ron does that I have never learned to do and where things are that he takes care of. Things like how to turn the digital thermostat to the new furnace down at night, how to work the new washing machine, where the house account cheque book is, and how to sort the garbage into boxes with only paper, stuff that is compost worthy and other stuff, and what days it all goes out.

Ron has been doing the housework since we retired in 2002 but for many years, while we ran the charity, we had a couple of women come in every two weeks to do whatever needed doing. When retired, Ron decided he no longer wanted strangers vacuuming our carpets, washing our floors and dusting things, and that he would do whatever had to be done around the house. Not being able to walk or even stand steadily, I couldn't do the housework. And, not being familiar with some of our new appliances, I had to learn in case he ended up in hospital … or worse.

Many years before, we had made our wills and have kept them current. At the same time, we appointed each other power of attorney for our finances and health needs. My brother Ronald had a major stroke in 2000 and this really brought home to everyone in our family the need for a will and power of attorney. He didn't have either. He also came out of the stroke unable to speak, read or write. It was very important that his wishes be known regarding his money and his health needs. After 34 years on the job, I had to retire him from General Motors. He has a way of letting us know what he wants but we have to have it in writing to get money from the bank for him, to sign for medical procedures on his behalf and anything else that has a legal slant to it. When he dies, we'll have to take care of his estate and his will tells us what his wishes are.

Ron and I had taken care of just about everything although it wasn't until just last month that he took me to his bank to have me made a cosigner on his bank accounts and I took him to mine to have his name included on my accounts. We've always kept our money separate, having a house account we put money into every month *that takes care of the house, car, insurance and everything else we use jointly. We both take care of our own personal credit cards and cheques and he never carries a balance on anything. That's just the way it is. I, on the other hand, splurge once in a while on a piece of jewelry or something I love and pay it off as quickly as possible and usually end up every year totally out of any kind of debt. We know that if something happened to me, Ron couldn't access my money easily unless he was a cosigner on my bank account … unless it was a joint account … and the same goes for me. So, we took care of that. We trust each other implicitly and I know he'll never go near my account and I wouldn't dream of touching his, so it wasn't too hard to decide to do this for each other.*

That night, we held each other as we watched Law and Order together … the dog lodged between us. I wanted to be close but we've found it just too uncomfortable in our years to get all wound up in each other. Holding hands, kissing, touching, being together almost 24/7 is what holds us together as well as mutual respect, love and kindness towards each other. We know we are partners in this marriage. We need each other for many reasons and we have come to realize this when we work through problems and answered the Ann Landers question, "Are you better off with him or without him?" We are better off, by far, with each other.

Friday came and Ron's urine was even darker and brighter red. I called the doctor's office and they told him to come in early. The office usually wasn't open on Friday after lunch but because the doctor was going away for two weeks, they were seeing patients that afternoon. Later that morning I called my insurance company to see if Ron was covered for hospital coverage and what kind of room he could have should the doctor order him to the hospital. He was covered for private insurance which also covered him for some drugs that the provincial seniors' drug benefit didn't and they might even take up the slack of what he had to pay before the government program kicked in.

The hour rolled around for Ron to go to the doctor. I had offered to go with him. I'd do anything for him, but he said no, he wanted to do it himself. He had a urine sample in one of my sterile bottles with him and Information from the internet on both of the prostate supplements he was taking. That morning we had logged on to see if either one of those could possibly be turning his urine red.

He kissed me goodbye and by doing this he knew I was very concerned and I knew he was concerned. He always kissed me good morning, after supper when we snoozed through the news from 6 to 7 and then again before I left his bed around 11 to go to my own, but never goodbye. Five kisses each time ... sometimes just little pecks if he was upset with me or something around the house was bothering him and sometimes four short kisses and one long warm lovely one followed by the backs of his fingers brushing over my cheek. I love those long, warm kisses. His lips are warm on mine and his nearness is so perfect. We read how we are by those kisses. They're like a barometer of our relationship. If I search him out for a hug or kisses, I need comforting. I think he usually looks for me because it is part of his routine. If there is trouble our kisses are pecks or don't happen at all. But in times of real trouble, like this time, we search each other out and our kisses are comforting and a confirmation of our mutual love.

Off Ron went to his appointment with my cell phone tucked in his jacket pocket. He had promised to call to tell me what the doctor said. Several other calls came and then Ron's. He was to go directly to the lab and pick up other tests while taking a sample in from home. He also said the doctor told him it could be bladder cancer.

To keep from going nuts until Ron got home, I searched bladder cancer on the internet. Everything said the main signs where blood in the urine and that there was usually no pain. I couldn't help looking for a mortality rate. Could Ron die from this? Would I lose my husband to something neither of us had ever thought of? Bladder cancer ... only 6,000 cases a year diagnosed in all of Great

Britain. I couldn't find any stats for Canada but it wasn't one of the top-of-the-list cancers. Usual causes: exposure to aniline dyes, smoking and drinking. Ron had done neither to any excess but he did say he had worked beside people when he was in his 20s and 30s who had a cigarette continually burning in an ashtray on their desk. The air was blue in most of the offices where he'd worked. Secondhand smoke is just as bad as firsthand and he was exposed for many years. And, he had smoked a pipe for about 20 years but only three times a week and never inhaled. Could that have caused cancer?

When I heard the van in the carport and the back door close, I shouted, "I'm in here." He came into the office and sat down ... a surefire sign that something was up. He told me about the tests he had to do: the next morning an ultrasound, no food after midnight and four glasses of water before the test. And another lab test where he has to drink a lot, empty his bladder and then pee into alcohol in a sterile bottle and take that into the lab. The doctor had also told him about one of his patients who had waited to come in, and when he did, there wasn't much they could do for him. He had advanced bladder cancer and was dead in three weeks.

Hearing that, I felt I'd been punched in the chest. My eyes began to tear up and I knew that this was the real thing. It was serious

200

as hell. Ron said he wasn't going to tell me what the doctor had said but we usually share everything from the fact that frozen dog poop is easier to pick up on his part to my enjoying zoning out while taking Chi Kung lessons at a local martial arts studio. Just about everything is fodder for dinner conversation. These constant exchanges of minute detail are the glue that holds us together. If we are talking and kissing, we are okay. If we are not, we aren't.

That night we shared a bowl of clam chowder, a plate of spaghetti and meatballs and a dish of Tartufo at a local Italian restaurant and then headed home with Venus sparkling above in a clear, cold sky. We didn't talk much. There was an elephant riding in the van with us, we just didn't know its name yet.

I had said to Ron while we were eating our dessert, "I guess if you've ever wanted to really do something, you'd better think about doing it soon."

His reply was, "Why, what difference would make ... to me or to anyone else?"

"You'll have had the experience," I said.

"I don't think of it that way," he said. "It doesn't make any difference to me what I do. There's nothing I want to do." And then a few minutes later, he said, "I was going to have my eyes looked at to see if I am a candidate for laser surgery to improve my vision in the new year but I guess that will have to wait." So, there was something he planned to do. It just wasn't something flamboyant like a cruise around the world or soaring in a hot air balloon ... the things most people think of when the unknown becomes a little more concrete. Ron had been born with nystagmus, his eyes constantly move, and he isn't able to focus on things. His world isn't sharp. Being a stickler for precision, a bookkeeper, and office manager all his life and a very neat buttoned-down type of fellow, I'm thinking having his world slightly out of focus all the time must sometimes drive him nuts. He was mustering up the courage to see if he could be helped.

The next morning, Ron was up, dressed and drinking water by 9 a.m. He had slept well and had actually stayed in bed until 8:30. He knew he had to fast for the test and couldn't eat, so why get up? Off he went for the ultrasound with a very full bladder and he was home by noon having gotten groceries for the evening meal, a video for evening viewing and wine for Christmas.

While washing my breakfast dishes, I noticed that every time my mind slipped into that neutral zone of contemplation where you aren't really thinking of anything, but your mind comes up with all kinds of things, usually solutions to problems plaguing you, I thought about Ron and his *dying. The unbearable pain of leaving him in a hospital bed or a gurney somewhere and going home without him, knowing I would never see him again, feel those warm lips, hear his voice or feel his hand in mine, would almost send me to the floor. My eyes would tear up and I'd have to actually force myself to think about something else … anything else. I was grieving and Ron had only had two tests. Cut it out, the worst is not in the cards yet and he's only 68, fit in every way, except whatever is wrong. I would likely have my man with me for many years to come. It was the not knowing that was the worst and when the doctor went on vacation for two weeks over Christmas and New Year's, we had 20 long days to wait. Christmas, New Year's Eve, our 25th wedding anniversary … all spent in suspended anxiety trying to go about our lives as usual, both being very kind to each other, realizing how precious our time together really is and how much we mean to each other. It was the worst Christmas we'd ever had.*

If all of this turns out to be just a scare and can be cured easily, we will have learned a huge lesson: not to take each other for granted, not to waste time wishing for something else and that love, shared, is so precious.

***

We somehow got through Christmas and New Year's and the ultrasound showed there was definitely something in Ron's bladder, probably polyps. With a positive ultrasound, he was sent to a urologist and the date was set for surgery.

Ron was told that he wouldn't be able to drive himself home from the hospital after surgery and it made sense that I take him, even though I was on my scooter and couldn't use the hospital bathroom.

On Ron's surgery day we arrived at the hospital on time. Ron was given a gown and told to undress, assigned a bed and told he'd be taken to the operating theatre when his turn came up. We talked and it was evident that he was very nervous. So was I, but I'd been through medical procedures many times and, at 68, this was his first.

When the attendants came to take him to the operating room, I vowed that I was going to stay exactly where I was so that when he came back I would be exactly where he'd left me. I had packed a lunch and a bottle of water and brought a book. I was prepared to be told to wait in the waiting room with everyone else but I propped my book up on the windowsill, turned off the scooter key, and just sat. I think I gave off some kind of "don't come near me" vibe because no one approached me, no one told me to move and I was adamant that I wasn't going to if they had; so I didn't.

I also didn't know that Ron had been in a

queue of patients being operated on, so even though he had left the room where I was, he was still waiting. I think it was a couple of hours later the man next to us came back in a groggy state, but no Ron. Finally I looked up and he was being rolled in beside me. He lifted his head and looked at me as if I was the best thing he'd ever seen. I couldn't wipe the smile off my face. I can't remember the words we said but we were both so relieved that it was over, he was alive, and we were together.

When the anesthetic had worn off enough for him to get up and get dressed, we went out to the parking lot and I got behind the wheel to drive us home. Everything went well until we were just past Brock University going down a long hill when he said, "I'm going to faint." Not more than five seconds later he was out cold hanging towards the door by his seat belt. I flipped on my emergency flashers, got down the hill as quickly as possible, and pulled off into a residential driveway. It took about ten seconds for me to put together what I would do if he didn't come to. It would take me forever to get out of the car on my scooter and every house in that residential area had steps up the front. I could sit in the driveway and blast the horn hoping someone would see me and come out to help, or I could head as quickly as possible

for the local general hospital, about two miles away. Fortunately he came to, asked me what had happened, said he was okay but had to pee, and we were on our way home again.

***

"You're cured!" were the words he heard from the surgeon the next time he saw him. There were quite a few cancerous polyps and all of them were taken out during surgery. The next thing Ron had to do was to go to the hospital and have a drug inserted into his bladder that had been developed for tuberculosis but had been found to work on stopping the reoccurrence of cancerous polyps. He was to lie on a bed while the drug was inserted into his bladder via his penis and every 15 minutes turn like a pig on a spit to coat his bladder with this drug. He twirled on the spit once a week for six weeks. After that he went for a bladder scope monthly, then bimonthly, then every six months, every year and every two years until the eighth year. He is still cancer free.

We now knew the name of that elephant and it had been banished, but we knew that there was yet another one lurking underneath the layer of relief from those horribly tense months. It couldn't be excised through surgery but, somehow, we had to deal with it.

26

Joan

When my father died in 1973, the entire family was shaken. We were all so young and he was only 57. After Dad's death there was a long period where no one in the family died and you get to thinking that you're almost invincible. But I don't think you ever get used to losing people no matter who or when and, as the years go by, it is inevitable that people you know and people you love are going to die.

My journal for May 28, 2006:

My sister's 52nd birthday, I'm 64.

I sit beside my cousin, Joan, and know she is dying. She knows she is dying, we all know.

When asked if she's comfortable, she says she is, her voice sort of a gravelly whisper …

soft … almost not there. She's sitting up in the hospital bed … almost up straight. Her head keeps flopping forward, she's barely strong enough to hold it up.

I've known Joan ever since I can remember. She is my cousin, my mother's sister's daughter. She's 73 and she's dying of heart failure.

When I was a kid, Joan and her mother, Madeline, and father, John, would be on our doorstep every Sunday night around 8 o'clock. My father liked to watch the Ed Sullivan Show. It was one of the few pleasures for a hard-working GM office employee: golf Sunday from 10 to 2, take the wife and kids for a drive or somewhere in the afternoon, a nice dinner followed by a snooze on the couch and then TV until 10 or so. Not a bad life really, but knowing that your wife's relatives would be showing up as regular as clockwork every

Sunday night must've been hard to swallow.

John, Joan's dad, sold life insurance and he collected every week. It was something like $2.11. It's hard to imagine nowadays but he and Madeline went out after dinner every Sunday night to collect and they always came to our place even though my father could have written him a cheque once a month, or for the entire year, and Joan usually came along.

I remember Madeline saying Joan had mastoid. I never knew what that was but learned later that it affected her hearing and it would put her in bed for weeks. Now she's dying at The St. Catharines General Hospital and she's skin and bones, likely 80 pounds or so, and everyone thinks she has cancer as well as a prolapsed heart valve.

They said they could fix the valve about six weeks ago but she had a blood clot behind her knee and they told her to go home, take a blood thinner, and come back, "We'll fix the valve then." Joan got thinner and thinner. She moved herself into a retirement home and ate voraciously but couldn't put on any weight. Eventually she was so weak she couldn't lift herself off the toilet. An ambulance was called and she was two days in intensive care. Now we're told she's not to have surgery and not getting better. She's dying.

"I'm trying to get my head around it," she said. "I thought I had more time," her head bobbing on bone thin shoulders. The doctor has told her that there is nothing they can do. She's too weak to withstand tests to look for cancer and her heart won't take surgery; it's on its last legs as well.

Joan has made her way in life pretty well alone. Someone once told me she looked like a bag lady. They didn't look close enough; didn't know her. She was a woman of intense privacy. She didn't gossip about others and gave no one anything to say about her. She was difficult to get to know because she wouldn't let you into her life. I know she collected miniatures and she loved cats, often referring to "pussies." We never knew if she was serious or pulling our leg. She made us laugh but she had a stubborn streak as well. If you said or did something that annoyed her she'd say, "I don't like that." And, she could be slow in the physical sense, not intellectually, but I think that slowness had something to do with her obsessive-compulsive disorder. Her brain was telling her to check everything over and over, again and again.

A close friend of Joan's told me that Joan kept her waiting in her car an hour and 55 minutes while she went back and forth to her apartment to get items she wanted to take to the cottage where they were going to spend several weeks. She was never finished and always had to go back to check on something or get just one more thing.

Finally, the friend's frustration got the better of her and I believe she told Joan that that was the last time, they had to leave.

No one ever got into her apartment. Even her best friend was asked to wait at the door. I did however see photographs that Joan took of areas of her apartment and they were a sight to behold. She had her grandmother's antiques and her mother's antiques and a few things that she had bought for herself but first, before her own needs, she was the keeper of all family things that came before her. One picture in my mind is of a beautiful Victorian antique dollhouse under an end table. But more about that later.

I remember my husband, Ron, pushing me in the wheelchair from the car to the entrance of a restaurant. Joan tagged along – way behind. Ron and I were talking and she thought we were talking about her. "I don't like that," she said. We weren't talking about her.

Joan and I used to go to craft shows together and she would get annoyed because I would stop and talk to the vendors, many of whom I'd known and bought from for years. I didn't know at the time that she had a dodgy heart because she didn't tell us. She was probably very tired. She never bought much at the craft shows and just about tied herself in knots trying to decide if she was going to buy

something that she liked. It was hard to watch. I realized that she was likely living on her investments made from the sale of the family home and that was why she was so frugal in every way, but I couldn't imagine a $30 necklace would place her in dire straits. I remember Joan buying moss when we were out together, just a small pad of beautiful green moss. That speaks volumes.

I can't help notice that while Joan is lying there dying, the world outside is being reborn. Pink dogwoods bloom on the trees in the back and front of our house, purple clematis climbs up the side of the garage and a light dusting of bright yellow pollen covers chairs, tables, leaves, and shrubs. The hemlock is doing what it does every spring along with the Scots pine, cedars and Shademaster locusts. Everything is blooming and there's pollen everywhere. Nothing else stops when we do.

Joan's parents were big in the Anglican Church and her mother held many positions in women's organizations there as well as worked on the bazaars to raise money for the church. I'm thinking those bazaars were the source of the many antiques that filled their basement. Madeline had a good eye for what was old and perhaps worth something and she had a front row seat because she would be there as people were setting up and could pick and choose before the public arrived. For years Madeline and John we're responsible for the Christmas decorations in the church proper and always did a magnificent job.

I remember Madeline as a strong, handsome woman - bigger, straighter than my mother, her husband, John, and Joan. She was imposing. She had nice hands and always wore Windsor Rose nail polish, her hair pulled back in a tight knob and she sniffed continually. I'm not sure why but I can still hear that sniff and she's been dead for more than 35 years.

After high school, Joan worked in an office but I believe she felt the stress too much for her and after that she worked as the church secretary. I'm not sure how it all came about but Joan eventually vacated her secretarial position. I suspect it was because of her obsessive-compulsive disorder, but she didn't leave the church. As the rector once said, "Joan slept at home but she lived at the church." She was involved in everything. The church was her life.

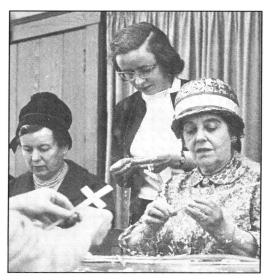

Joan (centre) making crosses for Palm Sunday with her mother, Madeline, (left) and another member of the church guild

May 30, 2006

The hospital called last night and asked if I could come up. Joan was in distress and wanted someone to be with her; I went. From 9 p.m. until midnight I sat with her and the Rev. Michael McKinley, the minister from St. Thomas's.

Joan was having a hard time breathing. We went from a cannula under her nose giving her oxygen to a mask that she did not like. Knowing what it is like to feel like you're suffocating, because I feel like that when I have pneumonia, I'm thinking the mask was hot and hurt and the cannula didn't give her enough because she is mainly mouth breathing.

"Help me … please help me breathe." she'd say and there wasn't a damn thing we could do.

The nurse said that end-stage chronic obstructive pulmonary disease usually ended this way; struggling to breathe. She lays there alternating between periods of sleeping and agitation. Her brain is likely telling her she is suffocating so she wakes up struggling for breath and complaining of a terrible headache. I wake up with hang-over like headaches if I sleep flat and my paralyzed diaphragm doesn't let me exhale enough CO_2. It builds up and the headaches don't go away until I'm up and breathing with the *benefit of gravity to help me breathe or I take several large breaths at a time while in bed but the relief by doing that is only temporary. When we tell her, "Joan, close your mouth and take a deep breath through your nose." She'd do it - three times, an hour later two times and then only one time.*

She looks like Jar Jar Binks out of Star Wars with the mask on and her mouth open. That's what I saw: Jar Jar Binks as she lay there dying.

But she didn't die. Robert McKinley stayed until 3 a.m. She was put on morphine to slow down her agitation and this morning she's still alive: responding to people and drifting in and out of consciousness. I find sitting with her quieting and also draining. Today I'm exhausted. It's in the high 90s out and terribly humid.

Monday morning the doctors decided to find out why Joan is so emaciated. Yes, she has a prolapsed heart valve but that shouldn't cause her to slowly fade away to nothing. She has always had a hearty appetite, as far as I know. When we would take her to restaurants, especially her favourite, Betty's, in Niagara Falls, after a hearty meal she would order the lemon pie with what she called 'mile high meringue.' She never had any trouble getting any of it down and neither did we.

The tests are ordered and some kind of medication given pretest. Joan reacts very badly. An antidote is ordered. She comes around for a while, then she becomes lethargic, really despondent, and can't wake up. That's what brought the phone call that she was dying. The doctors said that she just had to sleep it off. The nurses figured she was going to die. Sleep it off, indeed.

I read so often about elderly people being overmedicated ... so often. I watch Joan dying and I fear for myself, for my old age, for the next 20 years. Of being overmedicated, being shuffled off to a seniors' home, sitting in dirty diapers, being ignored, bathed twice a week, growing really fat and suffocating from over medication and no activity.

I'm not alone, hundreds of thousands must feel the same way in a province with too few doctors looking after too many old people in too often crowded and aging seniors' homes.

I see nurses who don't really understand the elderly because it would take too much time to do what they need if they truly owned up to the real needs of the aging individual. A perfect example of that is in my own extended family with my 52-year-old sister, Kathie, in the centre. Kathie has two teenage daughters. Paul, her husband, is an artist. She also looks after my mother, 91, who rarely gets out of bed. "I use my bed as

209

a couch. I'm warm in it and why should I bother getting dressed when no one sees me and I never go out." And, "How dirty can I get in bed all day?" she says when asked if she'd like a bath at least once a month. Her skin comes off in silver flakes. She ignores soiled sheets. Bed protection sheeting has to be changed daily – sometimes hourly – she really is incontinent but no one talks about it. The minute she stands up, she pees. Her short-term memory is shot but her mind still works pretty well. Kathie makes her food and tries to keep her from going insane from loneliness. Not easy when Mom doesn't remember if Kathie has been there three minutes after she leaves.

Kathie also looks after my brother, Ronald, 61, who was separated from his wife when he had a major stroke six years ago. He lost his ability to speak [except for six or seven words], read and write. He's trapped in his dysfunctional body. He's angry, frustrated and strong. I love him but I can't go near him as his anger shakes me to the core and his frustration is powerful. He grabbed me a couple of times and shook me because I couldn't understand what he was trying to get at. I would forgive him anything, unless he really hurt me, and that's what I'm afraid of. And, he drinks – a lot.

Kathie buys his beer, his groceries, looks after home maintenance [Mom lives in an apartment over the garage] in Ronald's home that used to be the family home until

Mom gave it to him after Dad died. As to the question of allowing him to drink when he is obviously an alcoholic. How do you reconcile keeping a man who has pretty well nothing left from the one thing that he wants? None of us could really answer that so we bought him his beer, his Chevas Regal and Bailey's Cream and hoped he wouldn't kill himself by falling down the stairs.

Kathie also has the responsibility of getting Ronald to doctors. His liver enzymes are not right. Is it his drinking? He tells the doctor two or three a day when it's really seven or eight every day, or more. His teeth were broken and loose and we couldn't figure out where the smell was coming from when he was in the hospital just after his stroke. Turns out his mouth was badly infected. Kathie has persuaded him to see a dentist but he's lost so many teeth that he can hardly chew and he won't wear his partial plate. Even his toenails, fingernails, hair and mustache have to be part of Kathie's concern.

Then there are Kathie's husband's parents. Barbara is in her early 80s and has Alzheimer's. She's due to go into long-term care this Thursday if they can figure out how to get her furniture there before she arrives. That is almost impossible. She'll know something is up when all her lovely pieces start disappearing.

Barbara's husband, Peter, has senile

dementia but is a lot better off than his wife. On the weekend he ran his car into the front porch steps at Kathie's place. She says the place now looks like a slum. He stepped on the gas instead of the brake, he says, but may have used the steps to stop the car ... sort of slid into it.

Peter doesn't cook, do a wash, clean the house, shop for groceries or do anything else like that. Barbara has always taken care of everything. Now, she's incapable of it and he doesn't know why he can't just pick up the phone and order take-out or call friends for a get-together. Barbara hardly knows what a telephone is for.

Kathie has Paul, her two girls Kitty and Julia, brother Ronald, mother Dorothy, mother and father-in-law Barbara and Peter, to look after. Homecare is so limited Barbara has to go into long-term care. My mother is waiting for long-term-care. Peter has lined up a retirement home and brother Ronald will live on his own with limited homecare until he drinks himself to death or drowns in his own swimming pool.

May 31, 2006

The phone rang at 8:10 a.m. The phone never rings at 8:10 a.m. I'm still in bed. Joan died at 1 a.m. this morning. The nurses called Rev. McKinley but she was gone before he could get there. Her best friend, Monica Stevenson, had been in around dinnertime and Joan wouldn't, or couldn't,

open her eyes. Who knows what was going on in her mind as she lay there being watched by those who loved her, wanting her to live, to be well, to thrive ... but it is not to be. The woman who walked everywhere with her shopping cart. The woman who dressed in sensible blue, navy, maybe grey and, surprisingly, sometimes bright red, who's smile lighted up the room, whose cheeks were like apples when she was well ... is gone. The woman who, when I asked Rev. McKinley to tell me what she did at the church said, "Let me tell you what she didn't do, she never gave a sermon." Everything else was fair game for Joan. The church was her life from childhood when she helped her parents get ready for bazaars and decorate the church for Christmas to everything else for more than 50 years.

I always thought she'd have made a good nun.

Monica, known as Stevie, and Joan had known each other for 64 years, and Monica is Joan's executrix. The obituary has been written. Who knows what's in Joan's will. Only Monica. I'm betting it will all go to the church as it should. The church was her loving family. We really couldn't get in, she didn't let us, and from what I know she didn't let anyone in, not even her best friend.

When I left Joan for the last time I looked into the room where the nurses stayed at the computer equipment that was attached to the monitors of the people who were dying. I asked if someone would be with her because I couldn't be there any longer. I was exhausted. They said they would. I couldn't read their minds but my thought was that, 'They are likely saying, why would they want to sit with someone who is dying when they could be sitting in front of a monitor that told them what her vital signs were and let them know if she was dead or not?' I wanted so badly for someone to hold her hand as she left this world but I'm told she died holding the little stuffed tabby cat I bought her on Monday. I figured if she loved cats, and I knew she had a big grey Persian named Smokey she adored when she was growing up, she'd loved them then so she'd likely feel comforted with one while lying there dying.

I called my mother this morning to tell her Joan was gone and I thought she was going to die. She was very upset and kept asking if I was coming up to see her and I kept telling her, 'I am Linda, I can't walk, and I can't come to see you.' Thinking about it, I likely shouldn't have told her at all because she'll forget and remember and forget and someone will tell her again and she'll be shocked all over again and then again.

I ordered flowers from the family for Joan. The memorial service is on Saturday at the church at 11 a.m. The florist says she insisted on yellow when she was in charge of the altar flowers so I said, "Make it yellow. Yellow and white. She'd like that." "She won't be there," he said, "You can get what you like." And he laughed and said he and Joan had a running joke: He was to find her a man. The last time he saw her he told her he may have found one – but he was Chinese. "Oh, dear, that would never do." she said. A man for Joan was not to be. She once had a boyfriend, Mom told me; a nice man and I knew him. He owned a nursery and his son did some tree trimming for me. One day, I met his wife and, no word of a lie, my mouth fell open. She looked so much like Joan they could have been twins.

Joan never really spoke of him but on several occasions I told her that I had talked to him. He always sent his regards. I like to think that there was a love there but it was quashed by Joan's father. My mother, at 91, called him a bitch last night. That doesn't really apply to a man but that's the strongest word Mom could come up with. "He was a bitch," she said, "He controlled every move Joan made, no man would ever have been good enough for her." Every time Joan was mentioned, Mom would say, "Poor thing – she never really had a life. That father of hers made sure of that."

Joan had a life: one she made for herself. She saw her mother to her death and about 10 years later, her father. That was about 25 years ago. She was free when he was gone. She inherited the family duplex that had eventually been converted into four big apartments. My mother was born in one side of the duplex and my grandmother died in the same one. Mom said people were always dying there. They came to die because my grandmother would look after them. "The big front bedroom was for visiting relatives and those who were dying," Mom said." I had to sleep with Madeline because no one from the family slept in the front room, it was for others." Madeline was about seven years older than Mom and really didn't want to share her bedroom. It must have been hard for Mom feeling insignificant as Madeline dated and grew into a woman.

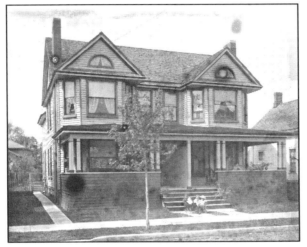

The duplex on Wellington Street around 1910

I remember back. I am about five or six I think. I'm staying overnight at my grandmother Clara's. I called her Nanny, and she was a large, strong woman who wore a big apron over a cotton print housedress, had large knuckles on gnarled hands and long white hair pulled back in a yellow bun at the nape of her neck. She had whiskers and her dentures clicked when she spoke but her large lap, soft bosom and an old rocker on the front porch were wonderful. She'd rock me and sing and tell me about the people walking by. She told me about Cecelia Rusnak, a little girl who was lured away as she walked home after buying milk from the local grocery store and was murdered in the canning factory right across the street from where we were rocking. Her body was found in one of the big old ovens. Every time I looked at that place I imagined Cecelia and saw glass milk bottles with cardboard lids.

Waking up in Nanny's big bed when she had already gotten up, had breakfast, and was moving about the kitchen, was wonderful. I could smell bacon and eggs, so strong, so good. But it wasn't bacon and eggs, I was smelling the huge blooms of purple wisteria hanging just outside the bedroom window. Wisteria still reminds me of waking up in a huge bed in a bedroom with brown art deco wallpaper and bacon and eggs.

My mother can't remember what the TV remote control looks like but she often tells me that her mother brought her flowers. Clara died 45 years ago.

Stevie told me that Joan has been extremely generous in her will and she left money to all of us but that was as far as she could go.

I've always thought her entire estate would go to the church but that was not the way Joan saw it. Yes, she left money to the church but she also left her money to her friends and relatives and another dear body who helped her anonymously. None of us knew who it was.

When Joan sold the family home about nine years ago, she received financial advice from the church and her money was invested. She had lived on the interest from that plus her government pensions and was content to live and work within blocks of each other, never owning a car, secure in the knowledge that the money would be there for her and now, for us. I can't deny that I'm delighted at the prospect of an inheritance. Whenever I begin to dwell on work or worry for my worn-out body, I switched gears to the day when I get the lawyers' letter.

Some years ago, a librarian living in Ottawa named Sophia Abarbanel bequeathed a small portion of her estate to me. She never married and, when she died, she had a stock portfolio that would choke a horse. My little bit was only a tiny portion but it started me on a search for a female investment advisor. I found a woman in her 60s and she told me that what I had wasn't really very much but she would do what she could. Some 17 or 18 years later I'm living off that money in my RRIF. Along with annual contributions it has grown to make all the difference

between constant worry and having enough. That is huge. Enough is the important word here for me. I don't need a lot but having enough love, care, hope and money helps. And one small inheritance can make the money part happen if you help and foster it along.

Joan's funeral was on June 10. The minister's painted Joan as a "character" and indeed she was, but a wonderfully loving, kind, and generous character. Her Rose Scottish family pin says something like Steadfast and True on it. She was incredibly steadfast and true. And, she was well loved and admired by many for her work, dedication and true love of Jesus and church.

At the reception in the church someone brought up the question of what Joan had in the two bags that she always had with her: one in her hand and another in a small two-wheeled shopping cart she pulled along behind her. The Rev. joked that she had lunch in there but Monica told me there was a bag of her medications in there as well as Scotch tape, a stapler and even the Parish list. She was prepared for anything and everything. I know that she had paper towels, disposable toilet seat covers, hand wipes and raingear in there as well. At the end of the reception Stevie gave me several bags and a case along with the stuffed cat I'd bought Joan – the one she had her hand on when she died.

214

The bags came home with us and included pictures of her mother, father and the cat, Smokey, pictures of my grandmother, Clara, and her grandmother on her father's side. Sister Kathie told me that Mr. Rose just walked out on the family one day, and John had to be the head of the family at God knows what age. So when he married Madeline he was strong and hard on them as well. Kathie said someone remarked at the funeral that they, Madeline and John, didn't treat Joan very nicely. We'll never know and I never heard Joan speak ill of anyone, ever.

In the smallest bag I was given, there was a modest string of pearls and an almost child-sized gold ring, the Scottish Rose clan pin Joan wore on her high school reversible pleated plaid skirt and Joan's watch, made in Japan, stainless steel with a sturdy, well-worn, black strap, and a Swiss made yellow lacquer bracelet with butterflies etched on it as is often done on silver. I wish I knew the story behind that bracelet ... maybe a gift from a boyfriend ... some long-lost love. I kept hoping I'd find something that told me that Joan did have a love at some time in her life.

I touched Joan's box with her ashes in it as I left the church to go down the elevator to the reception. I wanted to gather it up and take it down with me. She'd love to be there – to talk to everyone – to be serving sandwiches and above all, taking pictures.

The Rev. had her camera now, the one she lovingly used to record every move of the congregation. Olive, the minister's wife, told me that every time Joan took pictures of an event at the church she had 30 copies made. Thirty! I imagine many of them ended up in the garbage but she wanted to make sure that anyone who wanted a photo got one. That life is over – images no longer captured with love, and shared over and over.

Before she became ill, for a statement on the weather, a photographer at the local paper had taken a picture of Joan on a rainy day, trench coat neatly belted and buckled, plastic rain hat securely tied around her chin, umbrella overhead, bent forward just a little in her very determined walk as she pulled her little cart behind her, plastic all tucked in to protect the contents. He didn't know who the woman he had photographed was, but we did, and I thought that, as far as I was concerned, that exemplified Joan: all tucked in, everything taken care of. "They never asked me if they could use that picture," she told Stevie, but said she liked it anyway.

June 15, 2006

The lawyer's letter came today. I am to receive $10,000 from Joan's estate. How lovely of her to think of us. I'm sure we didn't deserve it but she thought we did. She never forgot us at Christmas or on our birthdays. She'd show up at the door a

215

couple of times a year on our birthdays, leave gifts with whomever answered the door, turn around and walk away. When we were older and began acknowledging her generosity in person, her face would light up in a huge smile. Thank you takes so little to say and can mean so much.

But that wasn't all – Joan's generosity had just begun to unravel.

July 18, 2006 – Hot and sunny

Last Saturday at 11 a.m., we put Joan's ashes to rest in the columbarium in the basement of St. Thomas's Anglican Church. Stevie said she's where she always wanted to be and she'd never be late for anything at the church again. I had no idea that she was always late for everything but that's what I was told. She'll always be on time for everything at the church from now on. There were nine of us and a man I didn't know held Joan's ashes and placed them in the little square opening about six feet off the ground. The plaques simply read: Joan Marilyn Rose 1932 – 2006.

August 20, 2006

Stevie called and said 16 people from the church had spent from 9:30 in the morning until 4:30 in the afternoon cleaning out Joan's storage locker. Most of it was paper, bags and bags of paper: family records, receipts, paid bills, advertisements, junk mail ... she kept everything. One whole load of paper had already gone to the dump.

She had also gone to Joan's bank and had her safety deposit box lock drilled. She had bunches of Joan's keys but none fit the safety deposit box. In it were four pieces of jewelry: a diamond and sapphire bracelet and three diamond rings. Stevie is giving those to us as well as Joan's miniatures and dollhouses. We have no idea what the jewelry is like.

This is fun ... you might call it sad fun. Joan is gone but what she has left behind carries on to give us a glimpse into the puzzle of her life and thinking. Stevie also says there are family pictures, some furniture and other family related items that we should have. Anything that we don't want has to be sold as the money goes to church.

August 31, 2006

Yesterday Kathie and I went to the storage facility – a long row of red-roofed white garages and a large main building. Joan's storage room was in the main building, down a long hall and into another hall. Stevie was there, down the hall, looking as usual, all neat and round. Rev. and Mrs. McKinley were also there as well as one of their sons. Stevie showed us the small storage space the church had rented, kitty-corner to Joan's much larger space. Kathie and I looked into the church space and there's a pile on the right for the church and one on the left for us. Stevie asks if either of us want an ornate sewing table, the kind with the big, U-shaped tapestry bag-like thing hanging from the bottom used for lady's fancy work and sewing. Neither of us really have a use for it. It'll go to auction.

There is a box of miniatures. We don't know if these are her good miniatures or just ones found in with everything else. Whenever people didn't know what to give Joan as a gift they gave her miniatures for her collection, consequently she had quite a collection. These ones turn out to be the dregs.

There is a lovely old doll and a newer Bye Lo Baby doll. There is a Limoges tea set - all green and white blossoms in see-through bone China. There are pictures of the old house on Wellington Street where Joan grew up before the big porch went on and then after, with all of its inhabitants standing on the front steps. We were told Joan used to go to yard sales and buy things. A lot of the things we found were not good – broken and chipped – but always curious and interesting. Something like Joan.

After looking at the room where the things for us were, I turned my scooter around to look at Joan's storage room. It was 15' x 20' and 12' high, I'd say, and although they had been working on it for two full days it was still half full. I could see a large old ornate bedhead at the back, the foot standing vertically against the wall, deep red couch cushions and green velvet pillows in the hall

waiting to go to Goodwill.

I remember those pillows on Madeline's couch. So much of her parents still alive in that dark storage room. To my right, a green hurricane lamp globe – the brass base somewhere nearby. That lamp could have been the same one that sat on top of the delicate mahogany desk in the big window that looked out onto that porch in the picture of the old house. Every Christmas Mom and Dad and we three kids would go up to Aunt Madeline and Uncle John's for a visit. It was only a mile or so and ten minutes but it seemed like another world away. An elegant little table stood in the hall and a brass stand held canes and umbrellas. Inside, there was a wine, satiny striped Victorian love seat that no one ever sat on, high white ornate ceilings, thick dark green carpet and a real old-fashioned Christmas tree with ornaments you couldn't buy at the store, like little Santas made of what looked like tapered red, green and brown pipe cleaners with white faces glued onto them, and bells and balls so thin and fine they looked as if they'd crumble at the slightest touch.

In the storage room, to my left: an oak washstand. In the middle, three plastic filing drawers. You could tell Joan tried to organize things but couldn't cope. File drawers gave way to stuffing everything into plastic bags likely out of desperation because everything had to be kept –

everything. Three large loads of paper and plastic bags had already gone to the dump and I'm sure more we're to follow. I just hope Joan took care of money as I hate to think that envelopes of money are being thrown out along with the five-year-old Canadian Tire catalog, receipts and bills and junk mail. There was even a bag of groceries from her apartment kitchen. The movers had just packed everything.

Stevie gave Kathie a little clear plastic envelope with four small white envelopes in it. We looked at each other as Kathie began to open each one. There was a lovely solitary diamond ring in platinum or white gold in one, another held a ring with a cluster of tiny diamonds surrounded by sapphire strips in an eight-sided deco setting. I think I was six or seven years old when I last saw that ring on Clara's hand. It was likely her engagement ring. The last of the rings had three large diamonds in it, flanked by two small ones on a white gold or platinum band. That was the one I thought I'd like to have. The last piece was a bracelet – surprisingly modern, with two diamonds and two sapphires - a very pretty bracelet. God knows why Joan just left these things in the safety deposit box for so long that the key couldn't be found, but out of sight, out of mind, and she wasn't much for jewelry, especially expensive jewelry. Kathie took two rings and the bracelet, the dolls and the china miniatures except for a few pieces I'm going to try to see if I can find on

google and she generously and graciously left me the diamond ring: the one with the three big diamonds that I liked. Kathie already had diamonds and emeralds and gifts of heritage diamonds from her husband's family or I wouldn't have asked for it but she asked me which one I wanted and I told her. I don't really remember that ring on Madeline, or do I? What I really remember is her Windsor Rose nail polish but I'll bet that ring was part of her overall look. One of the diamonds is yellowish. I'm thinking the three diamonds are from heirloom family jewelry. I'm still enjoying its sparkle.

September 3, 2006

Today, Kathie and I went to the U-Haul storage room to see the final leftovers of Joan's stuff. Four trips to the dump later the room was pared down to three piles: auction, family and church. We're told the entire stage of the church auditorium is covered with Joan's stuff to be sold at the next bazaar.

After three hours at a meeting of the Region of Niagara Accessibility Committee, (yes, I'm involved in that, too) discussing universal design, I pulled into our driveway and Kathie and her daughter, Julia, pulled in after me. We spend at least three hours going through everything they had loaded into her car from the storage facility but didn't finish, so after supper Kathie came back and we spent another three hours … most of it by flashlight … and it was like Christmas, one hundred times over. Every box, a hundred new things, and miniatures everywhere – hundreds of pieces. Family photos – thousands of them – going back to my grandmother's grandmother. So much stuff. I took the photos as I had more time than Kathie to put albums together. I took the silverware and some decent pieces of sterling that yesterday I spent an hour and a half cleaning. And there was my grandfather, Harry Collins' 25 year Odd Fellows pin: gold, enamel and his name engraved on the back and a very elegant oval photo of Clara taken in 1898 when she was only 15: her hair in a toned-down "Gibson", a long-sleeved, high-necked blouse and the long skirt of the day. By 10 p.m. Kathie and I were getting slaphappy, when we found one last basket we thought was empty. It would have to wait. We

simply couldn't go through one more thing.

Joan's death showed me a couple of things firsthand: death isn't easy – it is work, it is likely often done alone and it is frightening (for me and likely very much for her although her beliefs likely eased the way) and, when she said, "I thought I had more time," I thought, "Don't let time go by without enjoying life." I hope that Joan had enjoyed life in her own way. She certainly left a lot behind materially as well as much food for thought. I wish I'd gotten to know her better when she was alive but that had not been possible. I felt, however, that I knew her quite well after her death but it would have been nice to hold her hand as we laughed and to watch her rosy cheeks rise and her eyes sparkle when she was alive. It would have been nice.

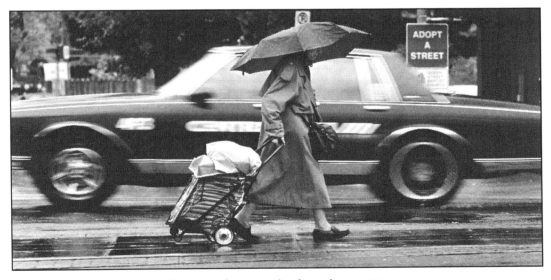

Joan, on her way in the rain *– pc26.1*

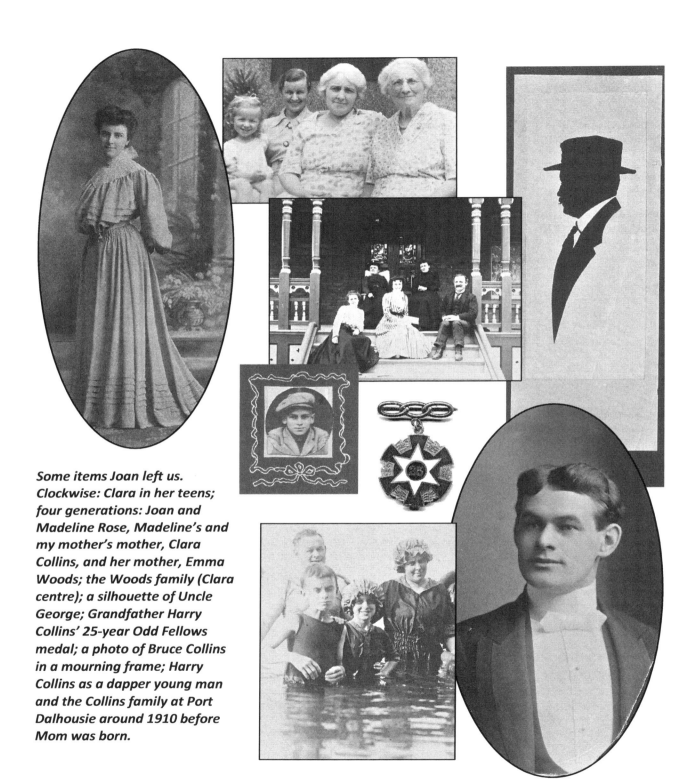

Some items Joan left us. Clockwise: Clara in her teens; four generations: Joan and Madeline Rose, Madeline's and my mother's mother, Clara Collins, and her mother, Emma Woods; the Woods family (Clara centre); a silhouette of Uncle George; Grandfather Harry Collins' 25-year Odd Fellows medal; a photo of Bruce Collins in a mourning frame; Harry Collins as a dapper young man and the Collins family at Port Dalhousie around 1910 before Mom was born.

27

It was time

After Joan's death, I vowed to look after myself better but as usual dove into more work volunteering to write about pain for the Hereditary Neuropathy Foundation in New York and to do public relations for Heartland Forest in Niagara Falls: 93 acres of provincially significant wetlands with Carolinian forest, frog and turtle ponds, and wheelchair/scooter accessible paths throughout. After much consideration and a lot of physical pain, because I write most things in my head before they ever get to the computer, I told the HNF that I couldn't revisit the sources of my disease as it was causing me physical pain. They understood. I think the work for Heartland Forest went well, since I'm still associated with them.

My work with people who have CMT was recognized by the Ontario March of Dimes, when I was given the Rick Hansen Award of Excellence in recognition of an outstanding contribution, nationally and internationally, to the cause of adults with physical disabilities. Rick Hansen's initial claim to fame occurred when he circled the globe in his wheelchair. He is now a serious mover and shaker in the world of disability issues.

I also received the Canadian Peter F. Drucker Niagara Regional Voluntary Sector Innovation Award for Community Leadership, The Zonta Club of St. Catharines Yellow Rose for making a difference to the women and children of the Niagara Region, The Joe Dinely Commemorative Award for exceptional leadership and commitment to furthering integration and accessibility for persons with disabilities in the Niagara community, and the T. Roy Adams Humanitarian of the Year Award from the chair and council of the Regional Municipality of Niagara in recognition of exemplary service to the residents of Niagara through community spirit and dedication to volunteerism (they said). Before receiving these awards, I didn't know that many of them existed and I certainly didn't expect them, but it was nice to be recognized for my work.

I also started taking Chi Kung, a gentle form of Tai Chi, and saw a nutritionist as well as an occupational therapist to help me figure out if it was possible to lose weight, since I could no longer walk or exercise without exhausting myself. And I saw an occupational therapist to figure out how to get myself up off of things more easily. Extensions under the legs of the chair that I used in my dressing room made it easier for me to get up off of that, and a VersaFrame, which connects onto the back of the toilet where the seat screws on and gives you armrests to push up on, made it a great deal easier to get off the toilet. A rehab specialist told me to stay away from doctors. He said he couldn't really help me and I realized years later that his tiny bit of advice was sound.

When it comes to my CMT, there really is no help but that doesn't stop most doctors from writing prescriptions. I wish I had the money that I've spent on prescriptions in the last 50 years, only two of which I take today for breathing and hormone replacement. I tend to experience what I call "doctor burnout." One doctor sends me to another, then another and on it goes. Eventually, I have to say enough is enough. I have seen perhaps 10 doctors for my burning pain and still treat it with cold packs I keep in the freezer. Sometimes there is no answer but I call us "Searchers" because we can't help trying and never give up hope that one day some doctor will write a prescription that will miraculously stop our CMT from progressing, calm our muscle spasms or quiet our pain. I'll bet the medical profession wishes they could do that as well.

Falls were commonplace when I was

younger and also occurred when I was working at the newspaper, but now that I was older and using an electric scooter most of the time, a fall was a traumatic experience. When I had experienced a bad fall that had injured my knees and was still stiff and sore after 10 weeks, I also realized that I'd lost my confidence. Every time I tried to stand up I would panic, absolutely sure that I was going to fall. When I fell, I was like a ton of bricks going down and nothing could stop me because everything was too weak; I couldn't grab onto anything, my hands were weak and my thumbs paralyzed. I would bruise my forehead, cheeks, shoulders, breasts, hips and knees, crack the fusions in my feet, take the skin off my toes if I wasn't wearing shoes, and tear out fingernails on the way down. No wonder I was afraid of falling.

***

To look into my constantly burning neuropathic pain, I had gone to the McMaster Pain Clinic in Hamilton. An MRI was ordered and I had it done. It was suggested that a nerve block might help my pain and I was eager to give it a try, so I went back to the clinic. Unfortunately, the doctor hadn't seen the MRI when I got there and had to be updated on my condition. I was transferred to a gurney and when the time came for the nerve block, I was told to turn over on my stomach. I have scoliosis in the neck area of my spine, they call it a dowager's hump, and lying on my stomach gives me great pain. The doctor poked and prodded my lower spine and continually asked me if I could or couldn't feel the pain. All I wanted to do was turn over to relieve the pain in my neck. He didn't understand that the burning pain I feel in the backs of my legs and across my buttocks isn't sharp or distinct like someone stabbing or hitting me, it is a constant burning and all of the MRI diagnosing and nerve block work didn't change a thing.

I also saw a social worker to talk about what I described as anguish, anxiety and despair. She agreed that I had seen far too many doctors with far too many suggestions. Rather than looking inward, I had searched outward for help. If I had simply quieted my soul and listened to my inner self, I likely would've done myself more good than any of those professionals. I knew that what went on in my mind controlled the pain. If I woke up in the morning pain-free and started worrying about a project I had to do or something that was going on between Ron and me or the family, the pain immediately came rushing back and would stay with me for the rest of the day. I'd fixate on a problem and go over and over it in my mind and, as I did, the pain burned even more fiercely. I had to try to learn to put my mind in neutral so I could have some respite from the pain for even an hour or two. Without that, I would start to feel desperate and when the pain got really bad and went on for days and weeks, I would begin to think about suicide. I had tried more than 30 drugs and, what I call, modalities – procedures like exercise, nerve blocks, chiropractic, acupuncture, the TENS machine, physiotherapy, nutrition and over-the-counter supplements – to try to make the pain go away. Nothing worked for any length of time. So, in lieu of driving our van into the canal or my scooter into traffic or even taking every pill from every prescription I'd ever been given, I had to find a way to do the work I loved and not hurt because of it. I must say though that the raised chair and VersaFrame helped for years. I was a work in progress and even drew my pain.

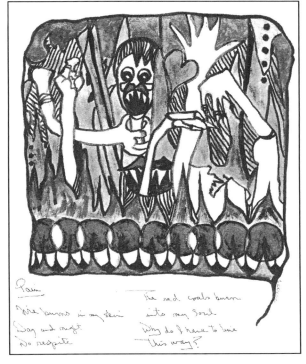

***

Kathie and I had been talking on the phone and the minute we hung up, Kathie got a call from a friend of my brother's saying that there was trouble. Because we had been on the phone, Ronald couldn't get us so he speed-dialed the next person on his list. Kathie immediately drove down. My brother's friend was there and my mother was being loaded into an ambulance. She had fallen downstairs and was badly injured.

At the hospital, when Kathie asked to see Mom, the nurses gave her a hard time and said it would be quite a wait because she was dirty and they had to clean her up. They had no idea the resistance Kathie had to deal with every time she suggested my mother take a bath or shower. You can't force someone to do what they should and it can be even more difficult if it's someone you love.

I saw Mom the next day in hospital and she looked like a corpse except I could tell she was breathing. She was lying there with her eyes closed and her mouth open and was heavily sedated because of the pain. The entire right side of her face was purple, blue and yellow, and her hand was bandaged. The nurse told me that she had severe bruising on her body, cracked ribs and vertebrae.

After ten days in the hospital Mom started to come around and was sent to the local rehab hospital, where she was to stay until a room could be found for her in long-term care. At one time she had made us promise that we would never put her in what she called an old folks' home. Later she softened and said, you will know when it's time. Kathie and I had visited three or four homes and had taken Mom to the one we thought was the best, but after about 15 minutes she told us to take her out of there; she couldn't stand it any longer. Now there was no turning back. We had to make a decision and after talking to Mom and trying to make it all sound sensible to her, we all agreed, it was time.

Following several weeks in rehab, where Mom was absolutely terrified of doctors and nurses who wore a yellow plastic gown and white face mask due to an outbreak of Severe Acute Respiratory Syndrome (SARS), we were told that a room in the long-term care home we preferred was available. Any longer in the hospital and I think Mom would have gone completely out of her mind. She was already delusional and paranoid; everyone who came near her was going to kill her, she was afraid of the person in the mirror at the end of her bed and any loud noise caused her to panic.

When she had been living at home she'd called the police several times because she said there was someone trying to break into her apartment door, when the door was on the stair landing of my brother's home. She also saw men's heads coming up from the floor looking at her. Of course, the police came, positioned their cruisers across the road so the perpetrators couldn't get away and then proceeded to scare the hell out of my brother, who was likely watching television downstairs and had no idea our mother had called the police.

The night before her move, Kathie and I searched the hallways at rehab for her as she'd been moved yet again, and as we neared where we were directed, we distinctly heard her voice offering $100 to anyone who happened to go by who would get her out of there. She had her feistiness back, that's for sure. She was to be moved by patient transfer the next morning.

Somehow, Kathie had worked her magic and Mom's room in long-term care was really quite lovely. Mom's blue denim wing chair, her cozy mohair throw draped over the back, a round pine table with its leafs folded down and an old pine captain's chair made the room look a bit like home. I contributed several pieces of framed floral artwork and we made sure Mom's television was on the pine dresser from home.

Kathie said that when she left Mom an hour

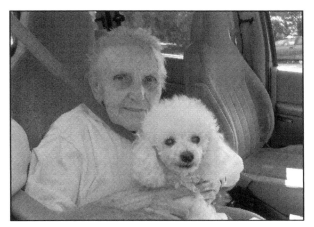

Mom with my poodle, Val, on one of her rare outings as she soon became disoriented and anxious when out and preferred the familiarity of her room

or so after she'd been transferred, she was sitting on the bed, her legs crossed, reading a magazine. When I went in the next morning, the side rails on Mom's bed had been raised. I'm assuming that in her effort to get out of bed, she had pulled herself up so she was sitting on the raised head of the bed; she was nude and she was trying to pull her catheter out. When she saw me, the look on her face was one of complete bewilderment. I don't think she knew what the catheter was for or why it was attached to her. She had likely been told many times but nothing really stuck. I was appalled that Mom had been left on her own long enough to do what she was doing.

Staff soon had her clothed and settled down but it was apparent that in her state of confusion and bewilderment, she had the potential to hurt herself if left alone, and alone she would be for many hours because there simply wasn't enough staff to keep an eye on everyone.

When Mom went into long-term care she could walk, but after a few sessions with a physiotherapist hanging on to the back of her belt trying to keep her balanced, it was decided that she would be better off in a wheelchair. Every morning at 7 a.m. she was awakened, washed and dressed, and put in her wheelchair and by 7 p.m. she was washed and ready for bed. She was given a bath twice a week and hated it. I had a feeling that she used to fight the attendants who gave her a bath, because one day we got a call reporting an "incident" and when we got to her she had a toenail ripped out. You don't have that happen during a gentle bath. For someone who had spent virtually every hour of the day and night in bed for the previous five or six years this was an entirely new, exhausting and likely frightening experience, although eventually she did learn to push herself around the halls.

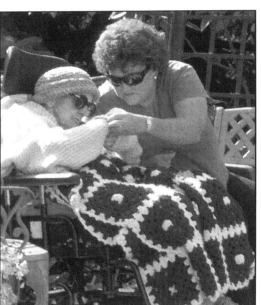

Mom and Kathie

Having Mom available was a new experience for me. When she had lived at my brother's in her apartment over the garage, to visit her a person had to climb three steps to get into the house and then another 11 or 12 to get up to Mom's door and another three to get into her apartment. I couldn't stand up much less climb stairs. I often thought about trying to

bum it up the stairs but knew my arms wouldn't hold up. Now I could drive to see her, park the car almost at the front door, go through the automatic lobby doors, up the elevator, down the hall and simply wheel into her room. I wanted so much to reconnect. During the years when I couldn't visit with her, we had talked on the phone two or three times a week and watched Antiques Roadshow together on the phone. Now I could spoil her rotten. I could buy her flowers and plants and magazines and clothes and anything she needed or wanted. I thought I could help her get on with her life in long-term care. Again, I was wrong.

My scooter would barely fit into the room and I had very little manoeuvring room but I could water her plants and get into her bathroom if she needed anything. But I couldn't get next to her bed if she was in bed and I realized fairly quickly that I wasn't much good to her. If she could grip the armrest of my scooter, I could pull her down the hall and she seemed to love that because she could go so much faster than she could on her own. But I had to ask someone else to help me get her into the elevator to go down to the garden and back up again, because I couldn't push her wheelchair and still steer my scooter. I wasn't strong enough to cut the stems off the bottoms of the flowers I'd just bought her and I couldn't lift or carry the vase full of water to put the flowers in it. It seems everything I did or wanted to do for her had to involve someone else. Yes, I could hold her hand, but other than that I think I was more a nuisance to the staff than anything else.

Speaking of holding her hand, Mom would grip mine with such ferocity that I had to get someone to peel her fingers away when I had to leave. She would beg me to take her out of there, telling me that she was alone all the time, that there was nothing to do, and that there was a big window she couldn't see out of while seated in her wheelchair. I knew that the recreation director was keeping an eye on her and that Mom was going to concerts and other events at least two or three times a week, but she'd forget she'd been to them. I tried to see her at least three times a week and she'd always ask me where I

Mom and her girls: granddaughter Kitty Gosen, Kathie, granddaughter Julia, and me

had been, because she'd forgotten I'd been there a couple of days before. In her mind, she was ignored and always alone.

I don't know how many times I left her only to hear her calling for me to come back as I drove down the hall with tears rolling down my cheeks. I'd go down the elevator, punch in the exit code on the big sliding automatic front doors, drive into my van and just sit there and cry.

Back at home, I wracked my brain trying to think of a way to be with her and not to feel so incredibly miserable every time I saw her. My body may have been living at home but my heart and soul was living in long-term care 24/7 with my mother. I was on empathy overload.

After talking the situation over with my Ron, I came to the conclusion that for my own sanity I couldn't visit Mom unless I had Kathie along. After that, visits became easier. Kathie and I would discuss everything from family life to what we read in the newspaper, what we'd seen on television the night before, how Kathie's two daughters and her husband, Paul, were doing, and if Kathie was involved in a new play, as she had been active in amateur theatre for more than 20 years. Mom would ask questions or sometimes just nod off. You could tell she was happy just being with her girls and I was able to enjoy my mother without the onus on me to do for her.

28

Closer and closure

Mom was well settled into long-term care when Kathie told me there was something wrong with our brother Ronald. Aside from the results of the stroke, she couldn't put her finger on what it was but he just wasn't the same.

Not long after that, Kathie called me and said that Bob, an acquaintance of Ronald's who had done some handyman work for him and stayed on to become a good friend, had called. He was passing Ronald's place and didn't see him in his usual chair on the front porch. On a whim, Bob pulled into the driveway, got out of his truck and while walking to the side door, heard my brother moaning. I'm not sure how Bob got in, perhaps he had a key, but he found my brother lying at the bottom of the basement stairs. He'd been there, unable to get up, for two days.

Mom and Ronald before her fall and after his stroke (2000) – the shoulder brace steadies his paralyzed arm

Off he went to the hospital. Nothing was broken but he was severely dehydrated. A visit by the attending doctor and several tests later, I was taken aside and asked to deliver the sad news that his calcium level was very high, which was one sign of possible cancer. A test for cancer had shown adenocarcinoma and a large tumor on his liver, although the cancer didn't originate there. They didn't know where it started. He would be put on chemotherapy to shrink the tumor and they'd take down the fluids that were accumulating in his abdomen and legs. How long did he have? Two to four months.

Ronald may not have had more than six or seven words but I know that the verdict hit him hard. "God, god, god!" he said, and shook his bowed head as if to say, what next? The stroke seven years before had left him unable to speak, read or write, and his right side was paralyzed. He could still program the remote control for the television so we knew he had his marbles, but to communicate, they were jumbled. He couldn't get the words out and couldn't comprehend the written word. It was sometimes difficult to get through to him and almost impossible for him to get through to us, although after a while with him you could almost read his thoughts. I had never felt closer to him in my life as I did that day when I had to tell him that he was dying.

After a week or so recovering from his fall, Ronald was allowed to go home and even though he said, "No, no, no!" to having someone be there for him, we knew he was going to need round-the-clock care. This was the man who had looked after himself for almost eight years with a paralyzed right side, very few words, and compromised vision. But, now, there was no way he was going to be able to go upstairs to his bedroom or take a shower by himself. He was very weak and, if the doctors' diagnosis was right, he was going to get a great deal weaker. He didn't have an appetite and we all agreed that not eating was going to make his time even shorter. His doctor said there was nothing he could do about his lack of appetite but I thought surely there must be something, so I got on the internet and found a drug that boosts a person's appetite and is specifically ordered for cancer patients. It worked wonders. If there was anything Ronald liked to do, it was eat.

Kathie was in a play at the time, her 24th I think, so I stepped in to do as much as I possibly could and that meant arranging patient transfer from the hospital to home, coordinating his care and putting his financial affairs in order. Since I had retired him from General Motors seven years before when he'd had his stroke, I knew what was where. So finances, updating his will and getting on with his stalled divorce were my jobs. Kathie had already done all of the sad work involved when shutting down a person's life three times: for her husband's parents and for our mother. Looked at realistically, caring for a person who is totally bed-ridden and dying can be a two-, three- or even four-person job. Community care supplied us with a hospital bed and everything else we needed for Ronald's care.

I took it upon myself to have the tiny washroom that was two steps down, moved up several feet so it could be accessed from the kitchen, thinking that he would be able to use it to do his business and to shower. Bob took this project on and worked like a dog so that Ronald could come home as soon as possible. The bed was set up in the living room so he could see the bird feeder out on the back patio and the front hall where most people came into the house. He also had a front row bed for his widescreen TV and a good view of what was going on in the kitchen. Years before, I'd had a ramp built onto Ronald's back deck so I could access the first floor of his house through the kitchen and patio doors. But what to do about round-the-clock care? His insurance wouldn't pay for someone to stay with him and he didn't require a full-time registered nurse, so what were we to do? I put an ad in the paper:

Wanted!
Housekeeper/Companion
Mature live-in person for male stroke survivor. Room and board in exchange for cooking/household duties in lovely downtown St. Catharines home.

Takers were scarce but I did get a call from a young woman who said she was definitely interested and could she bring her mother along to do the cooking. This sounded ideal and, when I interviewed her, I envisioned her doing the household chores and her mother cooking up delicious meals for the three of them. They were hired.

The first thing we needed to do was to buy groceries. Ronald had let things go and Kathie only bought what he wanted; the cupboards were bare. With my young caregiver in tow, we hit the supermarket and she began shopping like a woman possessed. When she had one cart full and began on the second one, I started to wonder but then thought perhaps her mother, being the cook, would be preparing meals that required ingredients we'd never had at home, so I let her go to it. The final total at checkout was more than $700. My antenna went up, this was kind of weird, but she was new to me and everything she'd bought was edible so I didn't think we could lose.

Mother and daughter settled in, each one taking a bedroom upstairs, and making the large master bedroom into a living area. Ronald couldn't tell us how things were going but Kathie checked on him often and things seemed to be okay; although when she'd ask him, he'd kind of shrug his shoulders as if to say "Whatever." She could tell he wasn't happy.

While shopping for a new electric razor for Ronald at Walmart I happened to bump into his wife, Lori, and her mother. Ronald and Lori had separated before his stroke. Of course, she asked about Ronald and I told her about his cancer diagnosis and what the doctor had said about only so many months to live. She asked me if it was alright if she visited him and I gave her a definite yes. I also told her that there were caregivers living there and that their job was to look after him.

Although they were getting room and board, we were also giving our mother and daughter team a small monthly cash allowance and at Christmas time we gave them both a bonus.

Lori began to visit and a week after Christmas called to tell me that she thought something wasn't right at the house. She said she couldn't put her finger on it but she really thought something was amiss. I couldn't for the life of me figure out what it was but I wasn't there as often as Lori. Then we noticed that the mother had a black eye. And Ronald seemed to be upset. He was on OxyContin for pain and before we could renew the prescription, we had to make sure that the old prescription had been used. Every pill had to be accounted for. Lori had been checking Ronald's medications and noted that he needed to renew his OxyContin prescription, but remembered that we had just filled it and the pharmacist verified that. I couldn't believe what I was thinking so I went to the house with Kathie and checked everything. One hundred OxyContin tablets were missing, worth $1,000 or more on the street.

Both mother and daughter were asked to be present while we checked Ron's medications. When I asked them if they knew about the missing drugs, they denied it, but I could tell that the daughter was getting very nervous. After a few more questions, I looked her straight in the face and told her she was fired and could leave the premises that day. "Me? You're firing me!?" she said. I didn't think her little mother had it in her to steal pain medications from a man dying of cancer and that black eye spoke to me.

I had to file a report with the police before I could ask Ronald's cancer specialist to write another prescription. An officer came to our home that evening and it was then that I learned that she was known to police. If I'd done a police check before I hired her I wouldn't have put brother Ronald in this regrettable situation and I wouldn't be preparing to beg his oncologist for another prescription. I felt like a damn fool. I had asked her if she had been in any trouble with the law and she said no and laughed as if it was a ridiculous question. Of course, she lied. I wasn't used to being lied to, always preferring to take people at face value until I learned otherwise, but this was different: it involved my brother's well-being. We let the mother stay on because we figured, and I believe rightly so, that her daughter had been beating her up, and she said she would do some cooking for Ronald. Lori asked if she could stay as well and that meant Ronald had someone looking after him who actually cared about him.

Before Ronald had the stroke, he and I were connecting like we had when he had come to Montreal before his first marriage. I would joke that I called him because I was wanting to hear his dulcet tones and then he would tell me what was going on in his life. He had said that he thought he could actually see himself with a woman again and that he felt like he was recovering from the separation from his second marriage that had left him bewildered and unsure of himself. Those months with him gave me a new insight into my brother and I liked what

I heard and wanted more, but the stroke took most of that away. Although I visited him regularly and we worked on his speech together during his rehabilitation, he made it quite clear to the rehab staff that he thought I was useless. That hurt.

Now, post-stroke and post-cancer diagnosis, I had been going to the hospital with Ronald every week while he received chemotherapy and paracentesis, a procedure to take the fluid that had collected out of his belly. Being there was something I could do and I wanted to spend time with him even though it meant getting up earlier than I ever did and being at the hospital by 9:00 in the morning to meet him as he was rolled out of the elevator on a stretcher by the patient transfer drivers. Every time they took him to the hospital it cost $140 and every time they took him home it cost $140. And anytime I had to use the washroom, I had to ask a nurse to help me get up off the toilet so I made sure I didn't drink. I think I only had to ask twice. Lori was able to go and see her ailing, aged parents while Ronald was with me.

Each time we went, Ronald had a blood test

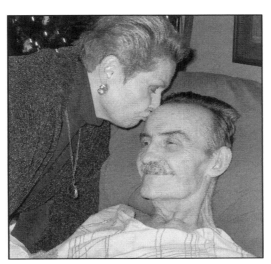

Kissing my thin, still smiling, brother

first, then chemo, and albumin, and then the paracentesis. The latter meant that a large hollow needle was put through his side into the area between his abdominal organs and his skin. The first time we did it, 7.5 litres of fluid were drawn off. That was more than two large orange plastic containers and he went from looking like he was carrying a basketball under his sweatshirt to flat. If I gently pushed on his abdomen, the fluid would drain more quickly and we could get the procedure done faster. While this was happening, I talked to him about our childhood, about his marriages and his children, and my marriages, and his job and my job, and I sang to him. At first he sang and laughed and we shared a delicious lunch that Lori made for us. Then, as the weeks went by, he rarely made eye contact. He slept and I closed my eyes and put my forehead down on the railing of his bed, all the while keeping the pressure on his abdomen, and prayed his death would be easy.

We talked about death and of our father who had died so many years before and Mel Torme and Louis Armstrong and all the wonderful musicians that had died. I said to Ronald that if whatever came after death was good enough for Dad and good enough for all those people whose talent had given us so much pleasure, then it was good enough for me. I told him that I wanted to go where dogs go and he laughed and shot an eyebrow up. He was an animal lover too. I brought him some prayers that I thought he might like to hear and he smiled during the 23rd Psalm: The Lord is my Shepherd. After I read it to him once, he asked me to read it again and then again. I asked him if he'd like me to read it at his funeral and he nodded and softly said yes.

As the months went by, spring turned to summer. Lori slept on the couch in the living room, so close to Ronald she could almost touch him and exhausted herself into a major bout of pleurisy, but showed her true devotion by staying with Ronald through everything. Ronald had lost about 60 pounds and was very weak; his old friends from GM would've done a double take.

Sam, Ronald's middle daughter, came home from Calgary where she was working, to see her dad – maybe for the last time. When she told him she was leaving, they both burst into tears. I told her to tell him that she'd be back and we'd arrange it so she could, but we all knew it was likely that he'd be gone very soon.

The mother of the caregiver that we had dismissed became quite forgetful and would leave pots of food cooking on the stove, go upstairs, and fall asleep. Ronald could see the stove from his bed in the living room and I can just imagine how helpless he felt knowing that a kitchen fire could easily speed up his demise. The caregiver's mom finally became so disoriented she was admitted to hospital. While there, her bags were packed, and although it may seem heartless, she was left to her own devices at the hospital. We knew she had a daughter somewhere and we simply could not take on any more.

On July 7, 2009, a Tuesday, I'd climbed into bed early, knowing that I had to get up at seven to meet Ronald at 9 a.m. at the hospital, our routine since November. But I had a funny feeling as the evening wore on that this time it wasn't going to happen. Strange as it may sound, sometimes I get a premonition like someone is going to call or someone is pregnant, but this time I felt very strongly that I wasn't going to be making my usual visit with Ronald for his paracentesis. Around midnight, Lori called. No one called at that time of the night unless it was an emergency. She couldn't get Kathie on the phone. There was something wrong with Ronald's breathing … something very wrong.

In the meantime, Kathie had heard the message and was rushing over. Ronald had had a great day: he'd been laughing and eating everything he wanted. But then he'd been sick to his stomach, had diarrhea and then started having trouble breathing. Lori said he had taken big, heavy breaths, gurgled a couple of times and then he just stopped breathing. He died quickly and quietly with no real pain other than his regular stroke pain and some muscle cramps. Was it a blood clot? A heart attack? Just the cancer? All three? Who knows.

Kathie described Lori as a basket case. She couldn't believe he was really gone. She hugged him, talked to him, stroked his hair and, when the nurse arrived and proclaimed Ronald dead, Lori asked to use her stethoscope so she could make sure in *her* heart that his heart had stopped. She said he was white, his head tilted a little and his mouth open a bit.

The mortuary service was called and about two hours later two men came. They gently placed Ronald in a maroon body bag. Kathie held the door and brother Ronald left his home, just as his father had 37 years before. I called the hospital to tell them we wouldn't be coming in that morning and cancelled his patient transfer service, took a sleeping pill and sobbing, went back to bed.

The finality of Ronald's passing brought a sad stillness to all of us who cared for him. Everything had centred around him for so long and now the core of our attention was gone. In one way it was a huge relief and in another there was incredible sorrow, for loving and looking after someone who is

helpless is emotionally all-consuming. I was in a strange position: I couldn't do the actual physical caregiving but I was with him every week at the hospital, had grown incredibly close to him, and was looking after all his financial and post-departure concerns. I felt like a hole had been bored into my soul.

When Kathie and I went to see Mom the next day, her attendants told us that she had said over and over again that something was missing … something was missing. We told her that Ronald had died and she cried but then she forgot and we never told her again.

That week, Carrie, the only daughter of my old friend, Bruce Hallett, had decided to take a ride with a friend on an all-terrain vehicle, had lost control and ended up breaking her neck when the ATV hit a tree. Her funeral was on Friday. Ordinarily I would've sent my condolences and not gone to the funeral but this funeral was in the church where I was confirmed, just up the street from where Bruce and his sister Joyce and Ronald and Kathie and I had been raised. It was familiar, safe territory and it was for the beloved daughter and niece of two of my oldest friends, and I so badly needed to grieve.

That afternoon my Ron let me off on my scooter in front of St. Thomas's Church and as I rolled into the door, Joyce rushed towards me, wiped the tears off her face with the palms of her hands and enveloped me in her arms. I cried like a baby. When we finally settled down long enough to look at each other, I told her Ronald had died Tuesday night. She had known Ronald almost as long as she had known me. We'd played together and he had chased her across our newly-seeded front lawn where she tripped on the rope my father had put around it to keep people out and broken off her two front teeth. My mother said she'd always regretted not having gotten Joyce's teeth fixed.

The service for Carrie was beautiful but some of the mourners appeared a little odd to the rest of the straight-laced Anglicans in attendance. She and her husband were members of the Biker's Rights Organization and the group had parked their motorcycles in Montebello Park, kitty-corner to the church, and were now seated in their leathers, beards and long hair, on the right side of the church.

After the service, which Joyce and I cried through, I went outside and happened upon Bruce in his car. He rolled down his window and said, "Do you see what I have to follow?" meaning the entourage of bikers; he obviously didn't approve. However, those people did something I will never forget. As the casket was being loaded into the hearse, the leader of the group positioned his motorcycle on the road in front of the church and others drove up behind him to form a procession, two motorcycles wide, and when he circled his arm in the air, they all began to move out. A police escort had been requested but was late and I watched the black and white speed down the street, siren wailing, lights flashing, toward the forming column of motorcycles and force its way through the left-hand side to the front. Then, following the cruiser, 60 or more motorcycles streamed past the front of the church, followed by the hearse and Carrie's extended family. I could only sit there on my scooter and watch this heartfelt scene unfold. I'm not sure why but I pounded my fist over my heart. There were more tears. I was grieving for the loved one of my old friends, hating to see them so heartsick, and grieving for my brother. I felt guilty that I, as I would eventually say, hijacked that funeral but it had served a need and I was so sorely in need.

Ron's funeral was held a week later. He had asked to be cremated. I wrote his obituary. His ashes in a green velvet bag were placed beside his father's. Kathie placed a bouquet near the ashes. I put a huge cream lily, my cousin had given me, on the bag and Lori read a beautiful poem. I read the 23rd Psalm.

Six people we knew, and some we loved, died that month: Harry, a bon vivant bachelor who had been a dear friend of my sister's in-laws for years and had worked with husband, Ron, at Eaton's in the '50s; Peter, my sister's father-in-law; Margaret, a neighbour; Ann, who had volunteered many hours with CMT International; Carrie, my old friend Bruce's daughter; and brother Ronald. Would it never end?

From my journal –

Six deaths

Harry was 100, welcome everywhere
Born when horses pulled the van
Went through life with a joke on his lips
And a dirty limerick in his pocket
A long-lasting man

Peter, born in Russia
A gentle, pleasant man from peasant stock
His wife an actress, far outshone him
His son loved him
That says volumes

Margaret, a nurse from Holland
Who walked by my kitchen window every evening for years
Said she couldn't sleep without it
Her head bowed in silent tears
For a lost son and husband

Ann, the farmer who taught children when she was young
Volunteered her time to help the cause
Shone her gentle smile on all
Celebrated her anniversary with her husband then died
No one had the heart to tell her they lied about the date

Carrie, so young at 30
No one could tell her so she lived as she wished
She died after her ATV hit a tree
Neck broken and her back in three places
Her father's heart, broken forever

Brother Ronald, my beloved brother
He lived hard, had lousy luck with women
Fathered three daughters, only one bothered
His big brown eyes spoke volumes when he couldn't
He lives in my heart forever

Six deaths within one month
Shocking, no matter how prepared
Teaching gratitude for what was given
Some for ages, some so little
We learn, we gather, we cry, a glimpse of what will be.

237

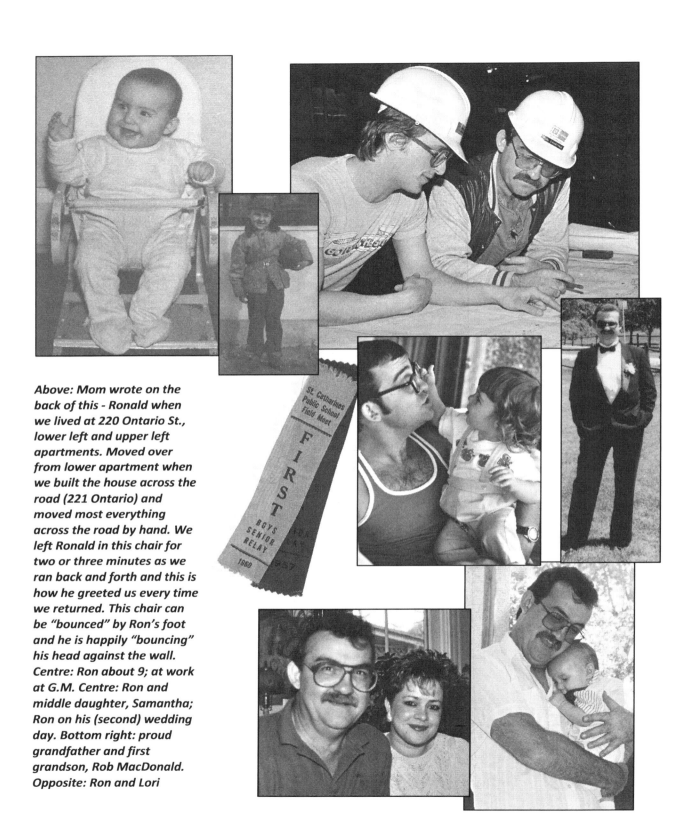

Above: Mom wrote on the back of this - Ronald when we lived at 220 Ontario St., lower left and upper left apartments. Moved over from lower apartment when we built the house across the road (221 Ontario) and moved most everything across the road by hand. We left Ronald in this chair for two or three minutes as we ran back and forth and this is how he greeted us every time we returned. This chair can be "bounced" by Ron's foot and he is happily "bouncing" his head against the wall. Centre: Ron about 9; at work at G.M. Centre: Ron and middle daughter, Samantha; Ron on his (second) wedding day. Bottom right: proud grandfather and first grandson, Rob MacDonald. Opposite: Ron and Lori

238

29

Goodbye Mom, hello marijuana

Life carried on while my brother was dying.

I had been chosen by my alma mater, Brock University, to be one of the 30 people lauded during their "Thirty from the Past Thirty" celebration that looked back over the years that Brock had been in existence and the graduates that had passed through its doors. For the occasion, I bought a lovely black velvet jacket, heavily embroidered in black

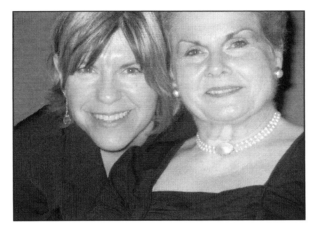

Sigrid Blake and me at the Brock celebration

with a black fur collar that extended down the front, and black fur cuffs. It looked like the designer had had a major affair with a Cossack, but the jacket fit me well and I was very glad that I had it because the conference room where the dinner and presentations were held was quite cold. The event also gave me an opportunity to wear a circa 1950 double strand choker of pearls with a huge mabe pearl and gold clasp that I bought at an antiques store simply because I loved it. Ron actually sewed me into my

top so my brassiere wouldn't show and sent me off with five of my lady friends to enjoy the evening. This kind of thing was not for him even though I wished with all my heart he had been with me.

Several months later I was maybe one of 100 people who were invited to have high tea with the Princess Royal – Princess Anne – at a hotel in Toronto. HRH had come to help raise money for the Ontario March of Dimes at a $500 a plate dinner after the tea.

Jocelyne Gagne, from the March of Dimes here in Niagara, had submitted my name and drove our van so I could attend. Once there, we noted there were no parking instructions mentioned for people using mobility devices in the underground parking. When we did find a spot, there was no curb cut to the elevator.

At 4:30 p.m. we were all seated in the bistro

in the Sheraton Centre and at 5 p.m. HRH Princess Anne began her walk-about. She was dressed in a Black Watch silk suit with a gold chain necklace, matching earrings, and a huge golden and diamond pin. She wore half-length black gloves. Her hair was in a French roll and needed something on it to make it shine. Very gracious, she spoke to everyone. Secret Service and Scotland Yard were everywhere. Jocelyn introduced us. She sat and talked for about 30 seconds.

The people from the March of Dimes were standing on the sidelines watching. Jocelyn was given one of the bouquets that had been presented to the Princess.

The little sandwiches of smoked salmon, cream cheese and cucumber, and brie and strawberry slices were hardly a substitute for supper and neither were the scones, clotted cream and tarts, but they were surprisingly filling.

The next morning, I felt used. It bothered me as much as Jerry Lewis did when he picked up the leg of a disabled child during one of his telethons and, shaking it, said something like, "We can fix this!" I didn't want to be on display and I didn't want to be labeled as disabled … I was and still am much more than that. I felt we were a photo op, showing her doing something before the big event. I guess her just being here was news or maybe I just didn't get my head right about the reason for the event. I actually felt sorry for Princess Anne having to go from table to table making small talk with people she didn't know. The only good thing about it was that she was likely very used to this kind of exercise and thought little of it.

The next spring my Ron celebrated his 70th birthday. His niece Cindy and her husband John invited the two of us over to their home for a meal. We hadn't expected a birthday celebration but barbecued lobster tails and steak were served, as well as Ron's favourite carrot cake with 70 candles on it. We all sang happy birthday to him and he told us that it was the first birthday party he'd ever had. It was then that I had a vague glimpse into his early years and that his upbringing had been nothing like mine. Perhaps the gulf between us was more psychosocial than anything else.

I had also been inducted into the Terry Fox Hall of Fame. Lincoln Alexander, the first black Canadian Member of Parliament, a cabinet minister and one-time Lieutenant-Governor of Ontario, received the honour the same day I did. He and I had crossed paths before and at one time he paid me a compliment that I've never forgotten: he told me he liked my hair, that it wasn't all gussied up. And the Tourism Industry Association of Ontario (TIAO) made me their volunteer of the year for my work developing and running AccessibleNiagara.com. That had been a huge job and the recognition was welcome.

Mom, in the midst of dementia, was terrified most of the time. When you can't remember past experiences, you can't reassure yourself that what you are presently experiencing is going to be okay and that you can get through it. Now that I am older, how many times have I faced a problem or situation and said to myself, I can do this … been there, done that? But if you can't remember that you'd been there and done that, every problem and every challenge is brand new.

When we put Mom in long-term care, the social worker there told us that we were the ones who were going to have a rough time with it, not Mom; that she'd be the same no matter where she lived. She lives in the now and doesn't remember what happened five minutes before unless it is lasting violence. The social worker also admitted that there *was* violence and people do get hit where she is, hit by other people living on that floor, but at least they didn't wander into each other's rooms and "borrow things" like they do on an Alzheimer's ward. A small thing to be grateful for.

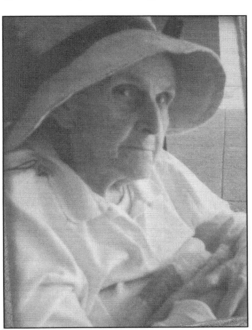

My favourite photo of Mom

The cost for a private room for Mom was $2,061.04 a month and her General Motors survivor's benefits paid for $1,756.87. She still got her government old age pension on top of that, so she was fine financially. She would get a ticket every month so she could go down and buy things from the tuck shop, but not being a candy or chip eater, I didn't think she'd be using that much.

Like me, Mom always had cold feet and I asked if she could have a heating pad or hot water bottle but they weren't allowed; however, microwavable hot packs were. So I took one of mine for her but was told that it couldn't go in the microwave because the microwave is used for food.

When you have CMT, you need an outside heat source because no number of blankets or layers of socks warm up feet that are simply not going to respond on their own. You need an exterior heat source to stimulate blood circulation, and once you've relaxed the veins and tiny capillaries they will stay open and your feet will stay warm until exposed to cold again. I sleep with a heating pad at the bottom of the bed and have one at the foot of the couch in the living room. I put the soles of my cold feet

241

against it and within 15 minutes my feet are comfortably warm. Then I can turn the heating pad off and they will stay warm for the rest of the night. I did get Mom a pair of fleece-lined bed slippers and hoped they'd be put on her while her feet were still warm, so they'd stay that way.

I had put together a story book for Mom, *The Life and Times of Dorothy Crabtree*, and in it were pictures and tales from the time she was a baby in a big fancy wicker carriage, popular in the late 1800s, to photos with my dad when they were courting and looked like fashionistas, and then to their marriage, my birth, the birth of my brother, and her journey into the world of antiques and art as well as the many conventions Mom and Dad went to together every year while dad was local secretary-treasurer of the musician's union. Pictures of Kathie as a baby went in and I touched on Dad's death and Mom saving the carousel several years before he died, and then her helping to renovate the house that they bought together for me. That book was her favourite and I think her only connection with her past life. The recreation director or anyone reading it to her would have her rapt attention and I know she'd go through it on her own because the pages became sticky with apple juice and smudges from ice creamy fingers. Two newspaper clippings about Mom and how she saved the carousel were framed and hung over her bed. She wasn't just a room number, she was our mother and we wanted everyone to know she had a name, she'd had a wonderful life, had accomplished much and she was loved. She became known at the home as The Merry-Go-Round Lady.

Occasionally Mom would descend into some kind of hell, throwing things, screaming and crying. She'd throw her teeth across the room, tear off her clothes and try to pull her catheter out yet again. She said she was cold, then hot, and nothing would put her right. The doctor prescribed a sleeping pill and an antipsychotic drug. We were told that Mom got agitated when she had too many visitors. "Don't visit so much … I know you love your mother but she doesn't know whether you've been there for 20 minutes or twenty years; it's all the same." On one of her good days, when she was more lucid, she looked at me and said, "I just have to hope today's a good day and tomorrow is a good day too." I felt exactly the same way.

On the mood-altering drugs, she was a bit calmer but still had episodes of violence. When asked if she was in pain she said, "No, more frightened than anything. I just wish I could die and get it over with."

Depressed and utterly exhausted from the 12 hours in a wheelchair routine that she was forced to endure, Mom became very quiet and unresponsive. We celebrated her

92nd birthday with flowers and gifts but she really wasn't with us. Soon after that we asked that she be taken off the antipsychotic drug and her sleeping pill. Take her off everything but keep an eye on her. Within four days, mom was lucid, talking and laughing, although she was still hallucinating and thought she saw a man standing by her window curtains and then cross the room. She told me her mouth fell open when it happened and she continued to be very upset. She said she was either going to go crazy or commit suicide. After that episode we spent about an hour together in the dining room with our foreheads together looking out over Martindale Pond as we watched the sun on the water.

Mom gained weight – 2.5 pounds after only six weeks – but she only ate puréed food because she'd spit out anything that had lumps in it and she never drank enough. Everyone figured that she became delusional because she was so dehydrated: her urine was very dark, her skin dry, her tongue looked like it was lined with clay and her eyes were scaly. Everyone said they would chart her fluid intake and make sure she got more liquids but no one really had the time to pay attention to what a 92-year-old woman drank.

She had one urinary tract infection after another and the medications for it made her even more confused and crazed. I

bought her two sippy-cups that she couldn't spill if she dropped them in her lap. She forgot what they were for and didn't touch them. I looked to the heavens and swore that the word "forget" should be erased from the English language after age 80. Mom said she felt ashamed that she was now the child and I was the mother. I told her she'd never be the child but she was … in a way.

***

For the past 15 or more years I had lived with chronic burning neuropathic pain across my buttocks and down the backs of both legs to just below the knee. Most of the time I felt as if I were sitting in a pile of hot steel wool. Pain affects everything: your work, your health, your relationships, and your family. And the stress from constant pain eats away at you. If I was working, my mind was off the pain and I could bear it, but seat me on my scooter at a meeting where I was listening to people for several hours at a time and eventually the pain would become almost unbearable. It seemed to burrow into me and grow hotter as I tired, as my back and shoulders began to ache, and I wished I'd never volunteered to be part of any committee, ever.

When the days were hard, the work demanding, and I'd leave my computer hoping to get some rest, it was then that the pain would just dig into me like rot into a log. I began to feel hopeless, to wonder if I could really live like this … if I wanted to live

… and then I started thinking about marijuana … again. It had been on my radar for years. Way back when I joined a local weight-loss clinic, the woman doctor there signed the government form that let me apply to use and grow medical marijuana. How hard could it be? I'd buy some seeds, start them under the same lights that foster my orchids and then put the seedlings outside in big pots in our little private fenced-in backyard. Easy-peasy … and I'd have my pot harvest.

But not so fast, little lady! I sent money away to Marc Emery, a marijuana seed dealer in British Columbia, and received 10 seeds for a strain called Dutch Treat that was supposed to be high in CBD, the properties that relieve pain, and low in THC that give one a high. I diligently started them under lights and, of the tenderly tended ten, six came up. During the last week of May, the six were planted in huge pots and placed in the sun in the backyard. During the summer, three died but the remaining three grew into huge, green, leafy bushes that sent the pungent odor of skunk wafting into my bedroom for four months. I put up with the smell, and even got to like it, because I still held out hope that these three plants could possibly yield the painkiller that had eluded me for so many years.

Into October the plants were starting to turn yellow and I thought to myself, "It's now or never." Did I have anything? I had huge seed heads but nothing that I would call usable – or were they? I didn't know what to look for. By the time my harvest failed, my license to grow had run out. I no longer had the option to go back to my weight-loss clinic because the doctor there had told me that she would only sign a renewal form for me to continue to try to grow it if I continued on with the clinic at a hundred dollars a week. I knew that I was getting weaker and weaker following the diet they gave me, so I quit.

Still interested in what medical marijuana might be able to do for me, I contacted a clinic in Hamilton and the person there said that he could set me up with the doctor who would sign the application for me for around $200. I thought that was a lot of money for a simple signature, and I knew that no one should charge for this, but I had run out of options.

So, when the doctor visited Hamilton, Ron drove me over and my contact was waiting at the door of a very modest hotel. We were directed to the elevator, which led to the basement. Once in the so-called waiting room, I saw more faded denim and long grey hair than I had in the last 30 years. It looked to me like every hippy within a 100-mile radius had come out to have their application signed. The only reasons I could think of for why they didn't buy it on the street was that you don't know who you're buying from and what you're getting on the street; and you have more control over what you ingest or smoke if someone is growing it for you, you are growing it yourself, or you are buying from the government.

What was supposed to be a medical examination, which went along with the signing of the application, was a simple form that I filled out saying that I have a neurological disorder and experience pain. When my name was called, I was told to go into a dark room and head towards the far corner. There, behind a curtain, akin to the Wizard of Oz, was a person I assumed was the doctor. He asked my name, signed the form, held his hand out for the cash, and that was it. Within months he was charged with indiscriminately signing copious numbers of marijuana applications right across Canada.

After I had my license to legally possess medical marijuana renewed, I contacted the clinic in Hamilton again. My contact there was going to send me some edibles to try. Within a week or so, a small package arrived and in it was a small jar of pungent, green marijuana butter. It sat in the fridge for a couple of weeks, but two nights before Christmas Eve, after a long week of meetings and deadlines, when my burning, aching body began to get to me, I thought, "Why not give it a try. What harm could it do?"

At 8:15 p.m. I spread some "butter" on a couple of rye crackers, topped them off with peanut butter and finished watching my TV program while eating. By 9:00 I was on my computer checking my email and I couldn't stop laughing. Everything was hilarious. I thought, "Wow, if this is what marijuana is like, it's wonderful!" By 9:30 I was in the shower and realized that I wasn't in control of my limbs or at least had less control than I usually did. I crawled into bed to watch TV and by 10:15 the screen was coming at me, every sound was magnified and I couldn't move my legs at all. I had never felt like this and it wasn't funny. I felt as though I had to go to the bathroom and was very afraid that I was going to wet the bed.

Somewhere between 10:30 and 11:30 Ron called the emergency department of the hospital and asked them what to do with me. I was seeing things, terrible things, and I was whooping, my speech was slurred and slow. I wanted to throw up everything evil inside me although I couldn't imagine what that could be. Questions were asked and answered. An ambulance showed up at the front door of the house and I was transported while shouting: up the street, left onto St. Paul Street (our main drag) and all the way down to the hospital.

After about an hour I still felt unattached from the world. My body didn't exist. I felt as if I couldn't open my eyes. Everything was moving and I became terrified that I was going to die. I recall a woman in the ambulance asking me to please stop shouting, but I felt so disconnected from my body that my voice was the only thing that made me feel alive; it was my umbilical cord. It was a terrible feeling and one that I'll never forget. I had visions of blue-booted troops marching through fields of fat, green cactus with long sharp yellow needles, their soles squishing the cactus pads as their goose-stepping feet pounded into the sand.

Ron had a hard time at the hospital trying to explain to them that I had Charcot-Marie-Tooth disease because no one knew what that was, but they seemed to know what a drug overdose was and they put us in a small dark room and told Ron that I simply had to wait until it was out of my system. I pleaded with Ron not to leave me alone with the horrors and the feeling that my body didn't exist. True, I had no pain, but what was my brain paying for it? Plenty.

During the hours we spent in that room, Ron sat beside me, held my hand and talked to me. When we stopped talking, the poor man would fall asleep. He had no terrors coursing through his brain to keep him awake. I asked where we were and he told me we were at the hospital because I was having an adverse reaction to marijuana. My only reply was an incredulous, "Nooooo!" I was mortified.

At 4:30 a.m. it had been eight hours since I'd had my crackers with the "special" topping and I knew where I was and why. I asked myself, how could this have happened? I took so little. I was ashamed of myself for abusing the medical system but also really ticked off. Had I been made aware of what ingested marijuana could do to me, I might have known a reaction like this was a possibility. Medical marijuana doesn't come with an instruction booklet. You're on your own.

Ron left me for an hour or so and I slept; there were no further horrible visions and I had my body back. At 7:15 Ron was back with my street clothes and my manual wheelchair out of the back of the van. I could feel my body but moving was another thing. It took two people to dress me and when I tried to stand, I collapsed. Even though I couldn't walk, I could usually stand to get my slacks up but this time I was a dead weight in Ron's arms. By 8 a.m. we were home, I took a quick shower and bed never felt so good. I slept until suppertime.

The next day I ate like there was no tomorrow. If this was what they call the munchies, I had them. It took two days for the effects of that little bit of green butter to wear off but during those two days I had absolutely no pain except that of trying to live down my little adventure the next day, which was Christmas Day.

Ron had called sister Kathie before the ambulance came to pick me up so she knew that I'd been carted off to the hospital yelling like a banshee and everybody at her Christmas dinner knew as well. Ducking all the wisecracks and silly jokes that came flying my way was impossible but I didn't really mind. I was okay and who on earth would ever conjure up the scenario of an almost 70-year-old disabled woman and Member of the Order of Canada being kept overnight in the hospital for a marijuana overdose? I couldn't help but smile.

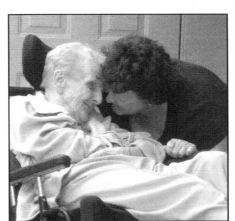

Mom and Kathie

Never one to miss an opportunity for a fun 700 words, I wrote my December *Access Niagara* column about it and my editor sent a photographer down to the house to take a photo of me with the offending edible. The paper gave me an entire page and titled the article, *Maiden voyage with medical marijuana a rough trip.* None of the many columns I had written before or since have received as much feedback as that one did. Several people with serious medical problems wrote to me and asked how they could begin to get medical marijuana as nothing else had worked and they wanted to try it. Many people found my adventure laughable, and I would've thought so too if it hadn't been so terrifying. One man, after

feeling bad because my article made him smirk, wrote: "Linda, please know we laugh with you, not at you! We have to find the humour in our situations or, besides being physically challenged, we will be insane!"

Many years later a complete stranger might walk up to me when I'm out shopping, give a little chuckle, and ask if I'm still using medical marijuana. I tell them yes but I know a lot more about it now than I did then. And I learned the hard way.

***

After four years in long-term assisted care, Mom finally decided she'd had enough. I can't imagine what she went through during those years: the anger, confusion, paranoia, the hopelessness, and confusion … everything that went with dementia. Sometimes you *can* live too long. When Mom went into care the doctor told us that the x-ray of her brain looked like lace. I can only hope that someday in the future my brain doesn't look the same way. I have learned that brain atrophy can be part of CMT 2A2. Was that what brought on her dementia?

Mom started refusing food and as she had never been one to drink much, began to go downhill quickly. The caregivers at the home no longer got her up first thing in the morning to plop her into her chair for a 12-

hour stint in the halls. She stayed in bed. Food was offered but declined and we watched as she slowly faded, until we were told the end was near. She was given morphine to keep her comfortable and after every shot she'd fall asleep but often woke up before it was time for another. She'd cry like a little child and rub her stomach, all the while looking at us with eyes pleading for help to make the pain go away. She could no longer speak. All we could do was hold her hand and, with a cotton swab, rub glycerin on her parched lips.

A week into Mom's decline, Kathie and I were spending afternoons with her. We were told the end was near and we could tell by her laboured breathing that she was shutting down. The home's policy was that her room had to be emptied of personal effects within 24 hours, but we had heard tales of staff simply throwing breakable items into a green garbage bag. We didn't want that to happen with Mom's things, so Kathie and her husband Paul had been taking furniture and personal items home during the past week. We decided to give her television to someone there who didn't have one. Sad, but some people there didn't have any visitors or anyone to go to bat for them except staff.

Kathie and I put together Mom's obituary for the newspaper and then stayed with her until 4 p.m. I couldn't get my scooter up to the bed because the nightstand stopped it. I hoped she knew we were there. I wasn't crying; I wasn't anything. We all expected this but it doesn't matter what kind of preparation you've had, when your mother dies I think a little of you dies too. I went home to Ron for supper and told him that I didn't think she was going to last the night but, if she did, I would go back the next day. At 7:00 that night the phone rang. It was Kathie. She had gone back after supper and spent an hour with Mom and when she got back, the home had called. Mom was dead. The Merry-Go-Round Lady was no more.

The newspaper asked me to write a final farewell for Mom. I felt so bad I didn't know if I could see through my tears well enough to pound it out, but figured it was the last thing I could do for this wonderful woman who had given me so much for so long and loved me unconditionally all of my life.

Mom's ashes were buried with her son, her husband, and her mother and father-in-law. It was a graveside ceremony, beautiful in its simplicity, just like her. When Dad died, Mom had put her name on the tombstone along with his. Now, some 38 years later, she was joining him. She was 96.

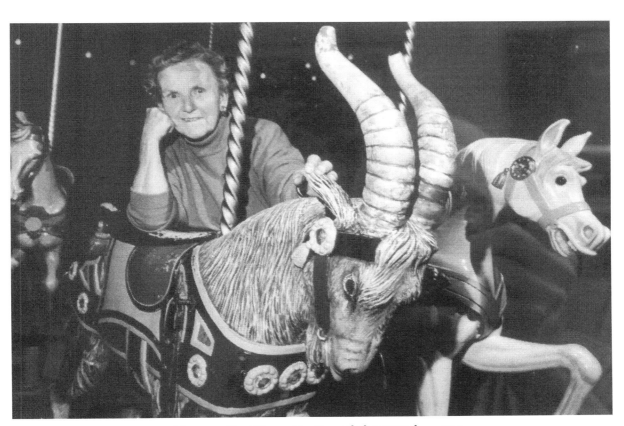

__Mom on the Merry-Go-Round she saved__ — pc29.1

I wrote this for Mom on her 78th birthday and it still applied until the day she died.

April 9, 1993

Dear Ma:

It concerns me that every time you look at a photograph of yourself you get upset. I know you are 78. I know your hair is thin and you have wrinkles and black circles under your eyes. But your skin is smooth as a baby's bum and I'll never forget the feeling when our cheeks touch as long as I live. I know that what you see isn't you, and believe me, what you see isn't what your kids see you either.

I can only speak for myself but I'll bet everything I have that if you ask Ron and Kathie what they see in your beautiful face they'll agree with me and add some.

Your beautiful face is a symbol of love and caring. It reflects an open-heart that cares so much for people that you spend most of your time trying to figure out how to help them.

Your beautiful face reflects the million times you have thought about us and cried over us and laughed for us and with us.

Your beautiful face reflects the millions of tears shed in loneliness and heartbreak for our father, your husband.

Your beautiful face reflects the strength spent surviving alone and making the very best of it.

Your beautiful face reflects the years spent with your grandkids watching them grow up under the watchful eye of your youngest daughter with the beautiful voice.

Your beautiful face reflects the love you have for your son and the renewed closeness you two have established.

Your beautiful face reflects honesty, a sense of fair play, a keen intelligence, a courageous heart and a loving soul.

Your beautiful face is never going to get any younger, but with every year we know you more, love you more and pray we'll have you here for many more years. So please hold that face up to the light, let everyone see it, smile and be proud of that face for it reflects what has made three people what they are. It has touched millions through you and your children and grandchildren. Be proud of it because we are.

Don't every despair that lovely, time worn face. For us it's the most beautiful face in the world.

I couldn't say this at your party but it is from my heart and my birthday present to you on your 78th.

~Linda

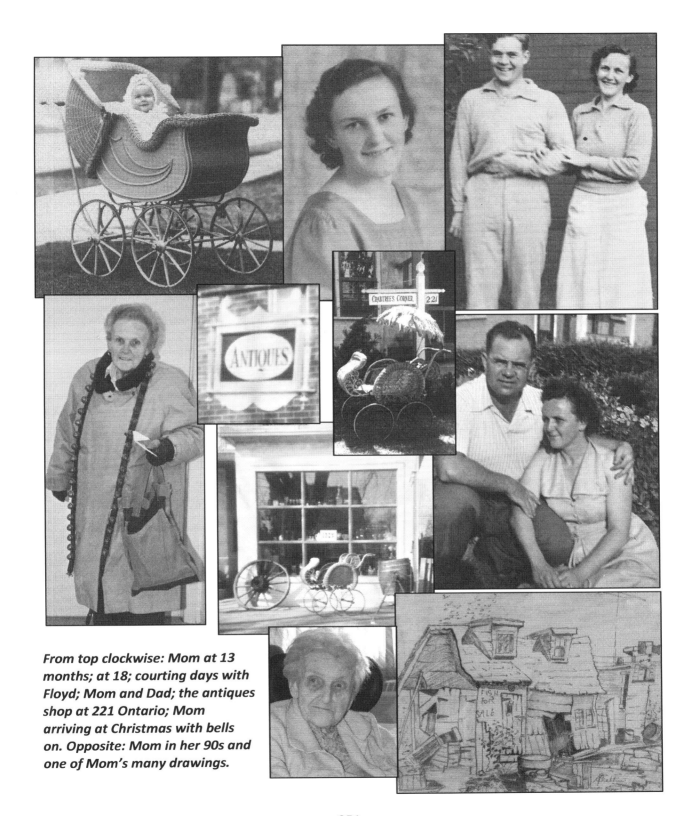

From top clockwise: Mom at 13 months; at 18; courting days with Floyd; Mom and Dad; the antiques shop at 221 Ontario; Mom arriving at Christmas with bells on. Opposite: Mom in her 90s and one of Mom's many drawings.

30

And along came Bill

When things get stressful I usually turn to my art for relief because it doesn't demand anything of me, there is no right or wrong. While I may have to make hundreds of decisions as I paint, those decisions are mine and mine alone.

Remember the thousands of photographs that I inherited when my cousin Joan died? Going through those and the boxes of small incidental family items that were left to me, gave me an idea. I had tintypes and old photographs going back to the late 1800s and I had small things like old watches, ribbons, stamps, wire-rimmed glasses, dried butterflies, an Odd Fellows medal/pin, and a beautiful ladies lace collar that must've come to my grandmother from some relative doing the grand tour of Europe. It was exquisite. I even had a snake-skin pouch with every document in it from

Harry Collins – my grandfather

the time my grandfather Harry was felled with appendicitis right up to his final arrangements, including the hymns that were to be sung at his funeral about a week later, all written in my grandmother Clara's fine hand. I could almost feel the tears on the pages as I slowly undid the case that probably hadn't been opened since the week after he died in 1931.

My thinking was that I would put a lot of the old photographs and bits and pieces together and let my artwork link it into one long lifeline collage. I was a founding member of the Niagara Artist Co-op and knew that members could exhibit there. I started dreaming about it. I don't know why I have such a strong internal force making me want to document my family, but as you can see by this book it remains with me to this day. It's not just my life I want to write about but that of my family, those I love, and my journey with this crazy disease that affects so many people but still runs under the radar.

Ron and I measured the exhibition space at the gallery and it turned out to be 32 feet. I decided that a 30-foot collage would be my goal. A local art supply store was going out of business and I picked up five boxes of double-sided sticky tape and a roll of heavy white paper about 40 feet long and three feet wide. As usual, my brain began working on the collage way

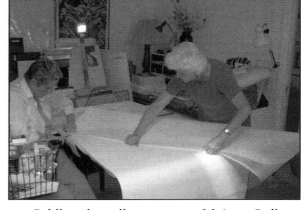

Folding the collage paper with Irma Bull

before I could get paper and paints in motion. There was no way I could manage it on one long piece of paper. I couldn't even fold it by myself because it was so long, so I set up an eight-foot table and asked my friend, Irma, if she would help me fold it.

First, we measured out 30 feet and a bit, and cut the remainder off. Then we folded the long piece in half and cut it so we had two 15-foot pieces. Then we folded those two pieces in half and cut them apart, which left us with four, seven-and-a-half foot pieces, which were then folded horizontally in half. My idea was that the upper 18 inches would be collage and the bottom 18 would read as a story. Viewers could follow the action through the visuals above.

Months before, I had joined the St. Catharines Art Association. Driving some of my artwork over to a local shopping mall for a show after supper one night, I parked and then rode my scooter into the mall and asked if someone would collect my paintings out of the trunk of the van because I couldn't carry them while on my scooter. A voice piped up and said, "Bill will help you, won't you, Bill?" A tall, thin grey-haired man in his late 70s came toward me with a big smile on his face and we went out to my van together, where he gathered up my canvasses and carried them into the plaza. From that night on, Bill Wenham and I were friends.

Several weeks later the arts group toured an old building in Port Dalhousie that we were thinking of taking over as our headquarters. After the tour, some of us congregated at the closest Tim Hortons coffee shop to discuss the project. As people began to leave I asked Bill if he would like to go for a walk, or in my case, a roll, on the pier with me. It felt strange

254

being with someone other than my Ron but since Ron was still very distant, and not usually there for me, I took a chance with my emotions.

It turned out that Bill's wife, Margaret, had suggested he get involved in something. "Get out of the house, volunteer for something, go help someone," she had said to him. So he did, he joined the art association and, after I told him what the 30-foot collage involved while we strolled along the pier, he volunteered to help me make my long paper dream become a reality. Both of us were struggling in long-term marriages. Neither of us wanted to leave our marriage but neither of us was happy. We had found, in each other, a kindred spirit.

One of my biggest problems was something I hadn't counted on: I couldn't manage double-sided tape. My fingers were so weak that I couldn't hold the tape and peel the back off, and I couldn't cut it small enough because my thumbs are paralyzed. Scissors were impossible, as was picking up the small pieces, if I was lucky enough to be able to cut them using a mat knife. I dreaded using rubber cement and I couldn't think of any other way to fasten the hundreds of pieces of paper that were involved in the making of the collage. If I had to struggle with each piece of double-

sided tape, the collage was going to take me years to complete instead of months.

Bill was the answer to my dilemma. From September until April, Bill and I sat in the reception room of my home, on opposite sides of an eight-foot table, as I placed photocopies of everything from watch chains to photographs of my great-great-grandmother camping in Algonquin in the 1850s, and Bill stuck them down.

Every week I took a file folder of photographs and small items, such as my Uncle Bruce's glasses, to the local print shop and every week the young woman who served people in the front of the shop grumbled because, "That isn't the kind of thing we do." I knew that mine wasn't the kind of job they wanted: it was finicky, she was always worried that my trinkets would scratch the glass on their photocopiers and they didn't make more than a few dollars from me, ever. They wanted me to order 10,000 of one thing, preferably 8 x 10 in full colour and give them two weeks to get it done. But I persevered and the colour photocopies of all my little knickknacks and photographs looked almost as good as the real thing, plus there was no way I could put the real thing on the collage without making it so heavy that it would collapse under its own weight.

Every Saturday, for three or four hours in the afternoon, Bill and I worked and talked across from each other. When the collage needed work or there was a question about something, we collaborated. Bill was, and still is, one of those artists who can paint anything he sees and make it very realistic. He has never had any formal training; it is just part of who he is, although he has turned his considerable talents to writing now and has some 50 mystery novels up on Amazon.

I know that some of my illustrations were pretty elementary but he didn't say a thing and just let me keep going as my vision, and life, unraveled on paper, Saturday after Saturday.

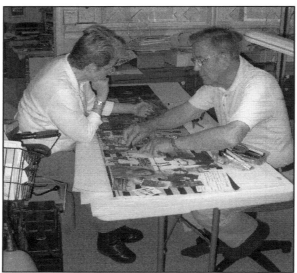

Bill and I worked on the collage together for months

We talked about everything and couldn't help commiserating with each other when it came to our marriages. Ron never said a word. Bill would arrive and often say hi to Ron, but that was it. I was so lonely that I felt if someone touched me tenderly or spoke a kind word to me, I'd burst into tears.

I remember when Bill looked across the table at me and said, "Our problem is, we both need someone to love us." The best Bill and I could manage were long, close hugs, maybe too close, and maybe too long, but they gave us that something we didn't get anywhere else and made us happy. And, don't forget, I couldn't stand up, but I did once and that hug was very special for both of us because Bill realized what it took from me to stand and I felt the warmth of a human body for the first time in many years.

When the collage was finished, I called it *From Good Stock: A Family. A Woman. A Disability.* That title might've been a bit ironic because the stock I came from was genetically riddled with CMT, but I chose to overlook that. My family was *my* family, CMT included.

Bill built a frame for it for the gallery wall and placed the four sections of the 30-foot collage on it. I had written my story, printed it out on beige paper and pasted it below on the black background. I'm not sure how Bill did what he did with it because I never could have mounted it like he did. He did such an excellent job that it looked better than I ever thought it would.

The opening was a Saturday afternoon. Ron said he would drop me off but didn't want to come in. This felt like yet another blow. I had arranged for him to come and pick me up so that I could come home to use the bathroom and have a bite of lunch. I actually talked him into coming back with me ... after all, he was a huge part of the last three or four feet of the collage. Maybe that was the problem.

The collage was covered in the newspaper. Before it came down, Charlie, Ron's best friend, took photographs

My niece, Samantha, looking at the 30-foot From Good Stock collage

of it for me and Cogeco, our local cable TV provider, filmed me reading it. Unfortunately, neither of those efforts proved successful. What did work was the photographs of Robyn Chew. A young professional, Robyn's photographs of the collage were exactly what I needed when I went to have two copies of the original made in vinyl. The original was not stable and I knew that within several weeks it was going to be in pieces.

I had approached several organizations requesting funding to have the collage duplicated and was lucky enough that

Bayshore Medical took on the project and gave me enough money to have two banners made. The replicas were excellent. You couldn't really tell them from the real thing except, of course, for the fact that there were no little edges you could pry up and pick off. Bayshore sponsored the banners so they could be used as a teaching tool and they were sent off to Hamilton, British Columbia, and several other places.

As the printing company was making the big ones, they ran off several smaller ones: one half-size at 15 feet long and another, half of that. I could hardly believe my luck when they gave those to me. My friend, Hannalore, a bookbinder, took both of those and put hardcovers on the front and back but left them so that they could be pulled out into a long banner format. I had seen books like this hand-made in Nepal and I thought it would make an interesting format for these banners because if you cut them up into pages you've lost the continuity of the graphics. The story could be cut apart but the graphics were all melded together in one long continuous stream.

Bill and I decided that we were going to go to lunch together just before Christmas, at the same local plaza where I had met him for the very first time. As I drove into the plaza and started looking for a parking spot I saw him standing in one, motioning me forward. Once in the restaurant we ordered and sat there knowing that, as much as we loved being with each other, it was impossible – but we could dream. We laughed and talked about what-ifs and finally finished our meal, then he followed me back to my place.

When Ron saw us, he told Bill that his wife had called; she was locked out of the house and couldn't find him. Ron had told her that we were having lunch together. Bill hadn't. He hightailed it home and things really got out of hand. Margaret decided that we were having an affair. I guess she was partially right. It was an affair of the heart but nothing else. We were in "deep like," or at least I was.

It was wonderful having someone to talk to, someone who listened and made me laugh and didn't give me a snide answer or criticize my every word or thought. I had labeled Ron a contrarian in my mind and found him to be very negative. I also found it exhausting trying to keep my spirits up when everything he said pulled me down. Something had to change.

"How could you?" was the question put to

Bill by his son after his wife told him that his father was involved with another woman. He wasn't involved with another woman the way she thought he was, but that meant Bill and I could no longer see each other as we had, could no longer commiserate with each other, and there were no more hugs. We did see each other once in a while at art association meetings and we spoke on the phone from time to time, but I couldn't live with the thought of hurting Ron any more than I had already. Ron never said a word, but he'd get a look on his face that told me he knew I was growing away from him and I don't think he knew what to do about it. Or did he not care?

And then a phone call came one afternoon from Bill. I can't remember his exact words but they were something along the lines that he was now single. My immediate thought was that he had left Margaret but, in fact, she had died. Her death was completely unexpected. Bill was now a widower. What he did every day, with whom and where and why, was all up to him.

Did we have a future together? No. I loved Ron far too much and couldn't bear to leave our marriage after everything we had been through and had worked for together: paying off one home and building and paying off another, trying to make a go of it selling antiques and then running CMT International for 18 years. And I had to be realistic: our home was completely accessible to me, our modified van was the only way I could get around, our yard was made for me and then there was the question of the dog ... how could I possibly look after him on my own? I couldn't. If I were with Bill, everything would have to be changed in *his* life to suit *my* disability.

I used to lie awake and wonder how I could possibly get away if I did leave, but even if I could get a suitcase and myself into the van, drive over to Toronto and put myself up at one of the better hotels, I still wouldn't be able to take a bath or even get myself fully dressed without help. Just turning the key in the hotel room door lock was impossible for me and those plastic hotel key cards, have you ever tried to pull one out of the lock slot with your teeth? That's how I have to do it.

I could sense Ron's resentment of me and the help that I needed but I couldn't do a thing about it. Leaving wasn't the answer.

Bill wasn't the answer. Transferring me to someone else or someplace else wasn't the answer. That person would likely end up resenting me as well and no place was like the home I'd designed specifically for my own abilities. And, yes, I also had very real everyday female yearnings, I guess you could call them. The same desires as any woman: the need for touch, for love, and for sexual gratification. But I also had so many other things that had to be done for me, things I needed help with, things that couldn't be ignored while my mind was twirling in sloppy pirouettes trying to figure out how I could fulfill my normal womanly needs and desires.

Was my husband going to be a caregiver or a lover or neither or perhaps a little bit of both? There was still something there, holding us together, I knew it, but was it something I could ferret out so that we could live together in some kind of harmony? That was the question.

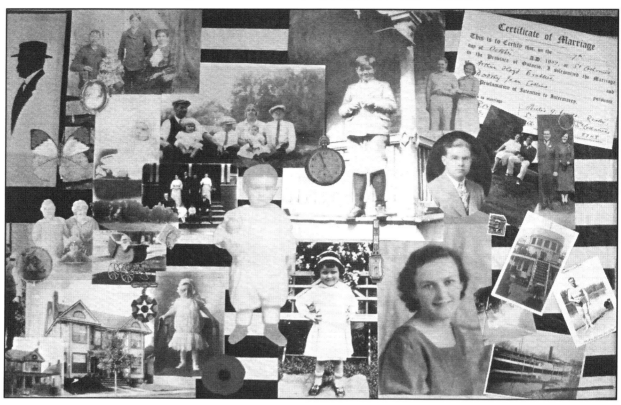

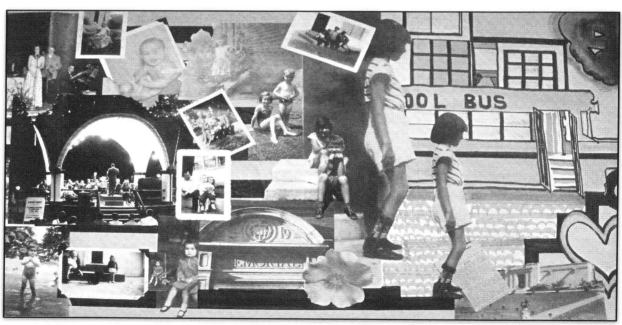

31

The good life

Mom being in long-term care and coping with her death saw Kathie and I become closer than we had ever been. She had driven me over to Burlington on a regular basis to attend a new weight-loss clinic, where my doctor was sure that if I followed their regime I would lose a great deal of weight. I thought that perhaps Kathie would join me in the clinic's program but she declined. She was gaining weight and even her husband was becoming concerned. After six months on the program I had only lost five pounds.

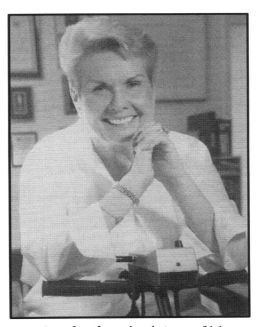

One of my favourite photos – pc31.1

The last time I was there, the director called me into his office and told me that he had reviewed my chart and I was not going to lose any more weight. The fact that my mitochondria, the energy producing part of my cells, was affected by CMT, on top of my age and my inability to exercise, meant I was wasting my time and that of the clinic. There was no need to come back. I had been following a strict 1,200 calorie diet and really didn't find it such a hardship.

Counting calories was far more tedious than what I was eating. I'd never been tossed out of a weight-loss clinic before and I found it almost laughable, but there was also a confusing side to it: if I couldn't lose weight under their watch, could I ever lose it on my own?

Yes, I was worried about what gaining weight would do to me but I was more worried about Kathie's weight than my own. She could walk and exercise but she didn't, and I couldn't figure out why. I remember one afternoon when I was driving her home from a shopping excursion. We pulled up in front of her home and I pleaded with her to look after herself because she was the only member of our family I had left. We were the last. I loved her and I told her so … many times.

Zoomer magazine, for those over 50, had included me in their issue 45/45, portraying

Canadians who were making a difference. Someone by the name of Beasley had said that alpha cities are the ones who realize that it is all about quality of life. I had been trying to persuade our area of the world that they should make life better for those with disabilities since I began writing in my 20s. The little blurb in *Zoomer* was nothing to write home about and I really disliked the photograph, but I got in touch with Paul Alexander, the photographer I had welcomed into our home to take my picture for the magazine, and asked him if he had one of me on my scooter and if so could I have a copy of it.

Several months later a large envelope arrived in the mail with two 11" x 17" prints in it and there I am; elbows leaning on the handlebars of my scooter and a huge smile on my face.

Being in the magazine was definitely secondary to having Paul take the photograph. I loved that in it I looked so happy because I rarely felt that way. I'd had my front teeth done in porcelain veneers, my hair was perfectly blonde and I felt like my spirit radiated from the portrait. In truth, Paul had massaged my ego to the point where I think I would've followed him to Africa if he had suggested it. He had a rakish handsomeness about him and I was very attracted to him, especially his muscular hands and the many string and bead bracelets he wore on his wrists. I

couldn't help wondering what stories were behind them and where his travels with his camera had taken him.

During that time, I began having problems with my voice again because I was using a speech recognition program and any prolonged use of my voice would have it reduced to a gravelly whisper. Losing my voice was the last thing I needed, so I registered for a 16-week course on speech at the local rehab center. We covered a great many areas but I think the thing that I really brought home from that course was a relaxation technique called grounding. The instructor told us that when we lie down most of us are still not relaxed. Relax, she said and let the surface you are on hold you up. That's what it's for.

She also drummed into us the fact that sipping water constantly throughout the day was the way to keep your voice in good shape. Dehydration can really do a number, not only in your body, but your vocal chords. I try to keep a bottle of water right above my computer keyboard and I take a mouthful every time I look at it. And, by drinking small amounts often, I'm not rushing to the toilet.

It was around that time, Christmas 2010, that I began to think that perhaps I would write my autobiography. I even had a title for it: *It Was Never Easy – My life with CMT*. Obviously, I didn't use the title, but it was a thought that would grow into what you're reading today.

In January 2011 Ron and I had to make the terrible decision to put our beloved dog, Val, down. I've written about that in the chapter about my dogs nearer the end, but it was one of the hardest things we've ever had to do. We were both heartsick and we talked to each other as we hadn't in a long time. Our emotions were raw and we needed each other. Believe it or not, the death of our dog brought us closer together.

Because I continued to search for ways to relieve my neuropathic pain, I was open to suggestions from anywhere and anything. I had heard about biofeedback and that it could possibly retrain the brain to relax and stop interpreting the nerve signals from the lower part of my body into pain when there was really no reason for pain at all.

Capped and buckled up for biofeedback

I found a local psychologist who was using biofeedback in his practice and he said he would work with me at our home. I'm not sure how many sessions we had, but the first one was something like a brain mapping. The results were sent away and the feedback showed that the pain center in my brain was indeed lit up bright green.

How many years had I been sitting? Twelve years at the newspaper where I did very little walking and then 18 years at CMT International, at which time my walking slowly came to an entire halt and I went from a walker to a scooter full-time. I have been sitting since 1970, more than 40 years; no wonder my behind and the backs of my legs feel like they are on fire. I learned that my spinal cord was compromised and I had chronic neuropathic pain because of it, but no one is ever really certain about anything when it comes to my CMT.

The psychologist told me that he thought I was manipulative, assertive and persuasive. I agreed to the last two wholeheartedly but as far as manipulative goes, I felt he really didn't understand me. When you have a disability and you need help for so many things, you're not what I would call manipulative. But you do learn to approach people in a different way, so that you don't come across as demanding but as someone asking in the nicest way possible that if they can see their way to help you do something, you would appreciate it. Most people understand, but unfortunately some don't and might feel used. I don't think this man really understood, or will ever understand, what it is like to be unable to do a great many things on your own and as a result be forced to ask for help whether you want to or not.

Heartland Forest, the 93-acre accessible woodlot in Niagara Falls, had received funding for a major build that would become offices, classrooms, party areas, workshops, and meeting and exhibition spaces. I was taken on as the accessibility coordinator. I worked with the architect and for almost a year was up to my eyeballs sourcing comfort height toilets, grab bars, adult diaper change tables, emergency eye wash fountains, sinks, automatic faucets, soap and paper towel dispensers, wall and floor tiles, door and drawer handles, automatic door openers – you name it. We all wanted the place to be as accessible as possible. We followed the Facility Accessibility Design Standards (FADS) developed for Ontario and exceeded them wherever possible. I'd never done anything like this work before although I had designed our home and taken courses on universal design, but who knew there were so many different types of garbage cans or soap dispensers? The catalogs came pouring in and I began learning.

Brock University asked me if they could put my image on a bus shelter. I laughed and said sure. The city put Crabtree on the list for possible street signs. They don't ask you if you want your name on a street but I

thought that having the family name on a signpost somewhere might be kind of nice.

Kathie and I would go to Buffalo to shop just to see what was offered in the stores in the USA compared to Canada. Clothing certainly is cheaper in the United States and we'd come home with enough cotton knit tops to last the entire winter.

I begged Kathie to make a CD so that we would always have something that captured her beautiful voice. She always said she would, but always put it off.

In the spring of 2012 I thought I'd like to get my hands into the dirt. I loved gardening but could no longer get down onto the ground. My idea was a large cedar garden box, something like a cradle on tall legs, but I found out it was going to cost $3,000. After I called the city to ask if I could put it a few feet north of our carport and they said no, as it would be on the city boulevard, I rethought my plan. If I had to keep my garden within our property line I came up with the idea of wine barrels, seven of them. Because we live in wine country, I was able to find barrels already cut in half for $50 each and Ron kindly offered to pick them up and bring them home in the van. Once in place, I found they were still too low for me to reach comfortably while seated on my scooter. Two eight-inch square by 20-inch long oak lengths placed under each barrel raised them up high enough so that I could slide up beside each one. When it was filled with Perlite and a light soil mixture, I could plant tomatoes, cucumbers, zucchini and flowers. That first spring started off with brilliant blue pansies and ended up with more tomatoes than we could possibly eat, so they went to our neighbours. I also had a rose garden dug and planted it with cream and yellow tea roses. There's nothing I like better than roses, except orchids, in the bathroom and kitchen.

By my 70th birthday in April 2012, I was still working on nine bathrooms for Heartland Forest and at the same time the biofeedback therapy sessions were trying to get me to relax my mind in the company of two strangers. I couldn't do both even though I would've liked to. I enjoyed the challenge of Heartland Forest immensely but the biofeedback, not so much. A tight cap with holes on it had to be put on my head, the skin under each hole was roughened with what felt like sandpaper, and then a conductor with sticky goo was placed in the hole. After 20 minutes or half an hour of trying to tell my mind to stop working, the cap was removed and my hair was an absolute mess and had to be washed. This was just one reason why I stopped the biofeedback sessions. Another was that I sensed it was a toss-up between letting go of the projects my brain enjoyed working on or having pain. I guess I chose pain.

I knew that when I worked really hard my CMT would worsen. An occupational therapist and I went to a huge trade show at the Exhibition Centre in Toronto, where I looked at electric wheelchairs, thinking that being able to relax in a reclining wheelchair from time to time might make it easier to work. I arranged to try a loaner at the house but the one they brought me didn't have a reclining option. I did use it often enough to know that my problems with one in the past were no different now – the protruding footrests seemed to be in the way of everything I wanted to do – and the chair I thought I needed was hugely expensive, as much as a small car. I was also thinking about a suprapubic catheter that would be permanent, which meant I might be able to travel again and wouldn't have to use the toilet during the day. But I had to be realistic, catheter or not, Ron didn't want to travel and I didn't want to go without him. I had to decide what would work best for me and for Ron. I decided to stay with what I had. I bought myself a new electric scooter and forgot about the catheter. I'm good for four hours between bathroom breaks and that'll have to do.

Ron always went along with anything I wanted to try but all this experimenting and indecision was hard on us. We needed predictability, stability and calm … something you can't always have with a progressive condition like CMT.

In the fall I decided to reorganize my office and other parts of the house that were cluttered. I knew I couldn't do it myself and Ron and I usually ended up arguing when we took on tasks like that together. I remembered reading about the late Judith Snow, a quadriplegic who used a wheelchair full-time, and her support circle of friends who helped her get through university and live a decent life when everyone else thought she belonged in long-term care doing nothing.

I wondered if I had enough friends who would help me get rid of the clutter and change things around, so that every time I looked at a wall I wasn't looking at something I had to fix but knew it was physically impossible for me to do. My office housed a huge carpenter's chest of drawers with nothing much in it but used computer parts, shelves full of books I was never going to read again, and files dating back 15 years. My hands were so bad I could barely open drawers or pull the files and I hoped that the people I asked to help understood. I could tell them what I needed and wanted but I couldn't do the work myself. I could barely hold a brush but I could buy the paint. I couldn't hold a screwdriver or hammer but I could buy the wood and brackets for shelves. I needed their time and generosity of spirit and I needed their strength and energy. Jasper, Eileen, Alison and Irma gave it to me in spades.

Within three weeks my office looked like a different place. My big teak desk that I'd used for 18 years working CMT International found a new home as well as my teak bookshelves and I had new shelving built on two walls in my office. My computer and printers are perfectly situated for me to just roll up in front of the computer on my scooter, stick a pillow behind my back, turn the seat and put my feet on a raised platform that has an electric heating pad on it to keep them warm during the winter. What more can a girl ask for?

In December 2012 the roof went on at Heartland Forest and finally the interior was safe from the elements. It had taken more than a year.

In January 2013 we bought a swivel seat for the passenger side of the van because I could no longer stand up from my scooter in the back and squeeze between the seats to sit in the passenger or the driver's seat. The swivel seat turned and I could transfer sideways from my scooter seat onto it and then turn it to face the windshield. If I wanted to drive, I could use my transfer board to slide between the passenger seat and the driver's seat. I would then clip my quad grip into its bracket on the steering wheel so that I didn't have to grip the actual steering wheel with my hand. With my entire right hand lying in the metal grip, I use my hand, wrist and arm to steer. The gas and brake are controlled with a very light touch of my left hand through the Sure Grip hand control below the steering wheel to the left. Driving for me is one of the few pleasures I have and, although it plays havoc on my arms and shoulders, I intend to drive as long as possible.

The spring of that year I was very depressed and simply couldn't shake it. I finally figured out it was the Clonazepam. Drugs like that, I found out, have a half-life, so taking it every day meant that it never really left my system. Through its overlapping, time and time again, I became so morose I was suicidal. I really couldn't see any reason for me being here. Thank God for spring.

When the ditches began to turn green, the frogs sang and a light green haze hung over everything, I felt I was ready to get going again. The office was organized. It was time to look at our backyard.

A trip to the builder's supply store in Niagara Falls saw Ron and me select an 800-pound granite boulder. I hired a landscaping company to come and take out our little pond at the back of the house and install the rock as a bubbler. Our big, beautiful beige boulder was drilled right up through its centre, a large reservoir was put in the ground and covered with some of the beach stone we have all over the property, and then four men manoeuvred our rock on top of the reservoir. A plastic tube went from the reservoir up through the drilled hole and a recirculating pump in the reservoir sent the water up through the stone, over the edge and then back down into the reservoir. Before the rock was put in place, the top surface was hollowed out just enough to hold as much water as that of a bird bath. The birds absolutely love it.

You may remember that when we moved into the house in 1989, I had designed a large pond out back featuring a granite waterfall. One summer our beautiful fat goldfish ended up as a midnight snack for raccoons and I had the big pond made into a smaller four by four-foot lily pond where an occasional pink lotus would leave me in awe. Through these transitions I began to learn that a water feature could be a lot of work and, in truth, I enjoyed the sound of it more than I did the visual aspect. This bubbling rock was going to be permanent and I was very happy to know that the sound of it was extremely pleasing and the birds plus all the squirrels, rabbits, moles and even an occasional groundhog made it their go-to oasis. It wasn't uncommon to see brilliant yellow goldfinches hanging in the hemlock above, waiting to float down and drink or to witness what I call an "argue" of sparrows, bickering full tilt with each other in the branches while they wait for bathing room on the rock below where they would once again fight until one pushed another off, only to fly again into the branches above. They always remind me of a bunch of little boys playing King of the Castle.

Test results around that time told me that my iron was low, which meant my red blood cells weren't working at their best to carry oxygen to my organs, including my lungs and heart. I had to do something to help myself and I eventually found everything I needed. Believe it or not, for many years I had eaten liver for breakfast. I love the taste but the smell finally did me in. An iron supplement was prescribed but I was so constipated on it that I couldn't use it. Then I found Lorna Vanderhaeghe's iron capsules and have been taking them ever since. I'm no longer anemic but have to watch it.

With my impaired capacity to breathe in and out, due to my partially paralyzed diaphragm at only 60% of normal lung capacity, anything that jeopardizes my ability to utilize oxygen has to be seriously considered. I see my respirologist regularly and have used a Symbicort inhaler, morning and night, ever since. I still take Coenzyme Q10, 400 mg a day. I'm convinced it helps my red blood cells carry more oxygen to my vital organs. Having said that, I know that we are all different; we all have our own thoughts on what works for us personally and our own vitamin regimes.

That fall I also decided to refurbish the two bathrooms. The guest bathroom had a new sink installed under a granite vanity top and a new larger and lower mirror put in place. Our en-suite bathroom glowed with a fresh coat of paint (Daybreak yellow), new cupboard and drawer pulls, strip light fixtures that feature huge Fat Albert bulbs, granite countertops with deep sinks tucked beneath them, and much larger, lower mirrors. All the shower tile was repointed, new thick glass shelves we're put in to hold soap and shampoo, and a new Moen handheld shower head with a built-in loop that went around the back of my hand (meaning I was much less liable to drop it) was installed. I figured if I didn't make the changes I wanted then, I wouldn't have the energy to do it later.

It seemed then that everything was going well. I was busy with work that kept my mind off of my pain and was excited by what I was doing. The house and yard had never looked better. Kathie and I were connecting regularly and I loved having her in my life. My pain was under control most of the time and Ron and I were closer than we had been in years. Life was good.

32

Why Kathie?

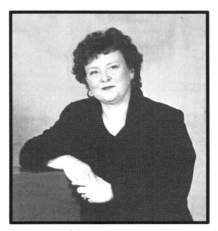

Kathie Gosen – pc32.1

Sunday, February 2, 2014 - 2:30 p.m.

Ron and I had been to Betty's Restaurant in Chippawa near Niagara Falls for brunch. When we got home I took to the couch to get warmed up. The telephone rang.

Ron answers: "Oh hi, Paul. Yes, she is."

He gives me the phone, saying "It's Paul."

Paul: "Are you sitting down?"

Me: "I'm lying down."

Paul: "Kathie's dead."

Me: "What?"

Paul: "Kathie's dead."

Me: "Oh, Paul, no. Oh God, no."

Paul: "I got up, you know how she likes to sleep in, and I went downtown. When I came back I looked and she was still sleeping, I thought, so I went up to Brock for a sauna and swim and when I came back I looked up at the house and the blind was still down on the upstairs (bedroom) window and I thought something was wrong. I went up to the bedroom and touched her. She was cold."

Kathie had obviously been dead for quite some time to be cold. Paul called his friend Berndt and he told him to call 911. An ambulance and the police arrived and, even as Paul was talking to me, a policewoman interrupted us and wanted to know if they had a good relationship. I said they were devoted to each other – and they were. One of their friends told me there was a little bouquet of pink rosebuds on the kitchen counter with a note – "Love you, I'm at Brock." Paul had, as usual, been dumpster diving behind The Watering Can florists on his way home from downtown and had brought them home for her.

My heart was broken. I loved her so very much. I kept asking myself why. At 59, why?

Kathie's girls came home: Kitty from Toronto and Julia from New York City. I can't imagine how they felt on their way to face the unthinkable. Somehow the girls and their father managed to arrange a funeral service and St. George's Anglican Church was bursting at the seams with people. Kathie was much loved by so many.

269

The eulogy was written by Paul and the girls, and although I can't remember any of it, I do remember wondering at the time how they ever pulled themselves together enough to write something so beautiful.

As everyone filed out of the church proper to the reception upstairs, I had a hard time leaving her ashes behind. I kept thinking, how can they just leave her there? I wanted to gather her up and take her with me.

At the reception I found myself surrounded by people that I barely knew. I had asked her theatrical friends from Garden City Productions if they would sing a tribute to her, either in the church or at the reception, but I suppose they found my request either distasteful or they were stunned by the fact that one of their own had been taken so young. In any case, nothing was done. At one point, when I found myself alone, I left the room and wound my way back down to the church. Her ashes were sitting there covered in green velvet surrounded by beautiful flowers. The organist was still sitting on the bench doing paperwork and I asked him if he would play *There's No Business, Like Show Business* for her. The service had been lovely but so solemn and I didn't think it represented my Kathie, but it wasn't my call. I was her sister, not her child or husband.

As the notes of my request bounced off the beams in that huge church, I leaned forward from my scooter, placed my hand on her ashes and tried to sing the words for her. Not much came out, but in my mind I could hear her pure voice singing along with me and she had a smile on her face. I've never seen anybody who could sing and smile at the same time like she could. Every word she sang came from her heart and soul and you believed it. She had her father's perfect pitch and she was genuinely a true spirit.

Twelve years younger than me, I had watched her grow up, play Daisy Mae through a wicked chest cold in a high school production of *L'il Abner*, date several brilliant fellows whom we all knew were gay but weren't sure she did, and then fall in love with Paul Gosen, who had just graduated with a degree in bilingual journalism. They bought a little century-old brick house on one of the nicest and oldest streets in the city, renovated it, and eventually filled it with the laughter of two beautiful little girls.

Their Christmas dinners were the stuff of legends and the beautifully decorated little house simply bubbled over with relatives, friends, and people on their own with no place to go on that special day.

Introduced to a local amateur theatre group by her mother-in-law, Barbara, Kathie took to the stage like a duck to water. When she died she was looking forward to playing Miss Hannigan in *Annie*. It was to be her

35th performance. When she got the part she'd called me all excited and pleased. "There will be three of us," she said, "one very tall and thin and two round." She considered herself round.

Thank heaven for habit. I was grieving so deeply that my mind was never on what I was supposed to be doing, but routine and habit saw me able to go about my daily chores fairly well although waking up every morning was like waking into a nightmare. My only peace was through sleep. I'd cry myself into an exhausted slumber every night and as soon as I woke up everything would come flooding back. I began taking Clonazepam again just to get some sleep but again found that it added depression to grief and I didn't need that.

It took months for me to stop crying. It would just happen out of the blue. One minute I would be fine and the next, tears would be running down my face. We never did get to bury her ashes. Paul still has them at the house. Nobody wants to let her go.

Kathie was the last member of my immediate family. She was my rock. She was the person I thought would look out for my welfare if Ron was gone. Now *she* was gone. I know that sounds selfish but there is often dependency amongst family members and I think it is justified. Kin should at least try to look out for each other. I still have my suspicions that her addiction to diet colas and hamburgers did her in and high blood pressure was also a real concern. You can't really change your genetic makeup and our father died the same way at age 57. She was a loving mother and, according to Paul, a partner beyond compare. As far as I'm concerned, she was a part of me and I loved her unconditionally.

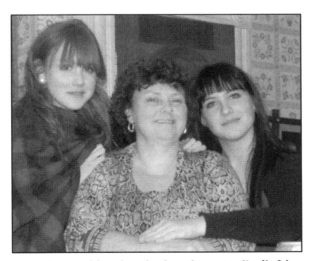

Kathie and her lovely daughters: Julia (left) and Kitty

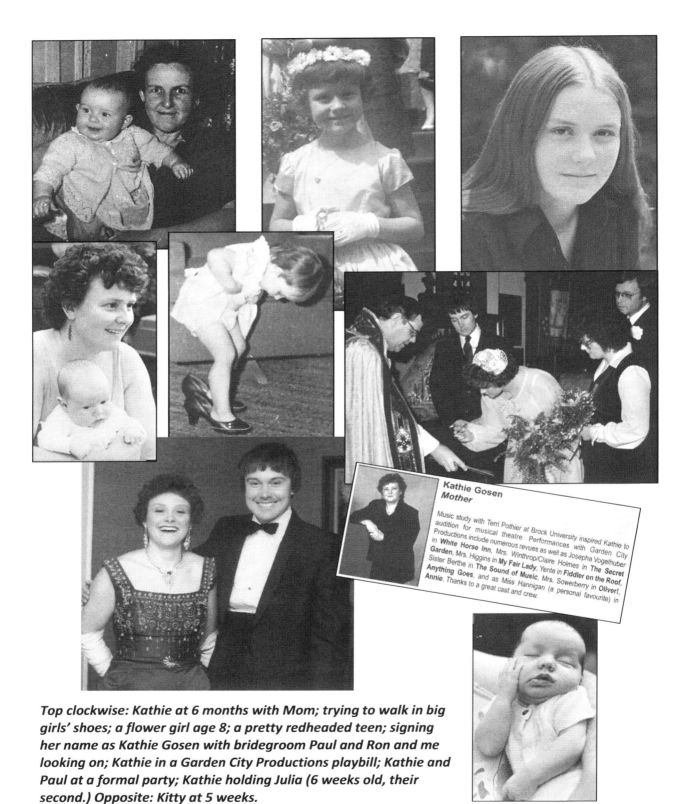

Top clockwise: Kathie at 6 months with Mom; trying to walk in big girls' shoes; a flower girl age 8; a pretty redheaded teen; signing her name as Kathie Gosen with bridegroom Paul and Ron and me looking on; Kathie in a Garden City Productions playbill; Kathie and Paul at a formal party; Kathie holding Julia (6 weeks old, their second.) Opposite: Kitty at 5 weeks.

272

33

CMT and All That Jazz

I remember writing in my journal, *"If I'm sick it must be December."* It never failed, every year around Christmas I would get that familiar feeling that I had learned throughout the years was my body fighting something off and not winning. I'd usually have a bad sinus headache, then a sore throat that eventually went south as bronchitis or even pneumonia. When things progressed down into my bronchial tubes and lungs, I was in trouble. First, I would cough so often and so hard that eventually I would lose my ability to cough. That isn't good because you can't get the gunk up. I'd also lose the ability to blow my nose after blowing it for the hundredth time. My diaphragm, the large dome-shaped sheet of muscle under your ribs that helps you push air out of your lungs, would simply give out as it is affected by CMT and the nerves that fire it to work would simply stop firing. Without the ability to cough or blow my nose I was in trouble: fluid would accumulate in my lungs and I'd have a terrible time breathing.

After spending hours waiting for help in the emergency department of our local hospital during one of these bronchial episodes, where I wanted to lay down so badly I was actually leaning up against the wall while seated on my scooter, I was finally treated using a nebulizer with Salbutamol in it. Inhaling the fine mist from the nebulizer let me breathe again and I asked my pulmonologist if there wasn't something I could do at home so I wouldn't have to go through that awful scenario at the hospital. He prescribed a nebulizer for me and vials of Salbutamol.

Now when I find myself headed for bronchitis or pneumonia, I take an antibiotic called Biaxin right away. I also take extra good care of myself, get plenty of sleep and hope for the best. If the infection progresses down into my lungs, the nebulizer makes it possible for me to breathe in spite of the congestion. I can't think of anything more terrifying than trying to sleep sitting up because I'm afraid that I'm going to stop breathing if I lie down.

Back in late January 2014 I was just getting over a three-week bout of bronchitis when Kathie came swooping into my bedroom with a vase full of beautiful yellow tulips and put them on the windowsill where it was cool. She was dead within days but those tulips didn't die. The cold kept them just the way they were when she'd brought them until they almost turned to dust. Now every time I see yellow tulips I think about my Kathie the way she was when she was happy and doing good for others, which was most the time.

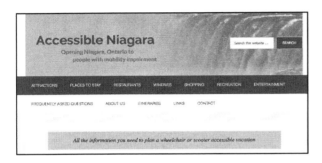

That January I followed up on my promise to myself to completely rework AccessibleNiagara.com, as now The Access for Ontarians with Disabilities Act (AODA) was asking everyone with a website to make it accessible for everyone. Being that AccessibleNiagara had been built expressly for people with disabilities who wanted to travel to Niagara, I thought it only right that the site be totally accessible. I mentioned this to Marissa at the Niagara Parks Commission and she got me in touch with someone who got me in touch with someone else and eventually I ended up with a Masters of Design student, Tom Pokinko, living in Ottawa, who was taking his degree online through the OCAD University in Toronto. He needed a thesis project and agreed to rework

AccessibleNiagara.com to fulfill its requirement.

Tom and I worked on the site for five months. I re-wrote all the lengthy hotel descriptions and, as much as possible, put everything in point form. Detail is important on a site like this because a simple thing like a lip on a shower can stop the person in a wheelchair from bathing. We tried to keep as much detail in as possible without going overboard with words. We used the WordPress format, which meant I could add, delete and rewrite anything on it. The new site was launched in June, but without photographs. There had been hundreds of photographs on the old site and I firmly believe a photograph of a shower that shows no lip on it says more than anything I can write, but all the photos came over in one huge clump and I had no idea what shower belonged to what hotel and so on ... so, no photos.

When I mentioned that I had always wanted to produce a video for the website to a young man who was visiting me for a completely different reason, he said, "Well you're in luck, I just happen to be a graduate of the Toronto Film School." I had never produced a video before but managed to raise about $5,000 and write a script. Jordan Fowler did a lovely job videoing the five couples, including Ron and me, who volunteered to go to a dozen venues in Niagara Falls and be recorded.

We made sure the resulting six-minute video, *Niagara Falls on Wheels: Seeing is believing*, was closed-captioned and I wrote a separate voiceover to describe the action for people who could not see it. It went up on the new AccessibleNiagara.com as well as YouTube. We stopped printing guides. It was just too much work raising the money

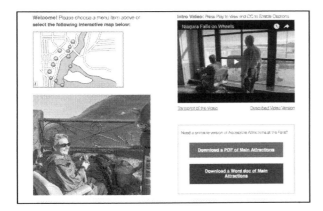

to have it printed, weeks of work to put it together and the delivery? Well, neither Eileen nor I were getting any younger and it was a tough job. Seeing the finished printed product was like giving birth to something after being pregnant for a year, but at what cost? The Accessible Niagara website attracts many viewers. It must be working because I now get a lot fewer private email queries for information than I used to.

On the home front, I took it upon myself to redo our kitchen. That sounds like I was going to do it myself, but with my hands quickly deteriorating everything has to be done by someone else; however, I'm a pretty good organizer. The counter was wearing out where I ate my breakfast every morning and I had a ball picking out a huge slab of granite for the kitchen counter. Shopping for granite is the ultimate buying experience for me. It's like choosing a huge mural painted by Mother Nature that you get to enjoy every day. After much deliberation, I picked a huge slab that had some life to it as it contains all shapes and sizes of translucent quartz flakes along with white, grey, beige, brown and black pieces of mineral. The rest of the kitchen is fairly plain; the countertop is the focal point.

I had no idea granite sinks existed but they do and we now have a beige one. A fresh coat of off-white paint matching the white in the granite on all the cupboards and drawers, which coordinated with the off-white tile backsplash that had various shades of brown, grey and black glass tile accents running through it, really spruced things up. We already had new stainless steel appliances. When we built the house, I had designed the kitchen with the wall oven high enough so I could reach inside from my scooter and I also incorporated a stovetop built into the counter. Because I can't bend over or reach very well, I also made sure that there were plenty of drawers and found out that I was using them for everything from paper towels and vitamins to dishes held upright in a dish rack, utensils for cooking and eating, kitchen linens and of course pots and pans. A Lazy Susan in the lower corner holds flour, sugar and condiments. I believe there are 23 cupboards and drawers and I've plenty of counter space for chopping and mixing or, rather, Ron does because he does 99% of the cooking.

The one thing I made sure of was that there was continuity of countertop surface from the stovetop past the sinks to the counter where I eat my breakfast and then to the microwave and beyond that to the refrigerator. With that long stretch of countertop, which is thin in front of the sinks, there is an area for me to slide a pot from the stove to the sink or slide a soft-boiled egg in an egg cup across in front of the sinks to where I have my breakfast. I call this the "slide factor" and what it means is that I never have to pick up anything hot, heavy or breakable as, nine times out of 10, I will drop it.

It is likely obvious by now that nothing really stops me from doing what I want or need to do. But after Kathie's death I found my CMT had progressed to the point where, and this is very personal, I could no longer wipe myself after a bowel movement. I couldn't hold the paper and in trying to reach back from the front, I had a chronic bruise on my arm where it was pressed and scraped up against the toilet seat. I began to worry that it might never heal; after all, I was making it worse day after day by simply going about my business. It was then that I remembered back to the days when we ran CMT International. A lawyer had gotten in

touch with me and asked me what she could do to make things easier for her as she was trying to regulate her bowel movements so she wouldn't have to use the washroom at work. She was having the same trouble with her hands that I had. I did a little research and found the Toto Washlet seat that plugs into an electrical outlet and is also connected to the water that goes into your toilet. It runs automatically; all you have to do is press a

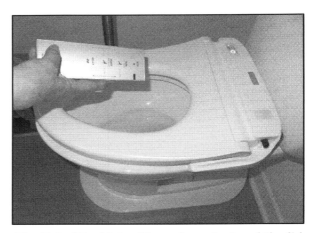

The Toto Washlet with push control and the lid off because it hindered a side transfer

button and it will not only wash but dry you, back and front.

I talked to Ron, after my doctor had agreed to write me a prescription for one, and we went to one of our local plumbing showrooms and, yes, they could get one for me but I would need to have the same make of toilet (bowls come in oval or round), so that it would all fit. It all had to be 22 inches high so I could transfer from my scooter to the seat, as I'd found that I could no longer stand up to sit down on the toilet. Having to transfer sideways meant we also needed a toilet riser that goes between the floor and toilet to bring it up to the needed height. The people where we bought the new toilet and Washlet told us where to get the riser. When everything was finally delivered we had a plumber come in and, in a matter of an hour, I had everything I needed to take care of my personal hygiene. It took me about a half an hour to read the instructions and set the digital controls and everything worked beautifully, except the seat lid would rise at the oddest times and was in the way when I tried to transfer sideways, so we took it off.

The entire project cost about $3,600, but the way I figured it, I didn't have to ask Ron to do something that neither he nor I wanted him to do. The Muscular Dystrophy Association of Canada, which I have been a member of for many years, helped us pay for much of it. That's why I tell people who have CMT to register with the Muscular Dystrophy Association in their province/state/country. You never know when you're going to need help and CMT, although it is a muscular atrophy rather than a dystrophy, is covered under their umbrella. Having them help us with the cost of this much-needed assistive device was very much appreciated. The Washlet continues to allow me independent toileting.

While we are on the subject of personal hygiene, I'll mention that I now slide from my scooter seat onto a shower bench that was built to protrude out of the shower. I can transfer onto the end that's out of the shower and then slide over to an open padded shower seat. My shampoo and facial scrub are within reach, as is the sisal Scandinavian-style back scrubber I love. The shower controls are easy to reach on my right. All of this means I can shower by myself.

How many so-called accessible showers have I seen in hotels with the bench at one end of the shower and the controls and showerhead at the other? If you can't walk to get into the shower, chances are you won't be able to get up off of the shower bench and walk to the other end of the shower to turn it on and off. I don't know where people's heads are when they design things like this but they certainly aren't thinking about people with real disabilities. The shower design and Toto Washlet let me be independent and allow me a small modicum of dignity. I guess you'd say that my motto is: "Let me do what I can until I can't" – and that includes looking after my personal hygiene.

For years I slept flat in bed with only a regular pillow under my head and then I started to wake up in the morning with a massive headache, something like a hangover, but it would go away after I been up for about 20 minutes. I'd been tested in the early '80s and knew my diaphragm was partially paralyzed. I'd also had a sleep test. Through that, my pulmonologist knew that if I sleep flat my diaphragm has to work extra hard to allow me to breathe out well enough. I wake up with a massive headache because I am unable to get rid of all of the CO_2 I should be breathing out.

To breathe better while in bed, I bought a new adjustable bed and that allows me to elevate the head to give my diaphragm the benefit of gravity while I sleep. This helps immensely. And, as I mentioned previously, I had read about Coenzyme Q10 helping red blood cells carry more oxygen to every part of the body and thought to myself, anything that lets me experience the benefit of more oxygen would be worth a try. I began with the lowest amount of CoQ10 they sold on the health supplements shelves and now, some 25 years later, I am taking 400 mg a day. Using the combination of an adjustable bed and CoQ10, the only time I have one of those terrible headaches is when I either overwork my diaphragm by talking, coughing or blowing my nose too much, or exhaust myself doing something I simply shouldn't be doing.

That brings me to pacing. Trying to learn to pace myself was, and still is, for me one of the most difficult things I've ever had to try to do. When I get an idea, I'm usually gung-ho on it because I'm excited. Sometimes I

feel as if my brain is on fire; I have so much enthusiasm. However, as I age, I find I am able to do less and am satisfied with what I can do without totally exhausting myself. I used to have a dozen or more projects going all the time, but not now. My weekly to do list has gone from 25 or 30 items to maybe a dozen and if I don't get them done, I carry them over to the next week. It doesn't really matter anymore. I have nothing to prove, but I do feel a certain amount of satisfaction in getting projects that interest me accomplished.

I've heard people say that they'd rather be dead if they couldn't walk. Personally, not being able to walk is nothing compared to losing the use of my hands and living in constant pain. Burning neuropathic pain is always with me. When at a meeting, I used to see people who use wheelchairs shifting and lifting themselves in their seats and I'd often wonder what they were experiencing. Now I know the pain can become almost unbearable when you have to sit in one position for any length of time and, when you can't walk or stand, you have no alternative but to sit, grin and bear it.

We all experience pain differently but we all try to relieve it in much the same ways. I had tried some 30 drugs and pain-relieving techniques, by which I mean acupuncture, massage, exercise, nerve blocks and biofeedback, to mention just a few. Nothing has worked well enough that I can keep using it. I began using marijuana but it really didn't help the pain, though it did help the muscle spasms I get in my biceps, triceps and those big muscles that run up and down the rib cage. It also helps me get to sleep. I can actually feel myself relaxing about five minutes after one deep inhale of an equally low CBD to THC ratio marijuana (THC 10.1% : CBD 6.9%), taken using a PAX vaporizer that I can easily work with my hands.

If I keep busy during the day I can bear the pain and I always use a thick gel pad on my scooter seat. I still get a pressure sore about twice a year but it usually heals in 10 days or so. Without the pad, sitting is agony.

It is always between 6 and 8:00 at night that I feel as if I'm on fire from the hips down. I remember back when Mom was in long-term care, she and the rest of the people on her floor would always be in worse shape in the early evening. The nurses called it the "sundown syndrome" and I wondered if that's what I was experiencing. After all those drugs and searching, I simply rely on the cold packs that athletes use to take down swellings and keep six at time in the freezer. I find the cold deadens the pain and I can actually relax with one under each knee and one under my right hip. Pain tightens me up and to be able to relax, to let go, is akin to heaven.

Slowly losing the use of my hands is one of the most difficult things I've had to face. Way back when Ron and I were painting the walls of the office at 34 Bayview, I remember acknowledging the fact that my thumbs no longer worked. Before that, my job at The Standard required that I type pretty well all day long and in order to do that, I wove a short pencil from the bowling alley under my index finger over my big middle finger and under the ring finger of each hand. That made my big fingers stiff and I could hit the keys with those two fingers. I typed like that for 12 years at the paper and for many years after until the muscles across the bridge of my hand got so weak that the stiff finger wouldn't point. That's when I began typing with the knuckles of my little fingers and looking into speech-activated software. I have dictated 95% of this book using the speech program that came with my desktop Mac.

Now my fingers will not straighten at all and I also have no grip as I cannot close my fingers into my palm. This plus my paralyzed thumbs make it very difficult to pick things up and I almost always have to use both hands to lift something. Without thumbs it is very difficult to undo tubes of paint so I look for tubes with flip-top lids. I ask my pharmacist to put my prescriptions in a bottle with an attached lid and a large overhang that I can get the side of the palm of my hand under. Ron has fashioned handles for the wide lids of stick and roll-on dispensers, so I can get them off by myself.

Just as I experienced foot drop as a youngster, I am now experiencing wrist drop. My wrists will no longer hold up my hands.

Many years ago, I had a wrist brace made that wound around my wrist and had a tongue that went out under the palm of my hand to hold my hand up. That brace was held on with Velcro and since I can no longer do up or undo Velcro, I had another brace made that is flexible enough to simply clip onto my wrist and hold my hand up.

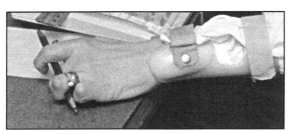

Wearing my old wrist brace with Velcro and the pencil woven through my fingers (1987)
pc33.1

And even though many years ago I said I would never wear a wrist brace to bed, I now find my wrist no longer aches during the day if I keep it in a neutral position at night. Since my natural position in sleep is to curl my wrists in, a soft fabric wrist brace that anchors around my left thumb keeps my hand from curling in. Since my mobility depends on my being able to slide my body from scooter to toilet, couch, bed and passenger seat of the car, it is imperative that I keep my wrists in good shape.

My right hand is almost totally paralyzed

and I can't flex my right wrist, but I can use it up against my left hand and wrist to pull and lift things. I can still brush my teeth using an electric toothbrush, and I still attempt to put on some makeup to make myself look as good as I can but it's not easy. Brushing my hair is a challenge

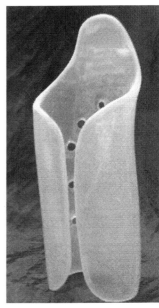

My present wrist brace – the tongue holds up my hand - no fastener

because the brush simply falls out of my hand as would the hair dryer if I hadn't figured out how to hold it balanced on my right hand. And eyeliner is something I used to wear every day but reality has hit home and I only attempt it for special occasions.

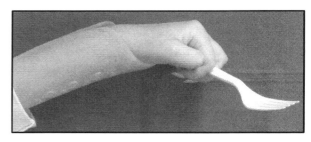

Mascara and a bit of eyeshadow followed by some yellow redness corrector under my eyes are about all I can manage. I recognized at an early age that I am fortunate to have my mother's soft flawless

280

skin and have moisturized day and night since age 15 ... that's 60 years! At my age, I think it prudent to wear less makeup because too much simply accentuates flaws and wrinkles. Most mornings when I look in the mirror I see an older woman with short grey hair, a nose and chubby cheeks that remind her of her father, her mother's eyes and complexion, and a firm resolve to take on the day no matter what it throws at her.

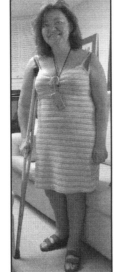

Iveta Leipa

In 2010, eight years after CMT International closed, I had a request from a woman who lived in Latvia but was visiting Ontario. She wanted to come and see me. I hadn't had a visit from anyone with CMT for years and I welcomed her and her translator, Agra, into our home. Her name is Iveta (pronounced Eveta) Leipa and from the time she began walking she has experienced what CMT can do. At 33, she went to university as a mature student and studied the Latvian language, graduating with a master's degree and a specialty in editing. She has always worked and, as a sideline, writes poetry.

Thanks to Agra, Iveta, now 45, and I spent three hours together and the conversation ranged from having jump rings on everything we owned with a zipper to, of course, our hands and feet. I featured Iveta and our visit on my lindacrabtree.wordpress.com blog in July 2010. Agra took some pictures that I think illustrate beautifully what CMT hands can look like and I'll add some photos I've collected throughout the years of CMT. As individuals, none of us experience CMT exactly the same way but it helps to know we are not alone no matter how the condition manifests itself.

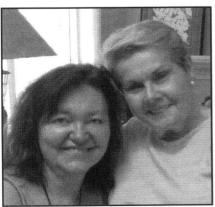
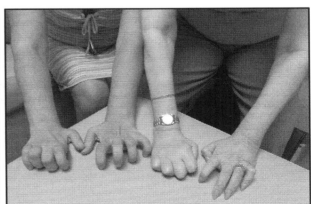

Comparing hands: Iveta's on the left and mine.

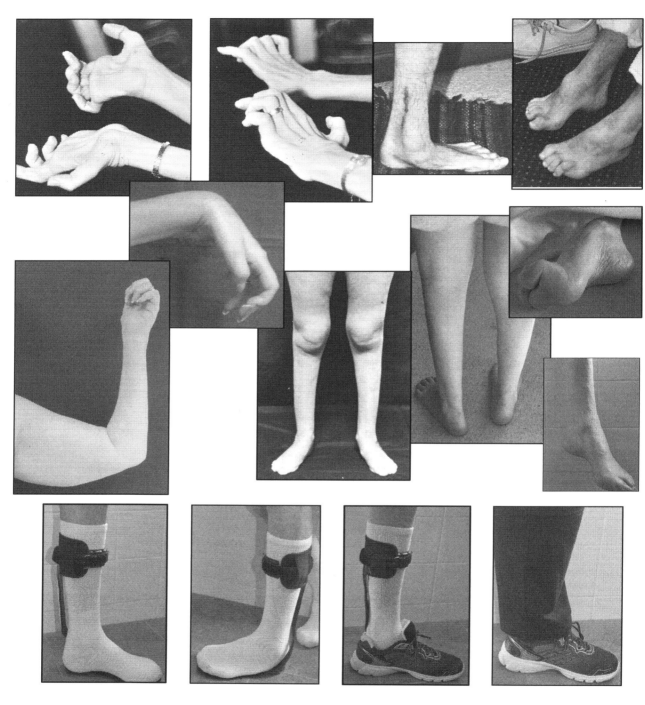

Top row: CMT can affect the hands leaving them with atrophied muscles and/or numbness, flat feet or very high arched feet. Second row: atrophied lower arm and hand, wrist drop, atrophied lower leg front and back, Mom's high arch foot and cocked toes, foot drop. Bottom row: foot in ankle-foot orthosis (AFO), other side, AFO in shoe, pant leg down, AFO invisible – pc33.2-6.

34

And then love

This chapter isn't about work or my CMT; it's about love.

Most of the people that I have loved throughout my life have died: my father, brother, mother and sister only exist in my memory and my heart, but in a way, they are also very real as they are in my thoughts daily. They have made me who I am and, very simply, they are part of me.

When Ron and I met and married there were no declarations of undying love for each other; it just wasn't our style, although I think I could've gotten into it if he had. In fact, there was no mention of love at all. We were obviously very happy with each other but displays of affection and the three little words never came into play.

As the years went by and our relationship grew distant, I began to feel the need for something more. It seemed we could talk about anything but love and intimacy. If I brought up the subject he would say, "*Please, let's not start that again.*" THAT was everything to me and I couldn't understand how he could be so unfeeling.

When we first met, I told him I liked to travel. He said he had been to Spain and travel wasn't out of the question. Running CMT International, we travelled across Canada several times together but after one meeting in the United States that he attended with me, I was on my own. I had to find someone else to go on vacation and to England and Scotland with me. Even a holiday in Florida was too much for him. I went with my niece or a friend. At one time he told me that he didn't like being called Mr. Crabtree. I always thought he was bigger than that, and he is.

When intimacy became nonexistent, I tied myself into knots that eventually undid themselves with the realization that he was doing everything he could. His bladder cancer and my painful muscle spasms sealed the deal.

And, when the dog died and Ron was insistent that we not get another one because he would have to look after it, I felt like that was the last straw. No travel, no sex, no dog. Those were the three things that I enjoyed in life and as far as I was concerned, he had taken those from me far too soon.

Selfish? Some people spend their lives searching for happiness. I knew what made me happy. I needed something to love and if it couldn't be Ron, it was a dog. I needed something besides work to look forward to and that was travel, and I needed intimacy to know that I, as a woman with feelings, existed.

I recall looking up at Ron one day and telling him that I needed something to love and, since we couldn't have another dog, I was just going to have to love him more. He said something like, "That's okay with me," and that was the end of it. But in truth, that was the beginning of it.

Over the months and years things have slowly changed between us. We have discussed his upbringing on the farm, where life was hard and there was no time or energy for displays of affection. No one had ever told him they loved him. Neither side of the family ever spoke of love and there was no hugging and kissing between them. Ron's grandmother, Estella, hung herself when his father, Ira, was only a year and a half old, so Ira never knew a mother's love. Affection was in short supply as Ron grew up. That made me think about the time that his niece made him a cake for his 70th birthday and he told us he'd never had a birthday party before. I had no idea. He had never brought it up.

He said he didn't know what love was. I realized that you can't give what you've never known. I told him that because he is the kind of man he is, he showed love in everything he did for me, every day, whether he realized it or not. And that I loved him for his steadfastness, for his desire to stay with me as my CMT worsened and his devotion, even though he couldn't understand what was wrong between us.

For some reason, I thought that perhaps if I told him in writing how much he was appreciated, it might help him see that love was giving from the heart. He already knew how to love. He just didn't know what it was that he was giving. For his 78th birthday, I wrote him a list that began, "Without you:" and listed the many ways he made my life better. I did the same thing for his 79th birthday, and as the list grew, I realized that this is a man who has devoted more than 30 years to my well-being. Yes, there was no more travel, no more sex and no dog, but we both have something far more precious than any of that: we have the realization that we love each other and we tell each other that we love each other.

During our first 30 years of marriage I think I heard "I love you" maybe twice, but now it comes easily after a kiss or a belly hug: because that's where my arms and head are when I'm sitting on my scooter. We love more and laugh more and life is so much easier even without travel, sex and a dog. I feel as if a large hole in my heart has been filled up with something soft and warm. I feel loved and I feel complete. I hope Ron does too but admitting something like that or even finding the words to express it, just isn't going to happen. You can't give what you don't have and I expected something that for a long time wasn't there.

Sometimes it takes a couple a long time to become truly comfortable with each other and it has taken us years, but comfortable we are and our greatest fear now is that one will lose the other. It's going to happen but it's something neither of us wants to dwell on, although it's often in the back of our minds.

***

In late 2015 I was nominated for the David C. Onley Award for Leadership in Accessibility by Katherine Fisher of the Niagara Parks Commission in Niagara Falls. In May 2016, she called me to tell me that, in fact, I was to receive the award the next month and it came with $5,000. How wonderful! David Onley had been a popular and successful broadcaster, a writer for

Receiving the David C. Onley Award for Leadership in Accessibility from The Honourable Elizabeth Dowdeswell, Lieutenant Governor of Ontario, with David looking on

years and been very involved in disability issues, as he had had polio as a child, was partially paralyzed from the neck down and a scooter user. From 2007 to 2014 he served as Ontario's Lieutenant-Governor, representing Queen Elizabeth II in our province. When his term was complete, he was given the opportunity to establish this award and I was fortunate to receive it in the Role Model category. It was the first time any award I'd ever been given included money and I thought it was a fitting way to likely finish off my award-winning days. As exciting as all that was, and believe me receiving this award from my peers was huge, I think the most gratifying thing happened when I told Ron and, before I even mentioned the fact that he might accompany me, he began talking about whether his suit would fit him or not. I was smiling all over.

My friend Alison drove Ron, Katherine and me to Toronto and I think we all enjoyed ourselves. I especially felt good because Ron was in the audience watching me receive an award for something that had evolved out of our lives together and for something that I couldn't have managed without his help. That award was just as much his as it was mine. Just as an aside, I invested the money in medical marijuana stock and it has done very well. Eventually we'll need a new modified van to take a scooter and, at $74,000 a crack, every little bit helps.

***

Now at ages 75 and 80, our days are quiet. Ron is always up by seven and I'm usually up by 10. Those three hours give him time to do what he needs to do for himself. He still works out on a big, black and chrome machine in his bedroom three times a week. He's strong and healthy, with no sign of cancer. His hair is thinning and white and I think he looks more handsome now than he did when I met him. He still does all the housework and most of the yard work although he has relented and actually hires someone to cut the grass during the very hot summer months. He grocery shops, prepares all of our meals and always seems to be nearby to help me with the many things my increasingly weak hands prevent me from doing. And, every evening when we kiss goodnight and go to our separate rooms we say, "I love you, see you in the morning,", or "anon" if we're feeling nutty, and hope that our wish that we have yet one more day together comes true.

I don't "do" mornings. My hours between rising and noon are precious and personal. I need Ron's help dressing and that ten minutes is intimate and always ends with a kiss. While I fix my face and hair, he puts together my yogurt with blueberries, ground flax and pumpkin seeds and makes sure there is an egg in the pot to be soft boiled on the stovetop. I have breakfast, read a catalog or newspaper while I'm eating, wash my dishes, take my vitamins and brush my teeth. Every day, even on weekends, I am in the office usually by noon. I sit at my computer on my scooter and from there flows my writing and my connection to the world, unless there's a Blue Jays baseball game on or the sun is shining, it's warm out, and the lounge on the patio beckons.

***

I've worn leg braces, had bone surgery, used crutches, a cane, two canes, a walker, a wheelchair and an electric scooter and now wrist and hand braces. If there's anything left to keep me mobile and working, I'll find it. I often tell others who hesitate to use a mobility device or helping aid like a cane or walker due to how it looks: it's not how you get there, it's *that* you get there.

35

My dogs

Dogs have been a very big part of my life, and I have to say, a very good part. I wrote about Gus in Chapter Two because he made such a difference in my childhood, but my other dogs are scattered throughout my life. Ron and I have been dogless for the last few years and will likely remain that way because he has made it clear that looking after me, the house and the yard is enough. Adding a dog on top of that, I think, would likely be the straw that breaks the camel's back or, in our case, Ron's resolve to keep everything going as it has always been. We also have to take into consideration our advanced ages, so a dog might very well outlive us.

TOBY

When I left my job in the morgue at The Standard at age 19 to begin a series of foot and ankle reconstruction surgeries, I was put on long-term insurance but first I was to apply for unemployment insurance. Because I wasn't doing anything, I had money to spare and I badly wanted a dog. I had experienced allergic reactions to dogs before – eyes, nose, mouth and lips itching – and had looked into various breeds that were said to be hypoallergenic. Poodles appealed to me for their intelligence and they were supposed to be okay for people with allergies to dogs.

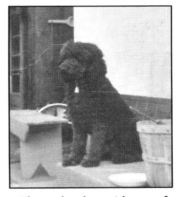

The only photo I have of Toby

I searched the pets for sale ads in the local and Toronto newspapers and found a breeder in Toronto who was offering black standard poodle pups, six weeks old. Liam drove me to Toronto. I took one look at the litter and immediately fell in love. A beautiful little curly-coated jet black boy slept all the way home with us that afternoon, tucked up in the sleeve of my winter jacket.

Exhausted from the trip to Toronto and back, I went to bed early and Toby, that's what I called him, curled up on the end of my bed ... but not for long. Very soon he was crying and had relieved himself on the newspaper, old bedsheet and soft warm towel that Mom had provided for him. She knew better than anyone that a six-week-old pup was going to take more work than I was capable of, especially in the state that I was going to be in very soon. I think I know why she let me have him: a combination of unconditional love and perhaps guilt. She had watched her firstborn daughter cope with CMT for 19 years and make the best of it. She would do anything in her power to make me happy and looking after a puppy was something she could do. Looking back, I think she certainly went above and beyond anything that a mother should have to do for her child. Looking after me and that dog as a puppy, and then as a looney adolescent, was like having two children needing her instead of one. I was asking a lot and she gave so much. I didn't appreciate how much that woman simply exuded love in her quiet, non-assuming way, but I certainly do now. She just gave, not in words, but every day, constantly.

Once the surgery started, I didn't have much interest in the dog. Mom raised him and he grew to be quite tall and elegant-looking even though she kept him in a puppy cut. He may have looked like a fit, lanky marathoner but mentally he was a randy piece of canine cunning. When the doorbell rang he went nuts and it took all of her strength to keep him from jamming his nose into the crotch of whoever was at the door, whether it be the paperboy collecting for the week or a very startled musician wanting to pay his dues for the American Federation of Musicians to my dad as the secretary-treasurer of Local 299.

Dad would come home from work at General Motors every day at noon and, after a quick lunch, settle down in the little brown loveseat in the corner of the living room, put his feet up on a stool, close his eyes, and try to catch a few winks. He'd always had a problem with gas and we'd always laugh like crazy when he'd let a roaring fart go across the kitchen or in the living room. When he was taking his nap and he'd let one rip, he'd either look up and exclaim, "Toby!" or announce to no one in particular, "That wasn't me." That was Toby's cue to walk over to Dad and stick his nose in his crotch, absolutely loving Dad's "odeur." Of course, we all snorted and howled with laughter.

We lived on a very busy street with railway tracks that crossed it just north of our house. Those tracks took freight cars down to the back of General Motors, where they would be loaded and then sent to whatever plant they were destined for. However, while the trains were dinging their way across the road, traffic was held up for 10 or 15 minutes.

One afternoon Toby broke out when somebody came to the door and ended up in the lineup of traffic. To all of our amazement, he looked as if he was trying to hump the back of a little green MGB. Mom had to go out, grab him by the collar and drag him off the car, whose driver was looking back in the rearview mirror with his mouth open in astonishment. Had he really seen what he thought he'd seen? Toby was one horny poodle.

I'd bought Toby in 1959. Two-and-a-half years later I was finally finished with my surgery and confinement in plaster and heading for Montreal to art school. By that time Toby was truly Mom's dog. She'd had him castrated in an attempt to try to calm his lovemaking urges but it hadn't really produced the results she'd hoped for. He was an opportunist, loving every leg he came across, and you had to be careful every time you bent over because he was so big that, in trying to mount you, he'd knock you over.

After I was gone, I think Mom was looking forward to getting on with what she wanted to do and Toby was too much of a handful. She never said anything to me, but looking back, those two-and-a-half years weren't easy for any of us. Mom pretty well devoted her time to me and the rest of the family, even though she had always had a huge love for antiques and was a very good artist. Dad had agreed to let her make the garage into a small antiques shop and I think that saved her sanity as she was coping with me. Don't forget she also had a seven-year-old in elementary school as well and my

brother struggling his way through high school. Her plate was full. Finally, she had her life back and I was doing well on my own. One long weekend when I came home from Montreal, Mom told me that she had given Toby to a farmer that she knew and Toby had made a cardinal canine miscalculation: he had tried to mount a cow. The upshot was the cow had kicked him in the head and that was the end of our beautiful black four-legged Casanova.

MIMI

Years later, after art school and after working in Montreal and Toronto, I was back in St. Catharines and for the second time working at the St. Catharines Standard, this time as editorial assistant. Part of my job was to handle a great many public service announcements. I'm not sure where I came up with the idea but I asked my boss if I could put together an Adopt-a-Pet column, so that the animals at several of the humane society's shelters in Niagara waiting for adoption would be brought to the attention of our readers. He asked around and something like that was being done in other papers. The answer was yes.

Now, knowing that I was an animal lover, especially of dogs, one of my lady friends, who was a window dresser for downtown businesses, told me that she knew of a little poodle who was tied up day and night in someone's enclosed front porch and was being badly neglected. How bad was it? She said the dog hadn't been groomed in years and was hard to recognize as a poodle but she knew that it had been used for breeding. We hatched a plan.

She knew the son of the dog's owner and I think it went like this: he said he would untie the dog and let it out of the porch if my friend would be available to "find" it. She would then take it directly to a pre-arranged veterinary clinic where its health would be evaluated and everything needed to be done would be. I'd pick it up from the vet after work. I had no idea what the dog's temperament was or what it looked like; all I knew was that it was in a horrible situation and I could give it a loving home. Was it theft? Likely. Sort of. Did it bother me? Not a bit. I was divorcing my husband Guy and living on my own. There was no one to say I couldn't have a dog.

It's a good thing Susan, my young friend from work, came with me to pick the dog up at the vet's because there were several steps at the front entrance of the clinic. I sent her in with a blank cheque and when she came out 15 minutes later, she had an almost bald pink poodle in her arms. The dog's coat had been so matted, the veterinarian technicians had to clip her down to the skin. She had nothing but a little white fuzz on her head and a little ball on the end of her tail. She was so stressed, she was vibrating. Susan passed her to me through the open car window and then she

drove us home to my little house on Canal Street.

Once in the door, Mimi (I'd found out that was her given name), who was still shaking uncontrollably from the stress of her great escape and then the vet's where she likely received more attention than she'd had in the last five years, began to devour the food I was laying down for her. Two minutes later she began to quiver, fell onto the floor on her side and was in what I soon learned was a full epileptic convulsion. I didn't even know that dogs could be affected with epilepsy. After another trip to the vet's and some medication to put in her food every day, she had only one or two convulsions during the rest of her life.

Mimi slept all day when I was at work and when I got home I fitted her with her little body harness (there was no way I was going to put a collar on a dog chained up by the neck for years) and we'd go out exploring the neighbourhood. She and I became like one. I loved her unconditionally and she was devoted to me. The hole that a dissolving marriage and alcoholism had bored in my heart was being filled by a little 12-pound bundle of white epileptic fluff.

One night my ex and I were taking a stroll on the beach not too far from the house and he was throwing sticks for Mimi to run after in the sand. She was having a wonderful time but when we got back to the house I noticed her eyes were running and she was pawing at her face. I went to bed and she climbed in but I was awakened around five in the morning by her restlessness and crying. One look at her and I knew she was in serious trouble. Her eyes were streaming water, swollen closed, and she was obviously in great pain. This wasn't going to be a work day for me; she had to go to the vet's fast. I called the vet's number and his service told me to bring her in the minute they opened.

I had her wrapped up in a towel, in the car, and at the vets before 9 a.m. It was just sheer luck that the veterinarian I had chosen for her was Dr. Featherstone, an eye specialist originally from New Zealand, who was escaping a broken marriage and had come to Canada to start a new life. The diagnosis was that she had sand under her eyelids and it had scraped her eyeballs. Whether it had damaged her corneas or not was to be determined but she had to be operated on and the vet couldn't say whether she would be blind or not. I couldn't help but think that all the enjoyment she had experienced the night before, running down the beach after a stick like a happy little abandoned soul, might result in her never seeing me or a stick again.

After surgery and several days at the clinic Mimi was able to come home and fortunately her eyesight had been saved.

She was very tolerant of me when I attempted to administer eye drops two or three times a day and after six weeks or so she was back to normal. What an experience ... who knew what a little sand could do!

Mimi also went through the automobile accident I had close to my 35th birthday that I described in chapter 12.

After being rescued from my upside down Honda, where she ended up on the interior of the car roof, it was at the hospital in Sundridge, sparkling safety glass all over her coat and tied to the railing of the stairs outside, where she had another epileptic seizure. She proved to be one tough poodle and also came through that terrible experience with flying colours.

TEDDY

Because I collected information once a week for Adopt-a-Pet, people at the shelters knew I had a soft spot for poodles and one afternoon I got a call from the local shelter telling me a small male poodle had just been brought in. I thought there was no harm in looking, so after work I pulled into their parking lot, went to the reception desk, and was directed to the small dog and cat room. I opened the door and slowly walked to the end, looking in all the cages. My heart fell; I couldn't see a poodle anywhere. Are you sure he's still here? I asked the girl at the front desk. Maybe he's been adopted. "No" she said, "I think he's in the cage behind the door." I went back and, sure enough, in a little cage behind the door was the fattest little bundle of white poodle I'd ever seen. The tag on the cage said his name was Teddy and, as I opened the cage door, he walked into my arms and ended up with his head stuck in my neck. I told him we were going home, he licked my chin, and that was that.

When I moved from the house in Canal Street over to the bigger house in the midst of being renovated on Bayview, the dogs came with me. Mimi was used to sleeping on the couch all day when I was at work, but now that she had Teddy for company, things were different. He was so fat (I learned that he was THE litter so he got everything his mother had to give) he couldn't get up on the couch even though he'd put his front feet up as far as he could get them and then huff and puff and give little hops trying to get the rest of his body up.

Some days I would go out the door leaving him on the floor and when I would return he'd be asleep somewhere in the house and Mimi would be on the couch. Other days I'd leave him on the couch with Mimi and when I got home he would be on the floor. I knew he'd fallen off and I was afraid he would break a bone. I had arranged for my mother to go in every day around noon to let them both out and give them food but it

wasn't an ideal situation.

Serious renovations were ongoing in the old house and the two dogs would sleep with me in whatever room was habitable that night. It was the morning that I woke up with the bedcovers dotted with spiders that sealed their fate. I couldn't stay in the house any longer and my only alternative was to move in with my then-boyfriend Graydon (Ron), but his apartment building didn't allow pets. I couldn't afford a hotel and they wouldn't let me have them there anyway and boarding the two of them for heaven only knows how many weeks and with Mimi needing medication for epilepsy, things didn't look good. I put the word out and also said that wherever they went, the two of them had to go together.

It wasn't long before I got a call from the father of a little boy who had muscular dystrophy and was in a wheelchair. They had a large dog but thought it would be good for him to have a dog that he could hold on his lap. I met with the mother and father and hesitated when they told me they were moving to Alberta. I knew it was very cold in Alberta, but no colder than Niagara at times.

Both the dogs had red turtleneck sweaters and both had experienced extreme cold. In fact, Ron and I had taken them out into the country where Ron had wanted to walk on a frozen creek. I suggested we take the two dogs along and he said he would take them with him on his walk and I would pick them up at the bridge several miles down the road. The only problem was, I missed the bridge and ended up driving back and forth, up and down the road until finally, there he was, carrying both poodles in their bright red sweaters, one under each arm. They had huge clumps of snow attached to their undercarriage and legs, but both were so happy and looked for all the world as if they'd just had the greatest adventure and couldn't wait to tell me about it.

My mother was there when the two dogs were picked up to go to their new home. I had said my tearful goodbyes that morning. I later received a card from the family, when they were settled in Alberta, telling me that Teddy was just fine and Mimi was in charge of everyone.

SID

In 1983, after my disability had forced me to leave my job at the paper and Ron and I were together in the fully renovated and quite beautiful house on Bayview Drive, I found myself deeply depressed. The job that had taken me from an obituary writer to art critic and all-round editor and journalist in 12 years had defined who I was – but what was I now? A woman who used to "bubble" was now face to face with her disability, had no place to go in the morning, and felt totally useless. For some reason my thoughts turned to a dog. I

wanted something to squeeze, to hug and to love when Ron didn't want to be squeezed or hugged. Unbeknownst to Ron, I told the humane societies in Niagara Falls and St. Catharines that I was looking for a poodle, about 10 pounds and preferably female. Because I had initiated the weekly

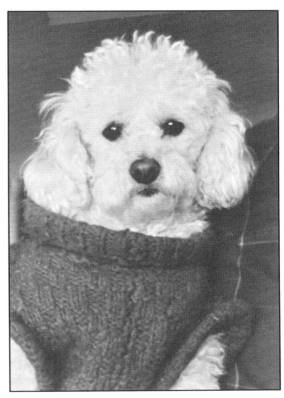

Sid in her favourite sweater

Adopt-a-Pet column at the paper, everyone at the pounds knew me as the one who had called for the adoptables list every week.

Late one Saturday morning I received a call from the Niagara Falls Humane Society: "Linda, we have a little white female poodle about a year old here we think you'll like. She's not even going to get as far as the cages in back if you can come down right now." I had told my mother what I was up to and after a quick call to her, we were both headed for Niagara Falls, about 15 minutes away.

The attendant asked us to wait in the reception area and in a few minutes brought out a little squirming bundle that she put on the floor at my feet. In her excitement, the first thing the dog did was pee all over my shoes then she sat down and looked up at me. Her bright eyes and sweet face said it all. Mom and I both laughed and looked at each other. "She's christened you," Mom said as she snapped a leash on her collar. In 20 minutes the papers were all signed and the three of us headed for home.

Ron wasn't exactly happy to see another dog but he let it go with one caveat: she wasn't to sleep on the bed. The first few nights she wandered the house and finally settled down near our door. We could hear her nails clicking on the kitchen floor and she'd cry, wanting to be with us. I wasn't getting enough sleep and neither was Ron, so my mother suggested that she put her in her little downstairs washroom for the night. Well, that just made everything even worse. As soon as she realized she couldn't get out of there, she'd start scratching at the door, crying and barking, and everyone in the house could hear her. I had no idea a dog that small could throw back her head and howl like a wolf, but she could, and she did.

Her name was Cindy on the adoption papers but neither of us could imagine calling a dog that, so we looked for something that sounded close and changed it quite quickly when we saw a sign for Siddeley Hawker, the airplane manufacturer, on our way to a tradeshow in Toronto. Cindy became Siddeley or, simply, Sid. Finally, Ron gave in and Sid spent the night quietly at the end of our bed, only sneaking up to get under the covers with me after he'd gotten up.

Sid was attached to me as if there was some kind of an invisible string from my heart to hers. She wanted to be with me all the time. At night, after supper, she would patiently wait for the last page of the evening paper to hit the floor. That was her cue. She would jump down from her chair ready to go, I would put her little harness on her, and we would go out together to explore Port Dalhousie. She looked, for all the world, as if she was pulling me on my scooter as she liked to run out in front of me, leading the way. She wasn't pulling, of course, but she liked to be the leader and I was okay with that as long as we weren't crossing roads. I could tell when she was tiring, as she would slow down. I would tell her to come up and she would hop in between my feet or, if she wanted to be closer, she'd climb up into my lap, sit on one thigh and lean into me.

She'd go anywhere with me. I once took her to a Grape and Wine Festival parade, where she spent the entire time tucked down in the front of my hooded sweatshirt with only her head sticking out. I could feel her little body startle when the bands with the big, loud drums went by. It poured rain and we were soaked by the time we got home. Ron pulled off my sweatshirt and our bodies actually steamed. We had kept each other warm through the entire afternoon. When she was out with me, whether she was prancing ahead, seated on my knee, between my feet or tucked up in my sweatshirt, she always looked proud as punch: she was with her lady and everything was right with the world.

I knew poodles were smart but this one was smart enough to teach me to ask questions that could be answered with a tail wag, or not – it's easy if you know how. I could ask her if she wanted to go pee. If I didn't get a wag, the answer was no; yes, was a wag, and out she went. "Go" and "run," as in "Go for a run," were the words she waited for all day.

Sid and I were featured in the local newspaper because so many people had seen a woman on a scooter being pulled by a small but very determined poodle or, at least, that's what it looked like. When she sensed danger, such as an approaching dog or a loud car, she would come very close to

Sid leading the way on one of our adventures around Port Dalhousie – pc35.1

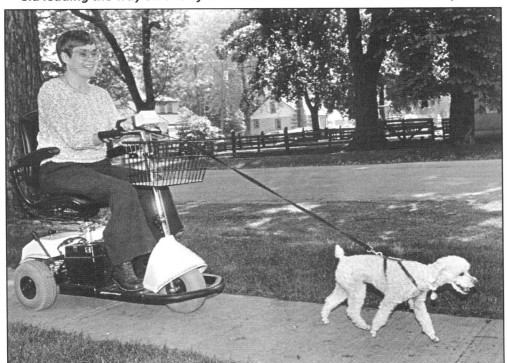

the scooter and, because she always wore a shoulder leash, I could help her up into my lap. I think some people thought it was magic when she put her front paws up on the scooter foot rest and then was suddenly transported into my lap. It wasn't magic: it was teamwork. She'd have her back legs ready to spring, I'd count one, two, three and say, Yes! She'd jump and I'd pull up on her shoulder harness at the same time and, before you could blink, she'd be up.

Everyone in Port Dalhousie knew us and we had great times exploring all the back streets and piers of that beautiful little village. Sid got me moving and she got me out where people, enjoying their summer evenings on the porch, pointed and laughed at the dog who thought it was a Husky pulling a woman on a scooter. I'd laugh, wave and shout, "Hi!" and away we'd go again. Because of her I met all kinds of people. I had learned that if you can't walk and you can't climb steps, many of the people you would like to talk to are out of reach. But in trotting around Port Dalhousie on an almost nightly basis, we became a familiar sight and people were very willing, almost eager, to talk to us. I also wrote an article about our life together that appeared in *Dogs in Canada*.

When we moved to the new house on Springbank, Sid was very excited about it all; she had a new house to explore, a nice fenced-in backyard with a big pond in it and

a whole new neighbourhood, which included the manicured grounds of Ridley College just behind us.

Sometimes members of CMT International would come and visit us at our office and Sid was the official greeter. Because she was used to riding on my lap, it wouldn't be long before our visitor was relaxed and at ease running their hand over Sid's head and down her back while they told me the story of the most traumatic thing that had ever happen to them. Sid was in her element.

The downtown area of St. Catharines was now only a mile from our home. Sid and I would cut through Ridley's manicured grounds always stopping to admire the roses, then we'd cross the Burgoyne Bridge which spans Twelve Mile Creek to St. Paul Street: the city's winding shopping area that used to be an Iroquois trail and saw its heyday in the late 1800s up to 1960 or so, when big shopping plazas pretty well took over. Sid would always either sit between my feet, where she was almost invisible, or on my lap. We'd visit the shops and I'd talk to people and often take photos. Around 1 p.m. we'd cut over to the farmer's market, where I'd buy some kielbasa and a loaf of heavenly smelling, homemade rye bread and we'd sit and eat lunch by the flower and vegetable stands … two old girls uptown together, enjoying the day.

Sid was 12 when I noticed that she was

shaking her head and, when she did, mucus flew everywhere. I took her over to the vet in the nearby plaza and was told there was nothing really wrong. However, as her condition worsened I noticed she was drinking copious amounts of water and lost control of her bladder on occasion, which wasn't like her. She was soon diagnosed with diabetes; Ron had to give her an insulin shot every day. The sinus and nose condition didn't clear up, so once again, we went to the vet's and this time a culture was taken and sent away. The verdict was she had a massive sinus infection. Because of the diabetes, her immune system wasn't taking care of it and antibiotics also didn't work. When the brand of insulin that she was doing so well on was discontinued, she simply couldn't adjust.

Added to that, our little girl couldn't smell her food because of the sinus condition so she wouldn't eat and that not only compounded the diabetes but caused her

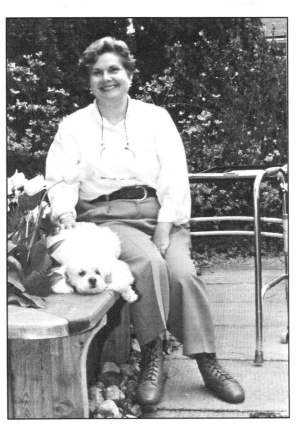

Sid and me on the side of the raised flowerbed where her ashes were buried

to lose a lot of weight and, at 12 pounds, she didn't have much to lose. We also figured that she must be in considerable discomfort. Unfortunately, it was time.

After much soul-searching and many tears, Ron and I took her to the vet's, knowing she couldn't go on the way she was and that letting her was cruel. The vet took her away just long enough to put a cannula in her front leg and then brought her back to my arms. He asked me if I was ready, I kissed her head and told her she was my girl for the last time, nodded, and then felt her little warm body relax into my arms.

Strange as it may sound, right after she died I felt a warmth descend over my head and around my shoulders as if she was telling me it was okay ... that she was okay. I wasn't going to explain it to Ron because I couldn't explain it myself, but that warm glow comforted me as we drove home in tears, dogless for the first time in many years.

For close to 12 years, Sid had raised me from depression and helped me move in a world that sometimes isn't very friendly to people who are disabled. She had been a loving companion and an ambassador for CMT International, putting a smile on the face of a disease that sees many of us unable to walk, and some unable to even do up a button. She'd pulled off my socks and sweaters when I couldn't manage, and sometimes even brought them out from under the bed. When I asked her to "get it," she'd diligently scrape any spider to dust for me. She made me laugh, she made me cry, but most of all she had shown me a love that didn't care what I did or how I had to do it, as long as I did it with her.

DAISY

Ron knew how much I loved having a dog and although he wasn't all that happy with it (he was raised on a farm where the dog stayed outside), he drove me over to Oakville where we took a look at a litter of poodle pups that wouldn't be ready to go for at least a month. There were five of them and from a jumbled pile of velvety ears and little pink noses and paws, I picked out a sweet little female. We went back to pick her up, receive her registration papers and pay for her ($600), when she was six weeks old. I called her Daisy although I gave her a much longer kennel name: SigmaChi's Lazy Days of Summer.

Having a six-week-old pup is like having a

baby in the house. She was very smart, learned quickly and moved fast when let out of her enclosure. I was using a walker around the house then and by the time I got to the patio door to let her out, she had zipped into the next room and done her business on the wall-to-wall carpet. I was always on tenterhooks because any

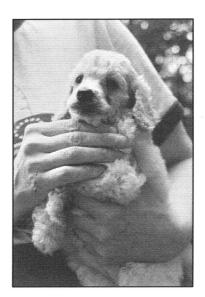

Daisy at six weeks

mistakes she made brought an I-told-you-so look from Ron and I so wanted her to work out.

The first time she got her first whiff of outdoor scents, the look on her face was something to behold. She stuck her nose up and caught it, looked at me in wonderment, and almost smiled. As we poked along the street she wanted to smell all the garbage cans and trees, flowers and lamp posts. The only things that seem to frighten her and had her cowering were big trucks. I can only imagine what they must have sounded like to her. For some reason she refused to pee on the grass and we couldn't figure out how to convince her it was okay to do that.

298

Ron and I had had several heated discussions about the dog and I was into my work more than I should've been with a tiny pup around the house. One night while Ron was making supper, I asked from the office, where I was on the computer, if he would pop the dog out the patio door. In an angry tone he told me he was busy and words were spoken, hurtful words. The upshot was, he grabbed his keys, got in the car and drove away. My heart sank. I was alone with the dog, pizza had been delivered because our discussion had ruined supper, and I pushed the pizza into the oven determined to have a meal with or without him.

Not being the cook in the family, I turned the oven up and in about 10 minutes, noticed flashing through the glass window in the oven door. When I opened it, smoke billowed out towards the ceiling and flames lashed the sides of the oven. I had neglected to take the pizza out of the box. Don't forget I was on a walker and couldn't carry. I phoned our neighbours two doors over and they came running with a fire extinguisher. Once the howling smoke detector had been turned off, the smoldering pizza box thrown out into the carport and a fan set up to blow the smoke out the kitchen window, they went home with my thanks. Without them I'd have had to bring in the fire department and heaven knows how that would've ended up.

I had forgotten I'd invited my brother Ronald and his wife Lori over. Just as they arrived a torrential rain began, with drops so big their pelting on the skylights sounding like one of those little Christmas drummer boy toys. I was sitting on the couch with the dog when Lori looked out

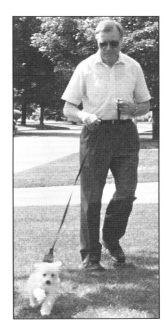

Ron and Daisy

the back door and exclaimed, "The pond is overflowing and goldfish are on the sidewalk!" She was right, the pond had filled to the top, spilled out over the walkway bordering it and large goldfish were trying to swim on the pavement. Ronald and Lori both went out and scooped the goldfish back into the pond and, once the rain stopped, the water went down enough so the fish couldn't escape again. I just sat on the couch, exhausted, holding Daisy, praying that she didn't have to go out because I didn't have the energy to get up. An hour and a half later I heard the key in the back door and Ron walked into the kitchen. He looked around the corner of the living room at me sitting on the couch with the dog and said, "Did I miss anything?"

It took a while before I told him what had happened and I found out that all he did was drive out into the country to cool down, but that night was a turning point for me. I realized just how much I couldn't do, how vulnerable I really was and how much Ron did and was needed, and that it wasn't fair for me to hold on to something that made his life so much more difficult.

The pizza fire, as I grew to call it, was on a Friday night and the following Sunday I took Daisy over to Ridley College for a run. For the first time in her little life she peed on the grass. I was so pleased with her I praised her to the sky and back and she almost turned inside out with happiness.

When we got home I told Ron about her success but I had a restless night; the pizza fire and what had brought that upset upon us, weighed heavily on my mind. The next morning I made a phone call to the breeder and asked if we could bring Daisy back. Very reluctantly, the breeder said that all her litter-mates had gone and that she would be alone, but she would try to find someone else to buy her and when she did I would get my $600 back. Ten days later no one had even looked at her and I couldn't stand the thought of that beautiful little 11-week-old pup all alone in a shed. I hatched a plan and called the Lions Foundation of Canada in Oakville that operate a Dog Guide Program, asking if they would take her. They said they would and they'd give me an income tax receipt for her full value. It was done and Daisy found a home with a family who looked after and socialized her in their Foster Puppy Program for a year until she went into full training to become either a guide for someone with vision impairment or a hearing ear dog for a person who was deaf, depending on her talents and aptitude.

It was perhaps two years later that I received a card in the mail with a picture of a lovely looking grey-haired lady sitting on a large rock with an elegant, small miniature poodle sitting proudly by her side. Daisy had become a hearing ear dog and was helping this woman live a full and happy life. That photo told me what I had wanted and needed to know. What a relief! Way to go, Daisy!

VAL

Later that same year, the only way I can explain how I felt was that I was waiting to exhale, I missed my dogs so much. I had joined an online poodle chat forum and met some very nice poodle people there who knew of my love for Sid and what had transpired with Daisy. I vowed I would never have another pup and was looking for a dog that was a year or 18 months old. After several months on the forum, I received an email from Marion, who lived not too far from us in Hamilton, saying that she knew a breeder in Acton, Ontario, who had a young male she would be willing to

300

sell. Thinking back to Sid, I preferred a female, but Marion suggested that she drive me up to Acton anyway – just to take a look.

The next day we piled into her car and Marion drove several hours to the breeder's home, out in the country west of Toronto. To keep from falling, I took my walker along on the trip for safety. We parked in the gravel driveway and a tiny woman, not more than 4' 8", with a halo of white hair wound around her head and a soft oval-shaped face, came out to greet us. Her name was Christine Davies but she went by

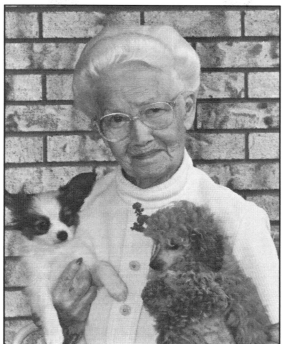

Christine Davies, dog breeder, with a papillon and poodle pup

Chris. She suggested we first go around back to the kennels so we could take a look at the dog she had in mind for me.

There were several poodles in the cement-floored kennels and all looked healthy and very well cared for. You could tell that the lady herself cared a great deal for her charges and she, herself, was as neat as a pin. She bred and raised show dogs, poodles and papillons, and the male poodle in question, who was cream, not white, and truly a beautiful specimen, was supposed to

have been *the* stud for her kennel, but as she put it, "The damn fool doesn't know what to do." She proceeded to tell us he had fathered one pup that had matured to be a small miniature and that she only bred and showed toys. The fact that *he* was a small miniature made me wonder what she was doing, but I expect she bred him with a small toy female hoping the result would be as good looking as he was but the required size. She also told me his name was Valentino, giving away her hopes that he would become the great lover that she needed for her girls.

We took a quick tour of the ground level of her tri-level home where she had a double line of screen-doored cages built into the wall. Each dog knew its own kennel and each one jumped into its own bed every night, knowing it would be given a goodnight doggy biscuit.

Back in the front garden area, Chris sat us down and began asking questions about me and my lifestyle. As the conversation warmed, the journalist came out in me and

I began asking her about herself. She told us she had run away from home at a very early age and, in New York City, amongst other locations, had been on the stage where she and her partner were adagio dancers, back in the era when a man flinging a woman about by her hair and pretending to treat her roughly was tolerated and thought risqué. The beautiful white hair she wore now had, at one time, been very long, jet black and part of the act. I couldn't help but wonder what she was chewing on, as every now and then I got a flash of white as she spoke. Somehow I managed to ask, in a way that it didn't offend her, and she told me that when she was growing up, people who found themselves without teeth or dentures chewed white wax and when they had to smile, they pushed the wax forward in their mouth and it gave them something other than their gums to bear. This was a first for me and I found Chris fascinating: a living icon reminiscent of a time way before me.

She suggested we sit down, served us cold drinks, and then said she was going in to get Valentino (registered name: Chrizrick's

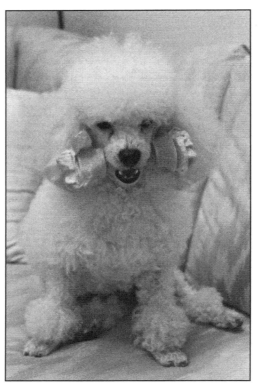

Val's first day with us

Valentino.) When she came back she gave him to Marion, while she and I talked business. I couldn't keep my eyes off him; he was beautiful and had obviously been bathed and clipped for my arrival. But she had put him in a full poodle cut with pom-poms on his ankles and one on his head and his tail. I knew I couldn't take him home like that; Ron would laugh him out of the house.

When he was finally given to me, I held him with his head on my shoulder. He had his front legs on either side of my neck, buried his head in my neck and stayed that way. He stopped shaking after I told him how beautiful he was.

Finally, after what seemed like many months, I exhaled, and tears began to run down my cheeks. I got my cheque book out to write one for $600 but Chris insisted I not write it until she took him out into the field that was her front yard. Using my walker, with the loop of his leash over her hand, she marched in the tall grass with the walker in front of her to see if he'd run along with her or if it would frighten him. Fortunately for me, he thought it was all great fun and although I couldn't see everything she was doing, I could see his head popping up above the weeds and her hands moving up towards her chest as she cleared the weeds with the walker's feet. He wasn't afraid and the deal was sealed.

I'd brought along a small animal carrying case and we popped him in it and left for home, but on the way stopped for something to eat. It was then that I asked Marion if she could shorten the hair on his ears so they wouldn't fall into his food and maybe tone down some of the pom-poms so he didn't look like such a dandy. She did what she could in the parking lot. I also asked her to work with me on ways I could feed him when I couldn't bend down and how I'd get water to him, as I was prepared to do it if Ron wouldn't. I know now that, in no time flat, he would have learned to jump up on a raised platform that was reachable for me, especially if food was involved.

After his ear trim, I couldn't bear to put him back in the cage again so he slept on my lap, with his nose in the crook of my arm, the rest of the way home. Every time he looked up and saw cars and trucks passing by the side of the car, he started to shake and then stuck his head back under my arm. I don't think he'd ever seen traffic.

It was dark by the time we pulled into our driveway. Marion went to the back door, rang the bell and Ron came out. She handed him the dog and then helped me out of the car with my walker. "Oh … my … God! What is this?" Ron said, holding the dog away from him as if it were covered with something awful. I'm not sure what I said next, but it didn't matter. Val was home, that was all there was to it.

Less than a week later, Ron asked if he could take Val out for a walk. This was truly a turning point. Ron is of German heritage and it looked like one German appreciating another, as the "pudel" originated in Germany, and I think there was a guy thing mixed in there as well. Val may have looked a bit strange for a male but he sure made up for it in his actions. He walked at heel beside Ron. No, he pranced. And he soon learned to sit, and stay … almost. There was no pulling and the two of them looked great together.

I called that my $1,200 dog summer. Expensive? Yes. But what price can you put on the kind of love, loyalty, and stress reduction that these beautiful little, white bundles gave me.

I had worried that a male dog wouldn't be as affectionate as Sid had been but Val proved to be a loving companion, reluctant to leave my side. Because he had been kept in a kennel he didn't know what a couch or a bed was, but he soon figured it out. When Ron was on the couch reading, watching TV or snoozing, Val was beside him or lying flat out on Ron's long legs.

When Ron and I were watching television he was usually beside me and when I'd stretch out he delighted in licking my toes, which was very special for me because very few people really went near my feet. I'm not sure what the attraction was but, as soon as the socks came off, Val got busy as if it were his only job in life. I know it sounds yucky but it felt marvelous. I wonder if he somehow knew there was something wrong with my feet, the way some dogs can find cancer, and that was his way of making things better. He certainly tried.

We had a big bamboo chair with comfy cushions, near the floor-to-ceiling glass

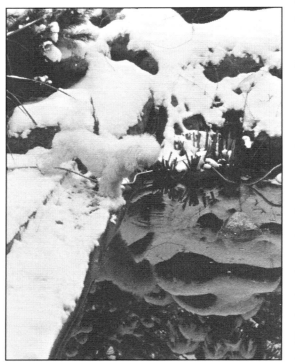

Val's first snowfall - checking out his reflection in the pond

patio doors just around the corner from my bedroom. For years Val slept there, after going round and round before settling into a big mohair blanket he just loved. That was also his chair during the day and he'd watch the birds out by the pond, only barking when the squirrels came for a drink. When you said the word "squirrel" it was as if you had injected him with some kind of sport performance drug: he would literally fly off the chair and bark and paw the glass like a mad fiend. Once out, if poodles could burn rubber, he burned it. The squirrels didn't have a chance unless they were close to one of the several trees in the yard. While he never caught one, he came mighty close several times, and upon his return would be panting, snorting and snuffing, as if to say, "Next time, you just wait, I'll get you next time." I rarely had to clip his back toenails because he mowed them down to nothing on the concrete while launching himself after the squirrels.

The same thing applied to the doorbell every time it rang. He never knew whether it was the front or the back door and began barking as soon as he heard the first ding, so we couldn't tell if it was one for the back or two for the front either. Once we figured it out and answered the door, he had to check out whoever was there. Thank heaven he didn't weigh much and Ron could pick him up so that whoever was visiting wouldn't get tripped up as he investigated.

Our first Christmas with Val was fun for all of us. Christmas day was a green one until around noon when a light dusting of snow began to fall and by dark there was a fine sparkle on everything. During the night it was bright enough to take a picture. A full moon, they said; there wouldn't be another one on Christmas night for many years. All day great big beautiful flakes came down, covering everything with a clean white blanket, leaving only the dark green boughs of hemlock, scotch and black pine snooping out from under the weight of it all.

Guess who was roaring to go first thing in the morning? Yup, Val. Picture it, if you will, everything is quiet, pristine white and ever so still. The kids next door are away and no one has started shoveling yet. It's beautiful, sort of God's main event. The mourning doves are plastered in the locust tree like some large tan mittens thrown by a playful kid and the sparrows are tossing the water in the pond around as though they are making a shampoo commercial; you know the ones where the women throw their hair over their heads when it's wet. The pond water is almost frozen because it is just cold enough to snow but not to freeze deep water yet. The big fat goldfish are clustered around the yellow immersion heater just in case; it's cool for goldfish and, after all, this is their home. It's a tranquil picture-book scene, the kind that seeps into your subconscious and stays there forever. But, carefully and very quietly, the patio door glides open and an absolute whirlwind of white fur hits the snow, sending the sparrows in a chirping flock into the sky and the doves wheeling backwards to the safety of the big blue spruce they call home. Val reigns!

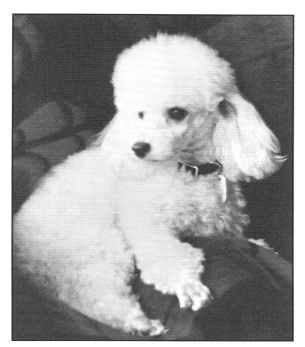

A mature, happy Val

For the next half hour he charges and flails, whirling the snow as he turns and plays, shoveling piles up his nose, carrying on like a little madman in a polar bear suit, and enjoying all that is his. What a guy! Nothing is safe, the rocks of the waterfall become a mountain he climbs with speed and grace, jumping off halfway down, landing on his feet like a little mountain goat ready to charge again, but this time it's up into the garden box to stand in rosemary, parsley and thyme; all frozen soggy and soft, wearing little snowcaps. Those herbs are mine. "Get out of there," I yell, and scold him loudly. He jumps from the box, "Hey lady, I'm not too proud, hey!"

Finally, his zip seems to lag, his zoom is all frittered out. He comes to the door and draws lines on the glass with his nose. If he could write he'd probably tell me to hurry up. The glass door glides open and he hops in, covered with snow from head to foot. His topknot sparkles with snowflakes and his body quivers, more from excitement than cold, I'd say, and we spend the next 20 minutes combing the snowballs out of his undercarriage, fetlocks and toes, so he can get on with his day of chewing his rawhide bone, snoozing and looking adorable.

Later that week, the doorbell rings. "Hel-lo! Someone is here! Got to check it out!" He flies off his chair, slides across the kitchen floor on barely dry pads and, hello, who should appear but groomer Holly and her big black portable table. Oh, dear!

Before he knows it, it's up and brush, clip and comb, ears and nails, bath and scissor, fluff and puff. He looks at me as if to say, "When will it ever end? Please rescue me!"

Then Holly's gone and you can tell he thinks he's gorgeous. When you ask him if he wants to go out he looks at you as if to say, "And mess all this up? You've got to be crazy lady. You want me to get wads in my pads and balls on my legs, my beautiful topknot sopping wet and my tail pom split?" And then, just like that, they're back, the wretched little varmints are drinking from the pond. He's probably wondering why they don't eat snow like he does. Does he want to go out? Yessiree, Bob! And away he goes like a bat out of hell, his furry buns driving his little body to accomplish yet another squirrel mission. He's the closest we'll ever get to watching a child experience his first snowfall. Tons of fun!

Ron and I used to joke that the only way you could tell which way he was going in the snow were the black dots: two if he was coming toward you and only one if he was going away from you. In a good snowfall, he was virtually invisible out there if he wasn't moving.

Every now and then he would take off around the house and do something we called interior jogging. I now know that it is simply a way for a dog to burn off excess energy and steam but back then, even though we had our suspicions, it was great fun to watch him fly off his chair and roar through the living room, down the hall, through the bedroom and back again. Every room in our home has two doors, so he could race in a big circle around the house until he was exhausted, then he'd jump back up on his chair and flop down, totally spent.

I would often take Val over to the Ridley College campus grounds when there was no one around, unclip the leash from his shoulder harness and let him run freely beside me. He always kept about four feet from me, no matter how many turns I made or where I went. Again, as with Sid, it was as if we were connected by an invisible thread. One word from me and he was sitting on the scooter between my feet. How wonderful it felt to have a dog love and trust you so much that he would do whatever you asked without the slightest hesitation. It was almost as if he understood English.

Val was almost 13 when he began to slow down. He no longer wanted to go with me on the scooter and he would lie on the stool by the couch, asleep all day, and then spend the night with me on my bed. He had cataracts and, for all intents and purposes, was blind and deaf, but I think that as long as he could smell my presence he knew he was okay. Ron had to take him outside, place him on the sidewalk and then wait while he did his business. If we left him alone outside he would wander off, following his nose, but inevitably bump into something again and again. Many times he came very close to falling into the pond and once had to be rescued by Ron from the water and then bathed to get him free of duckweed. Ron and I knew that there was no longer any quality-of-life for this little guy. Once the decision was made, the appointment booked and many tears shed, I was holding him in my arms while the vet proceeded to push the drug that would stop his heart into the cannula on his leg. I felt his little body jerk and then relax, his chin fell forward onto my arm and I knew he was gone.

We had his beautiful little body cremated. His ashes, along with a framed portrait of him, sits amongst a small collection of bronze and china dogs, I've put together since he died. As much as I would give everything to have another dog, I respect and acknowledge Ron's limitations. As I grow older and more disabled, he is my only caregiver and adding a dog to the mix is simply not fair. I also don't think either of us could survive having to put down another little being that we had grown to love and that loved us both unconditionally.

I've made Ron promise that if I am the first one to go, he'll take Val's ashes off the shelf in my bedroom, mix them with mine, and then place us in our plot in the old cemetery near his family farm in Silverdale. Ron likes to walk the perimeter of the huge field out behind the cemetery and, whether he knows it or not, Val and I will be with him every step of the way.

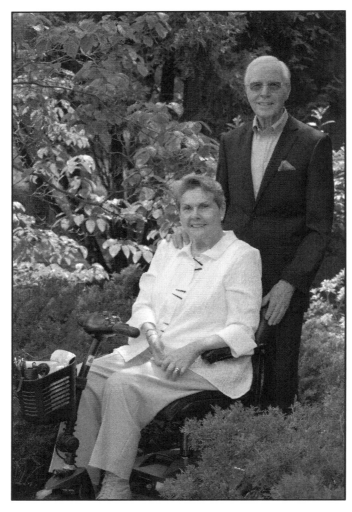

Linda and Ron 2017 – *pc35.2*

Epilogue

I'd like to leave you with some of the things that I've learned throughout the years while coping with my CMT and life in general. I'm no one special and don't pretend to be, and I know you've probably come to some of these conclusions yourself, but I thought it might be an interesting way to close.

Now in my 76th year, or as I sometimes jokingly call it, the final quarter, I can look back with some experience. If you've been keeping track as you've read this tome you'll know what most of them are. You know that I haven't been able to walk and have lived with chronic burning pain for the last 20 years, and am now losing the use of my hands. Believe me, losing the use of your hands is a lot harder than not being able to walk. Be thankful for what you have that still works and do the very best you can each day with what you have left.

Choose your battles wisely. You can easily get caught up in many causes. Everyone needs volunteers. If you want to make a difference, choose one or two areas that you feel passionate about and let that passion sweep you to heights greater than you ever imagined. You'll work harder than you ever thought possible but the results will be amazing.

When I was young, no one knew much about CMT and no one really knew what might be possible for me in the future so I just kept on doing my very best whenever and at whatever I could. I learned as I went and my disease progressed, taking with it my independence but little else. But now, we know what parts of the body various CMT types can affect. If you know what type you have, you'll have an inkling of what to expect. I recommend genetic testing.

Have you ever thought, Why me? I have. And my husband counters with, "Why not you?" He's right. Being diagnosed with CMT isn't the end of the world. If you look around, you will see people who are coping with all manner of disabling and even terminal disorders. Many of the conditions are invisible so you can't tell what other people are dealing with. If CMT happens to be your lot in life, then it's up to you to make the very best of it.

I've learned to never assume. And I'd like to extend that to physicians as well. I have learned that no doctor or medical professional should ever assume simply because you have CMT, that you can't do something and a physician should never attempt to predict your future. People tend to believe what medical professionals tell them and sometimes that belief turns into a self-fulfilling prophecy. You stop yourself from doing things you could do because someone has suggested you can't do them. Listen to your inner voice.

A good education will see you through life far better than anything else; it is an investment of time and money in you and what better place to put it than in your future.

Open your mind to everything while knowing that, in the grand scheme of things, you know nothing, no matter how much you learn. That should keep you learning for life. And, learning from experience beats anything you can read in a book. Don't tell me how to do something, show me, and then let me do it myself and, if I'm old, be patient while I write down the steps, especially if it's something to do with the computer!

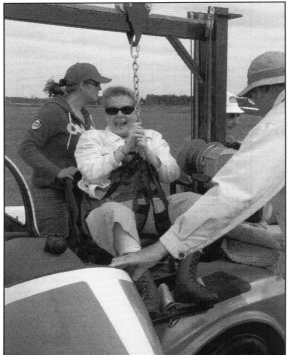

Being lifted out of a glider at the York Soaring Club in 2010

As you gain experience and years, when seemingly insurmountable challenges come your way, you can say, "I can do this...been there, done that." Because you have.

Don't put things off. If you keep a list of things you want to accomplish every week, and I keep mine on a Post-it stuck to the bottom of my desktop computer, you can tick things off as you do them and see that you are actually accomplishing something. For many years, I did the same thing with a five-year plan and amazed myself by finishing most of my five-year plans in one or two. Focusing on the job at hand can accomplish a great deal and loving what you do makes work fun.

Every time you say can't, counter it with a can, and pretty soon you won't say can't anymore because you'll realize how positive thinking can turn your world around. If I'd have listened to people who told me I couldn't, I would never have found a job, gone back to school, started CMT International and designed our home or written this book. I even went soaring, having no idea if I could get in and out of the plane, but thought I'd give it a try. We managed and it was beyond wonderful. You'll be surprised what *you* can do when you try.

310

Put money away as soon as you possibly can. The interest will compound and you will have a retirement you can be proud of because you worked and planned very hard toward it. Even $20 a week adds up to many thousands over 30 years. Learn about money. It, health and love can be the keys to a happy retirement.

I've learned that if you just put your head down and focus on the work at hand, while doing your best, you will usually succeed.

Try to balance work and play. It can be difficult, especially if you love what you do, but your brain needs change and you'll surprise yourself how productive you can be after some time away from the everyday routine. I've always preached pacing oneself but it is the most difficult thing I've ever tried to do except lose weight and I'm still not very good at either. Which brings me to something I keep reading over and over: Live each day as if it's the last day of your life. I laugh at that because if I knew it were the last day of my life there would be so many things I'd want to cram in, I'd be a blithering idiot. Talk about stress! My advice for me is to just to live each day as best I can, helping others as I go and trying not to make anyone else's, or my world any more difficult than it already is.

I travelled while I could. I wish I had travelled more.

I read anytime I have spare time: newspapers, web posts, journal articles and books. I read about people and I love discovering how others manage their world. My digital reader doesn't demand that I hold it, I can prop it up on a pillow, and a touch will turn the page. Those features eliminate the frustration I have trying to hold the written word and turn pages with weak wrists, and hands and fingers that don't work.

Buy land and plant trees on it because at least that way you will leave something lasting for others to enjoy and the planet will breathe a little better because you were here.

Surround yourself with beauty. I like orchids in the bathroom and enjoy art on the walls.

Don't be afraid to risk. Some of the most fulfilling thing I've ever done have scared the daylights out of me.

Don't be afraid to love, even if it doesn't come back to you. Someday it might. Love changes lives.

Be grateful for what comes your way and use it wisely.

Be thankful you're alive, CMT or not.

Held by Golden Threads
by Linda Crabtree

My atrophy progresses
While all about me,
life dresses
As a fancy woman.

What next will I lose?
My eyes? My ears?
Already my legs, feet,
Arms, hands,
My breathing, my voice.
I don't get to choose.

I wake up one morning
And something else is gone.
Is it God's plan
That I go on clearly and
slowly watching myself die
Or just a simple quirk
of nature?
Probably a little bit of both
The former to keep me modest
the latter to keep me humble

But I keep going and,
As I become less,
I am more
Only threads hold
what is left
They turn to molten gold
Mixed with iron
And harden to keep me strong
in soul
If not in body.

Each morning a gift,
Each experience savoured,
each kind word
hangs in my mind
until it drops
and spreads
into the crystal pool
that is me.

Symptoms of CMT

There are 90+ known genetic causes (subtypes) of CMT. Clinical signs and symptoms can vary depending on the type of CMT as well as the severity of disease in the individual. Symptoms may range from barely noticeable to severe and can appear in early childhood or later in life. No two people experience CMT the same way. Even those in the same family with the same type of CMT may be affected quite differently. Below is a list of the more common symptoms a person with CMT may experience as well as other less commonly reported issues.

Common symptoms of CMT
- Muscle weakness
- Chronic fatigue
- Chronic pain
  - Muscle cramps, spasms, twitching, tremors (in feet, legs, hands, torso, etc.)
  - Nerve pain (e.g. pins/needles, burning, stabbing, itching)
  - Pain in joints, spine, tendons, or other structures (often due to weakness, strain, muscle imbalances, frequent injuries or surgeries)
- Physical challenges
  - Balance issues and clumsiness (e.g. frequently tripping/falling, dropping things)
  - Difficulty running, jumping, climbing hills/stairs
  - Difficulty standing still (e.g. need to touch something, standing with knees bent)
  - Difficulty with fine motor skills (grasping/holding objects, opening jars, handwriting)
  - Difficulty with proprioception (ability to sense the position of one's body)
  - Difficulty performing the same level of activity every day (due to some days being worse than others and need for post-activity recovery time)
- Physical changes
  - Deformities (e.g. very high arches or flat feet, clawed toes, hand contractures, Achilles' tendon contractures)
  - Muscle loss in extremities (usually beginning in lower legs/feet and hands)
  - Thin ankles/calves (or calves may be typical size or large)
  - Unusual walk (high-stepping, feet slapping the floor, limping)
  - Reflexes that are often reduced or absent (or sometimes brisk)
  - Toe walking (early sign in children) or unable to walk on toes/heels
  - Foot drop and wrist drop (difficulty lifting foot/wrist)
  - Hip dysplasia (and hip replacements)
  - Scoliosis or Kyphosis (curvature of the spine)
  - Sleep disorders (sleep apnea, Restless Leg Syndrome, Periodic Limb Movement Disorder)

- ➢ Decreased nerve sensation (with increased risk of calluses, ulcers, and infection in feet)
  - ➢ Poor tolerance to hot/cold temperature extremes
  - ➢ Chronically cold feet and hands
  - ➢ Poor circulation (discolored or reddish/purple coloring or swelling in extremities)
  - ➢ Hearing impairment & processing issues
  - ➢ Enlarged nerves (in Type 1)
- Emotional challenges such as anxiety, depression, loneliness, social isolation, chronic grieving over progressive losses, etc.

Other reported symptoms of CMT
- Breathing difficulties, especially when lying flat, due to diaphragm dysfunction/paralysis or other muscle weakness or curvatures of the spine
- High residual lung volume (can't empty lungs fully, CO2 retention)
- Vision impairment
- Speech, swallowing, or chewing issues
- Inability to cough or blow nose effectively
- Vocal cord strain or paralysis
- Dizziness
- Pain due to areas of hypersensitivity (hyperesthesia) and hypersensitivity to touch, clothing, bedding, etc.
- Bladder issues (urgency, frequency, incontinence, etc.)
- Gastrointestinal issues (gastroparesis, constipation, reflux)
- Sexual dysfunction
- Exercise intolerance
- Joint hypermobility
- Nerve compression issues (due to enlarged nerves in Type 1 or HNPP subtype)
- Upper limbs involved more than lower limbs
- Patella (kneecap) dislocations
- Complete loss of use of hands
- Inability to stand or walk from a young age
- Lower leg amputation
- Autonomic nerve involvement
- Central nervous system involvement
- Cognitive impairment
- Life-threatening complications
- Worsening of symptoms with certain medications
- Other symptoms specific to a subtype or an individual or family

Resources

GENERAL INFORMATION ABOUT CHARCOT-MARIE-TOOTH DISEASE

- **US National Library of Medicine Genetics Home Reference**
  This site houses a significant amount of detail about CMT, including common symptoms, basic CMT subtypes, inheritance patterns, and links to many other resources.
  www.ghr.nlm.nih.gov/condition/charcot-marie-tooth-disease

- **Pub Med GeneReviews**
  Pub Med maintains a general overview of CMT as well as detailed reviews of many of the CMT subtypes. These may be found in the GeneReview section of their website.
  www.ncbi.nlm.nih.gov/books/NBK1358/

- **Neuromuscular Disease Center, Washington University, St. Louis, MO, USA**
  This Neuromuscular Disease Center maintains an in-depth CMT web page that details all the various CMT subtypes and associated symptoms.
  http://neuromuscular.wustl.edu/time/hmsn.html

- **CMT Medication Alert List**
  There are medications that are potentially toxic to those with CMT. Listings of these medications are maintained by CMT patient organizations. A list may also be found on the Pub Med GeneReview site.
  www.ncbi.nlm.nih.gov/books/NBK1358/bin/cmt_and_medications.pdf

CMT ORGANIZATIONS
CANADA

- **Muscular Dystrophy Canada**
  2345 Yonge Street
  Suite 900
  Toronto, Ontario M4P 2E5
  Phone: 1-866-MUSCLE-8 (1-866-687-2538)
  Email: info@muscle.ca
  Website: www.muscle.ca
  Facebook: www.facebook.com/muscle.ca/
  Note: There are regional and community offices across Canada that provide services,

including assistance with the cost of aids for daily living. Registration is free.

USA

- **Charcot-Marie-Tooth Association (CMTA)**
  PO Box 105
  Glenolden PA 19036
  Phone: 800-606-2682 (toll-free); 610-499-9264
  Email: info@cmtausa.org
  Website: www.cmtausa.org
  Facebook: www.facebook.com/CMTAssociation/

- **Hereditary Neuropathy Foundation, Inc.**
  432 Park Avenue South
  4th Floor
  New York NY 10016
  Phone: 855-435-7268 (toll-free); 212-722-8396
  Email: info@hnf-cure.org
  Website: www.hnf-cure.org
  Facebook: www.facebook.com/HereditaryNeuropathyFoundation/

- **Muscular Dystrophy Association - USA (MDA)**
  222 South Riverside Plaza
  Suite 1500
  Chicago IL 60606
  Phone: 800-572-1717
  Email: mda@mdausa.org
  Website: www.mda.org
  Facebook: www.facebook.com/MDANational/

EUROPE & AUSTRALIA

- **European Charcot-Marie-Tooth Consortium**
  Department of Molecular Genetics
  University of Antwerp
  Antwerp Antwerpen B-2610, Belgium
  Email: gisele.smeyers@ua.ac.be

- **TREAT-NMD**

Institute of Genetic Medicine
University of Newcastle upon Tyne
International Centre for Life
Newcastle upon Tyne NE1 3BZ
United Kingdom
Phone: 44 (0)191 241 8617
Email: info@treat-nmd.eu
Website: www.treat-nmd.eu/cmt/overview/

- **European Neuromuscular Centre (ENMC)**
  Lt Gen van Heutszlaan 6
  3743 JN Baarn
  Netherlands
  Phone: 31 35 5480481
  Email: enmc@enmc.org
  Website: www.enmc.org

- **Charcot-Marie-Tooth Association Australia (CMTAA)**
  Building 22
  Concord Hospital
  Concord, NSW
  2139 Australia
  Phone: (02) 9767 5105
  Email: cmtaa@cmt.org.au
  Website: www.cmt.org.au

- **Charcot-Marie-Tooth Austria (CMT-Austria)**
  Gersdorf 82
  Spielfeld, 8471 Austria
  Phone: 0676/660 18 51
  Email: office@cmt-austria.at
  Website: www.cmt-austria.at

- **Association Française contre les myopathies (AFM)**
  1 Rue de l'International
  BP59

Evry cedex 91002

France

Phone: +33 01 69 47 28 28

Email: dmc@afm.genethon.fr
Website: www.afm-telethon.fr

- **Charcot-Marie-Tooth France (CMT-France)**
  BP 70513
  35305 FOUGÈRES CEDEX
  France
  Phone: 820 077 540; 2 47 27 96 41
  Website: www.cmt-france.org
  Facebook: www.facebook.com/cmtfrance/

- **Associazione Italiana Malatta di Charcot-Marie-Tooth (AICMT)**
  Via Castelli Romani 6
  Rocca di Papa, Rome
  00040, Italy
  Phone: 39 800 180 437
  Website: www.aicmt.org
  Facebook: www.facebook.com/Associazione-Italiana-Charcot-Marie-Tooth-Onlus-62829197115/

- **Associazione di Volontariato per la Malattia di Charcot-Marie-Tooth (ACMT-RETE)**
  Via Giotto 34
  Sala Bolognese Bologna
  40010, Italy
  Phone: 39 340-2278680
  Website: www.acmt-rete.it
  Facebook: www.facebook.com/acmt.rete

- **Muscular Dystrophy Campaign (UK)**
  61A Great Suffolk Street
  London SE1 0BU
  United Kingdom
  Phone: 0800 652 6352 (toll-free); 020 7803 4800

Email: info@muscular-dystrophy.org
Website: www.muscular-dystrophy.org
Facebook: www.facebook.com/musculardystrophyUK/

- **Charcot-Marie-Tooth United Kingdom (CMT UK)**
  3 Groveley Road
  Christchurch, BH23 3HB
  United Kingdom
  Phone: 0800 652 6316 (toll-free); 01202 474203
  Email: enquiries@cmt.org.uk
  Website: www.cmt.org.uk
  Facebook: www.facebook.com/CMTUK/

CMT CENTERS OF EXCELLENCE

The following organizations have created international lists of CMT "Centers of Excellence" or COEs. These COEs are multi-disciplinary CMT clinics, staffed by some of the highest quality CMT clinicians and researchers in the world. Many Muscular Dystrophy Associations also sponsor MDA Care Centers (Clinics). Check with your local MDA organization for more information.

Inherited Neuropathies Consortium (INC)
https://www.rarediseasesnetwork.org/cms/inc/centers

Charcot-Marie-Tooth Association (CMTA)
https://www.cmtausa.org/resource-center/finding-help/cmta-centers-of-excellence/

Hereditary Neuropathy Foundation (HNF)
http://www.hnf-cure.org/centersofexcellence/

GENETIC TESTING LABORATORIES

There are many laboratories around the world doing genetic testing for CMT. Here are two in Canada and three in the USA. In Canada, genetic testing is covered by provincial insurance.

Molecular Genetics Laboratory,
London Health Sciences Centre
800 Commissioner Road East
London, Ontario N6A 5W9
Phone: 1-519-685-8500 ext.56495
Email: lab@lhsc.on.ca
Website: https://www.lhsc.on.ca/palm/labs/molecular.html#main-content

LifeLabs Genetics, GRL
175 Galaxy Blvd, Unit 105,
Toronto, Ontario Canada M9W 0C9
Phone: 1-844-363-4357
Email: ask.genetics@lifelabs.com
Website: www.lifelabsgenetics.com

Invitae
1400 16th Street
San Francisco, California, United States 94103
Phone: 800-436-3037, +1-415-374-7782
Email: clientservices@invitae.com
www.invitae.com/

GeneDX
207 Perry Parkway
Gaithersburg, MD 20877
Phone: 301-519-2100
Fax: 201-421-2010
Email: genedx@genedx.com
www.genedx.com

Athena Diagnostics Inc, ADX
200 Forest Street, 2nd Floor
Marlborough, Massachusetts, United States 01752
Phone: 8003944493
Email: genetics@athenadiagnostics.com

www.athenadiagnostics.com/

The US National Center for Biotechnology Information (NCBI) also maintains a Genetic Testing Registry of laboratories around the globe doing CMT testing.
www.ncbi.nlm.nih.gov/gtr/all/labs/?term=charcot%20marie%20tooth

PATIENT CONTACT REGISTRIES (FOR CLINICAL RESEARCH)

- **Inherited Neuropathies Consortium (INC) – RDCRN Patient Contact Registry**
https://www.rarediseasesnetwork.org/cms/inc

- **Global Registry for Inherited Neuropathies (GRIN)**
http://www.hnf-cure.org/registry/

INFORMATION ON PREIMPLANTATION GENETIC DIAGNOSIS (PGD)

- **USA:** https://www.cmtausa.org/resource-center/learn/genetic-testing/family-planning-for-cmt-part-1/

- **UK:** http://www.nhs.uk/Conditions/Charcot-Marie-Tooth-disease/Pages/Diagnosis.aspx

- **Australia:** http://old.mda.org.au/Information/Clinical/IVFTechniques.asp

ADDITIONAL RESOURCES
- **CMTCanada** – Linda Crabtree's Facebook group for Canadians with CMT.
www.facebook.com/groups/CMTCanada

- **CMTus** – An international group for individuals with CMT and those interested in learning about it.
https://www.facebook.com/groups/cmtus

- **Accessible Niagara** – Linda Crabtree's website with all the information you need to plan a wheelchair or scooter accessible vacation to Niagara Falls, Ontario, Canada. This site may in time become part of a province-wide site for travellers with disabilities.
www.accessibleniagara.com

- **CMT and Me** – Linda Crabtree's personal blog.
  www.lindacrabtree.wordpress.com

- And, finally, **Linda Crabtree's personal website and email** – On my website,
  www.lindacrabtree.com you will find additional information about my interests such as
  photography and art. You will also find archived articles covering a variety of CMT
  topics. This information was originally published in the CMT International Newsletters
  from 1984 to 2002. While the articles haven't been updated, many remain relevant and
  are posted for informational purposes for those who may find them of interest. You may
  also contact me directly at linda@lindacrabtree.com. Please let me know if you'd like to
  be notified about my future writings. I'm already working on my next book!

Acknowledgements

I want to thank longtime friend and editor, Heather Stonehouse, in Toronto who encouraged me to keep going when I had doubts that I could keep throwing my life out there, including the rawest of emotions, for everyone to see. And, when I wondered, would anyone want to read anything I'd written about my life and CMT, she assured me that what I had gone through would strike a chord with so many people, disabled or not, that I should keep going. I can't thank her enough for the hours we spent together pouring over chapters, correcting punctuation and trying to make sure that what I had in my head and heart got translated to the written word. Heather worked with me for almost 2 years to get this book to the point where another wonderful woman, who asked to remain anonymous, came on the scene to lend her expertise and another set of eyes to what we were doing. She and I worked to the end.

David Sharron, MA, CA, DAS, Head of Archives and Special Collection at Brock University for agreeing to take my ephemera and medals upon my demise and encouraging me to write this book.

Dr. Robert Gledhill for his advice on some of the surgical areas.

Author, reader and enthusiastic supporter, Alison Galvan, creator of Chubby Art colouring books for adults, published on Amazon.

Authors Bill Wenham, Lisa Bendall and Michael Clarkson, who gave me the benefit of their experience publishing with Amazon.

Cindy Osborne, Ron's niece, did some typing for me while I figured out the speech program on my iMac.

And the people on my Facebook page and blog who have encouraged me along the way.

And to my husband who listened to my highs and lows night after night at the dinner table and kept putting up with me.

Thank you all.

The book *Painter, Paddler: The Art and Adventures of Stewart Marshall*, written by Andrew Scott is out of print but, with little trouble, I found one on Amazon.

Dennis Geden's artwork can be found online and in major galleries.

Photo and Art Credits

- 2.1   Snow Church clipping – St. Catharines Standard
- 2.2   Bruce Anthony's Orchestra – Don Sinclair, Staff photographer, St. Catharines Standard 1950
- 5.1   Dancers at Port Dalhousie – Alan Walker, St. Catharines
- 5.2   Mom in living room and carousel horse – photo/clipping St. Catharines Standard
- 8.1   Linda Crabtree drawing from collage
- 8.2   Linda Crabtree linocut of Mountain Street, Montreal
- 10.1   Artwork by David Low
- 10.2   Filming on beach – St. Catharines Standard
- 10.3   GM skit – St. Catharines Standard
- 11.1   Plain and Fancy, watercolour by Linda Crabtree
- 11.2   Rubber Stamp, John B. Boyle
- 11.3   The Standard logo – St. Catharines Standard
- 12.1-2   Linocut of herself by Linda Crabtree
- 14.1   Wedding photo – Lee Paterson
- 16.1   Photo of Linda and Sid and clipping – St. Catharines Standard
- 16.2   CMT International logo designed by B. Bedell
- 16.3   Graduation photo of Linda – Brock University
- 17.1   Linda at computer – Mike Conley Staff photographer, St. Catharines Standard photo
- 17.2   Ontario Medal for Citizenship – courtesy of Province of Ontario, photo by Ray McFadden
- 17.3   Brock University logo – courtesy of Brock University
- 20.1   Concorde – Photo by Eduard Marmet, British Airways Concorde G-BOAC, May 1, 1986, www.airliners.net.
- 21.1   Order of Ontario insignia – courtesy of Province of Ontario
- 21.2   Order of Canada insignia – Sgt Johanie Maheu, Rideau Hall © OSGG 2016
- 22.1   Order of Canada presentation – Sgt Bertrand Thibeault, Rideau Hall © OSGG, 1994
- 26.1   Joan umbrella walking in the rain – St. Catharines Standard
- 29.1   Mom leaning on Merry-Go-Round goat – St. Catharines Standard
- 30.1-2   Photo of FGS collage – Robyn Chew
- 31.1   Photo of Linda – Paul Alexander
- 33.1   Portion photo 17.1 – Mike Conley Staff photographer, St. Catharines Standard
- 33.2-6   Graham Photography
- 32.1   Kathie head and shoulders – courtesy of Garden City Productions
- 35.1   Linda and Sid – St. Catharines Standard
- 35.2   Ron and Linda – Natalie Stickles Five by Five Design Studio
- Back cover head & shoulders of Linda – Natalie Stickles Five by Five Design Studio

Credit for photos are given wherever possible. Apologies for any photographs not credited.

Life Experience Summary

Linda Dorothy Crabtree

Birthplace/date: St. Catharines, ON   April 16, 1942

Married to G. Ronald Book since 1980, no children

Language: English

Education:

- **State University of New York at Buffalo** – online learning – Visitability – Anthropometrics/Biomechanics Jan./Sept, 2011
- **Sheridan College School of Science and Technology** – Universal Design Studies – Jan. 2004 – completed April 2004 (audited).
- **Brock University** – St. Catharines, Ontario – General Bachelor of Arts degree (B.A.) with distinction, majoring in psychology – graduated spring 1987
- **Sir George Williams University School of Art**, Montreal, Canada – three-year diploma in fine and commercial art – graduated 1966
- **State University of New York at Buffalo** (S.U.N.Y.) – Master's Ivy Training (counselling) – 1987

Honors:

- **David C. Onley Award for Leadership in Accessibility** – role model category – June 2016
- **Queen Elizabeth II Diamond Jubilee Medal** – June 2012
- **Zoomer Magazine: Canada's Top 45 over 45** – Leading our world – Reinventing our lives – 2010.
- **Community Action Award** (Ministry of Citizenship and Immigration) – Dec. 1, 2009
- **Terry Fox Hall of Fame** (Canadian Foundation for Physically Disabled Persons, Toronto) – Oct. 2008
- **Tourism Industry Association of Ontario (TIAO) Volunteer of the Year** – Oct. 7, 2008
- **Thirty from the Past Thirty**: an award commemorating Brock University's 30 years. Honoring 30 graduates who exhibit Brock's core values: imagination, innovation and commitment – March 3, 2007
- **T. Roy Adams Humanitarian of the Year Award** – from Chair and Council of Regional Municipality of Niagara in recognition of exemplary service to the residents of Niagara through community spirit and dedication to volunteerism – presented Aug. 11, 2005
- **Joe Dinely Commemorative Award** – for exceptional leadership and commitment to furthering integration and accessibility of persons with disabilities in the Niagara community; May 31, 2005
- **Zonta Club of St. Catharines Yellow Rose** in recognition of professional and volunteer work and making a difference to the women and children in the Niagara Region – March 2005
- **Canadian Peter F. Drucker Niagara Regional Voluntary Sector Innovation Award for Community Leadership** – March 4, 2005
- **Ontario March of Dimes Rick Hansen Award of Excellence** – October 2004

- **King Clancy Award** – (Canadian Foundation for Physically Disabled Persons) – Feb. 2004
- **Golden Jubilee Medal** (Governor General of Canada) – August 2002
- **Paul Harris Fellow** (Rotary International) – May 6, 1996
- **International Honorary Member Beta Sigma Phi** – March 6, 1995
- **YMCA 1994 Canada Peace Medal** – Nov. 22, 1994
- **Honorary Doctor of Laws (LL.D.)** (Brock University) – June 10, 1994
- **Member of the Order of Canada (C.M.)** – April 13, 1994
- **Toronto Sun "Women on the Move" award** – Nov. 25, 1993
- **Canada 125 Commemorative Medal** for service to country, etc. – Sept. 1993
- **Niagara Centre for Independent Living Breaking the Barriers Award** for journalism regarding disability – May 1992
- **Order of Ontario, (O.Ont.)** April 1992 – the highest recognition my province can give.
- **Premier's Award for Accessibility** – March 1990, Honorable Mention for design of home and offices.
- **Canada Volunteer Medal** – Sept. 1989
- **YWCA Biennial Award to Women** for work on disability awareness – April 28, 1989
- **Ontario Medal for Citizenship (O.M.C.)** – June 1987

Boards/Committees:
- **Member ARCH Disability Law Centre** – 2016
- **Tourism Partnership of Niagara Tourism Workforce Training Program advisory group** – 2012
- **Heartland Forest Nature Centre** – Universal Design (access) consultant – **Sept. 2011 through build**
- **Tourism Industry Association of Ontario (TIAO) and Restaurant Hotel and Motel Association (ORHMA) EnAbling Change Partnership Program Advisory Committee** – 2010 – 2011.
- **Mayor's Advisory Committee on Accessibility for the City of St. Catharines** (MACOA) – co-chair – Sept. 2002 to Feb. 2006
- **Region of Niagara Accessibility Advisory Com.**, May 2002 to 2004 – Vice-chair 2005 – May 2006
- **Brock University Crown Foundation** board of directors – 1994 to 2000

Initiatives:
- *Niagara Falls on Wheels: Seeing is Believing* – produced, wrote a 6-minute video in 2014-15 for YouTube and sponsoring websites: HOCO, Niagara Parks and Niagara Falls Tourism plus AccssibleNiagara.com. Also voice over, embedded described video and closed captioning.
- Founder/President, **Phoenix Counsel Inc.** – (1987 to 2012) a not-for-profit publisher of information for and by people with disabilities – published *It's Okay* Magazine on sex, sexuality, self-esteem and disability from 1992 until 1995.
- AccessibleNiagara.com – a website for tourists who are disabled and want to visit Niagara and the *Accessible Niagara* printed guide published for the first time in June 2003 (20,000 copies) and again March 2005 (30,000 copies). Ontario Trillium grant to update website 2009-10, include auditing tools and produce a DVD, *"Access is More than an Open Door: Accessible Tourism in Niagara,"* that went out to 200 tourism providers in Niagara. *Accessible Niagara*

brochure – 40,000 copies June 2011. **NiagaraShares.com** – a website providing a caring and sharing venue for seniors, people with disabilities and caregivers living in the Niagara peninsula. Given away May 2011.

- Also produced a 30' collage *"From Good Stock: A Woman. A Family. A Disability."* – a timeline of family and life used to inspire those who think their life is over when they become disabled. Exhibited at the Niagara Artist's Centre in St. Catharines; Vancouver and Hamilton at McMaster.
- Founder/President, **CMT International** (world-wide organization for people with Charcot-Marie-Tooth disease, a progressive neuromuscular disorder) (1984 - 2002)
- Co-founder, **St. Catharines Craft Guild**, 1976 – 2008.

Published in:

Access Niagara column in The St. Catharines Standard from Feb. 1987 until 1990 and then again from Feb. 1999 to present (articles also appear in Niagara Falls Review, Welland Tribune and online), Living Niagara supplement of The St. Catharines Standard 2008-2011; Hereditary Neuropathy Foundation, New York City – website – regular columnist 2008/9; West Side Story, St. Catharines 2008 - 2011; CARP Niagara Chapter News; Ontario March of Dimes Friendly Visitor; DisAbled Dealer; WOW - Windows on Women 2004; CMT...today 2002-3; March of Dimes Dimeline – 2003-6; Canadian Rehabilitation Counsel for the Disabled (CRCD) Rehabilitation Digest – reviewed books, wrote articles, took photographs for them for many years – several covers; Arch Phys Med Rehabilitation 1998; 79:1560-4 – article on neuropathic pain; Sexuality and Disability Journal, N.Y., NY – Winter 1997-98; What's Up Niagara – disability, accessibility; Disability New Zealand; Dogs in Canada; Healthfit; Caliper (Canadian Paraplegic Association (cover story, etc.); Abilities Magazine, regular column sex and disability 1994-95; Bridges, magazine for intellectually impaired, article on dating, Alberta; Senior's Review (columns on disability 1992-1994). March of Dimes Advocate; Canadian Women Inventors Magazine; Canadian Family Physician – Charcot-Marie-Tooth Disease as a disabling disorder – Feb. 1989; Canadian Builder – MacLean Hunter Ltd. – integrating aids for daily living into new home design, published June 1990; Focus on Abilities: Career Guide for Students – U. of Alberta; 50 Plus in Niagara 1987-88 – column on health and ability; The Standard, St. Catharines, editorial asst., family editor, features, art critic 1970-82.

Video, DVDs, websites, small publications:

- *Niagara Falls on Wheels: Seeing is Believing* – a six-minute video featured on You Tube and AccessibleNiagara.com showing or mentioning 24 venues or services in Niagara Falls that are accessible to travelers with mobility impairment – began June 2014, finished May 2015.
- *Access is More than an Open Door: Accessible Tourism in Niagara* – an eight-minute DVD for tourism providers to better understand access and how it can affect the bottom line – Oct. 2010.
- *Tips on Making your Bed and Breakfast Accommodation Accessible* – for bed and breakfast proprietors – small publication incorporated into AccessibleNiagara.com website. – 2005
- *Charcot-Marie-Tooth Disease: A Brief Overview*. 18-minute DVD and did introduction, voice over and end of video used for education and awareness, produced by Niagara College, filmed by Jon Ohlman. Bought by hundreds of people with CMT and sent gratis to many libraries in schools and teaching hospitals in many English-speaking countries.
- Wrote *cmtint.org* website that received 138,000 hits worldwide from 1996 until it was closed

down in 2002. ***WWW.CMTNEWS.com*** website opened in February 2002. Took six months to write and put up, closed in January 2004 but now continues on lindacrabtree.com.
- Write and maintain ***AccessibleNiagara.com, LindaCrabtree.***com that includes the best from the CMT Newsletters 103 copies and a personal blog at ***lindacrabtree.wordpress.com*** plus CMTCanada Facebook group page.

Produce(d) and edit(ed):
- **Accessible Niagara** – Opening Niagara to people with disabilities – (see **Initiatives**) brochure with more than 170 accessible venues on it for tourists with disabilities – 40,000 in June 2011– raised $12,000 to do it; a 32-page guide for the 60,000 people with disabilities who live in Niagara and those who'd like to visit Niagara as tourists. Raised $20,000 and 30,000 copies printed June 2003. Again, produced Accessible Niagara for 2005-6 (40 pages) (50,000 copies). Auditing, production, marketing – raised $52,000 which included help from The Ontario Trillium Foundation. Publication online since 2002 but went entirely to the internet in 2007.
- **CMT International Newsletter** – total production – bimonthly from 1984 until 2002 – 103 issues began with 8 pages and grew to 32.
- **It's Okay!** – Founder Dec. 1992 – an international consumer written quarterly magazine on sexuality, sex, self-esteem and disability. Subscriber base could not support production costs – lasted 2 years.

Previous work experience:
- **CMT International** – Founded 1984 – Executive Director; Newsletter Editor from 1984 – 2002.
- **The Standard in St. Catharines** – 1970 - 1982, a daily newspaper circulation 45,000. First introduced to newspaper work in 1959 when I was 17 and worked at my first job in the newspaper morgue (library.) At 19, I had five major operations on my feet and ankles lasting 2 ½ years and then returned to school for three years to study art, then rejoined the paper in 1970 as editorial assistant writing obituaries and typing letters to the editor, progressed to art critic and edited art page for seven years as well as public service items and other regular columns. Did much feature writing mainly on health and ability but I also covered many other topics from finance to dance. I was the assistant family editor when I retired after 12 years due to weakness and lack of energy from disability. More than 700 articles published in The Standard in those 12 years.
- **Arnott-Rogers and Batten, Inc. Montreal**, 1966-67 – (commercial art studio) production assistant for audio-visuals for Expo 67. Other positions in the art field, mainly commercials and photography.
- **Instructor** – Taught children art for two years on the 60s in St. Catharines at the old YMCA.

Art exhibitions and production:
- Over a lifetime: Work in batik, lino, acrylics, watercolours, mixed medium, assemblage, collage and box art.
- Co-founded St. Catharines Craft Guild and St. Catharines Folk Arts Festival Craft Show.
- Ontario Arts Council exhibition assistance grants, Molson's Awards, numerous one woman and group shows, juried and non-juried art/craft shows and workshops – still painting.

Featured in:
- Who's Who of Canadian Women – from 1995 to present
- Who's Who in Canada – 1995 to present

Consulting on access and Universal Design (UD) ongoing from 2004. Audited more than 200 venues including 40 hotels, 20 restaurants, 40 wineries, etc. for AccessibleNiagara.com website, worked with Heartland Forest, Niagara Parks Commission, George Darte Funeral Home – St. Catharines. Write about access, Universal Design and Visitability at every opportunity.

Public speaking/TV/Radio:
A full page of public speaking, radio and TV appearances in Canada, the United States and the U.K. including CBC Morningside with Peter Gzowski, Rogers Cable Toronto – Sex with Sue (Johansen) one hour live call-in on sex and disability 1993 and Brock University Convocation address, 2,000 people, 6/10, 1994. Now that I'm getting older, I'm being featured in various magazines for seniors. Love it!

Advocacy:
As a writer/artist with a severe disability, I am a natural advocate for the rights of people who are disabled. I consult and I enjoy bringing awareness to those who can make change happen i.e. Universal Design and Visitability. This includes making all public buildings (old and new) accessible and all new homes built with access and aging in place part of the design. And accessibility is a must for a tourism-related area such as Niagara. Through AccessibleNiagara.com, I regularly answer travel related queries from tourists with disabilities.

Looking back, my life seems to have been one big advocacy project. Now 75, I am more focused on end of life topics such as physician assistant death and pain management through the use of medical cannabis. I also continue to write my newspaper column and am also endeavouring to bring Canadians with CMT together through Facebook.

Until people with disabilities can go anywhere everyone else can and we can request, and be granted, a humane death, my work is not finished. All of my administrative, journalistic, publishing, art and photographic experience is helping me accomplish much.

My disability is progressive. I haven't walked in more than 20 years and my hands are very weak.

My mandate remains constant: *to do my best each day with what I have left.*

Linda D. Crabtree, C.M., O.Ont., O.M.C., B.A., LL.D. (hon.) *December, 2017*

linda@lindacrabtree.com One Springbank Dr., St. Catharines, ON L2S 2K1

–30–

Printed in Great Britain
by Amazon

82310929R00188